AF774607

Uterine Fibroids

Uterine Fibroids

Edited by
John C. Petrozza, MD
Reproductive Endocrinologist, Reproductive Surgeon, and
Chief, Division of Reproductive Medicine and IVF
Director, Massachusetts General Hospital Fertility Center
Co-Director, MGH Integrated Fibroid Program
Boston and Danvers, Massachusetts, USA

CRC Press
Taylor & Francis Group
Boca Raton London New York

CRC Press is an imprint of the
Taylor & Francis Group, an **informa** business

First edition published 2020
by CRC Press
6000 Broken Sound Parkway NW, Suite 300, Boca Raton, FL 33487-2742

and by CRC Press
2 Park Square, Milton Park, Abingdon, Oxon, OX14 4RN

© 2021 Taylor & Francis Group, LLC

CRC Press is an imprint of Taylor & Francis Group, LLC

This book contains information obtained from authentic and highly regarded sources. While all reasonable efforts have been made to publish reliable data and information, neither the author[s] nor the publisher can accept any legal responsibility or liability for any errors or omissions that may be made. The publishers wish to make clear that any views or opinions expressed in this book by individual editors, authors or contributors are personal to them and do not necessarily reflect the views/opinions of the publishers. The information or guidance contained in this book is intended for use by medical, scientific or health-care professionals and is provided strictly as a supplement to the medical or other professional's own judgement, their knowledge of the patient's medical history, relevant manufacturer's instructions and the appropriate best practice guidelines. Because of the rapid advances in medical science, any information or advice on dosages, procedures or diagnoses should be independently verified. The reader is strongly urged to consult the relevant national drug formulary and the drug companies' and device or material manufacturers' printed instructions, and their websites, before administering or utilizing any of the drugs, devices or materials mentioned in this book. This book does not indicate whether a particular treatment is appropriate or suitable for a particular individual. Ultimately it is the sole responsibility of the medical professional to make his or her own professional judgements, so as to advise and treat patients appropriately. The authors and publishers have also attempted to trace the copyright holders of all material reproduced in this publication and apologize to copyright holders if permission to publish in this form has not been obtained. If any copyright material has not been acknowledged please write and let us know so we may rectify in any future reprint.

Except as permitted under U.S. Copyright Law, no part of this book may be reprinted, reproduced, transmitted, or utilized in any form by any electronic, mechanical, or other means, now known or hereafter invented, including photocopying, microfilming, and recording, or in any information storage or retrieval system, without written permission from the publishers.

For permission to photocopy or use material electronically from this work, access www.copyright.com or contact the Copyright Clearance Center, Inc. (CCC), 222 Rosewood Drive, Danvers, MA 01923, 978-750-8400. For works that are not available on CCC please contact mpkbookspermissions@tandf.co.uk

Trademark notice: Product or corporate names may be trademarks or registered trademarks, and are used only for identification and explanation without intent to infringe.

Library of Congress Control Number: 2020939180

ISBN: 978-1-4987-3920-7 (hbk)
ISBN: 978-0-429-15573-4 (ebk)

Typeset in Times LT Std
by Nova Techset Private Limited, Bengaluru & Chennai, India

Contents

Contributors

Tejumola Adegoke
Department of Obstetrics and Gynecology
Boston University School of Medicine/Boston Medical Center
Boston, Massachusetts

Elise Bardawil
Minimally Invasive Gynecologic Fellow
Baylor College of Medicine
Houston, Texas

Bryann Bromley
Department of Obstetrics & Gynecology
Division of Maternal Fetal Medicine
Massachusetts General Hospital
Harvard Medical School
Boston, Massachusetts

Eden R. Cardozo
Division of Reproductive Endocrinology and Infertility
Women & Infants Hospital of Rhode Island and
Warren Alpert Medical School of Brown University
Providence, Rhode Island

Kamaria Cayton
Department of Gynecology and Obstetrics
Johns Hopkins University School of Medicine
Baltimore, Maryland

Victoria Fitz
Department of Obstetrics & Gynecology
University of North Carolina School of Medicine
Chapel Hill, North Carolina

Gary N. Frishman
Department of Obstetrics and Gynecology
Women & Infants Hospital
Brown University
Providence, Rhode Island

C. Scott Gallagher
Department of Genetics
Harvard Medical School
Boston, Massachusetts

Antonio R. Gargiulo
Department of Obstetrics and Gynecology
Northwell Health Fertility
and
Northwell Health
Donald and Barbara Zucker School of Medicine at Hofstra/Northwell
Manhasset, New York

Jeffrey M. Goldberg
Reproductive Endocrinology & Infertility
Cleveland Clinic
Cleveland, Ohio

Randi H. Goldman
Center for Infertility and Reproductive Surgery
Department of Obstetrics
Gynecology and Reproductive Biology
Brigham and Women's Hospital
Harvard Medical School
Boston, Massachusetts

and

Reproductive Endocrinology & Infertility
Northwell Health
Manhasset, New York

Karissa Hammer
Department of Obstetrics & Gynecology
Division of Reproductive Medicine & IVF
Massachusetts General Hospital
Harvard Medical School
Boston, Massachusetts

Amy L. Harris
Department of Obstetrics & Gynecology
Wright State University
Wright Patterson AFB
Dayton, Ohio

Holly R. Harris
Program in Epidemiology
Division of Public Health Sciences
Fred Hutchinson Cancer Research Center
Seattle, Washington

and

Department of Epidemiology
Boston University School of Public Health
Boston, Massachusetts

Anthony N. Imudia
Division of Reproductive Endocrinology and Infertility
Department of Obstetrics and Gynecology
University of South Florida Morsani College of Medicine
Tampa, Florida

Zubin Irani
Department of Radiology
Vascular Center and Interventional Radiology
Massachusetts General Hospital
Harvard Medical School
Boston, Massachusetts

Eleni Greenwood Jaswa
Department of Obstetrics & Gynecology
Division of Reproductive Endocrinology & Infertility
University of California San Francisco
San Francisco, California

Jovana Kaludjerovic
Senior Medical Science Liaison
Abbvie
Boston, Massachusetts

Anatte E. Karmon
The Fertility Institute of Hawaii
Honolulu, Hawaii

Zaraq Khan
Division of Reproductive Endocrinology & Infertility
Mayo Clinic
Rochester, Minnesota

Louise P. King
Department of Obstetrics & Gynecology
Division of Minimally Invasive Gynecologic Surgery
Brigham & Women's Hospital
Harvard Medical School
Boston, Massachusetts

Whitney A. Leonard
Department of Obstetrics and Gynecology
Section of Reproductive Endocrinology and Infertility
University of Oklahoma Health Sciences Center
Oklahoma City, Oklahoma

Annie Leung
Department of Obstetrics and Gynecology
McGill University
Montreal, Canada

Michelle Louie
Department of Obstetrics and Gynecology
Division of Minimally Invasive Gynecologic Surgery
University of North Carolina
Chapel Hill, North Carolina

Shruthi Mahalingaiah
Department of Obstetrics and Gynecology
Boston University School of Medicine/Boston Medical Center
and
Department of Epidemiology
Boston University School of Public Health
Boston, Massachusetts

Joan M. Mastrobattista
Division of Maternal-Fetal Medicine
Baylor College of Medicine
Houston, Texas

Stacey A. Missmer
Department of Obstetrics, Gynecology, and Reproductive Biology
College of Human Medicine
Michigan State University
Grand Rapids, Michigan

Evelyn Mok-Lin
Department of Obstetrics & Gynecology
Division of Reproductive Endocrinology & Infertility
University of California San Francisco
San Francisco, California

Cynthia C. Morton
Department of Obstetrics, Gynecology, and Reproductive Biology
and
Department of Pathology
Harvard Medical School
Boston, Massachusetts

and

Broad Institute of MIT and Harvard
Cambridge, Massachusetts

and

Manchester Academic Health Science Centre
University of Manchester
Manchester, United Kingdom

Janelle K. Moulder
Obstetrics & Gynecology
Wake-Forest Baptist Health
Minimally Invasive Gynecologic Surgery
Winston-Salem, North Carolina

Roni Nitecki
Division of Gynecologic Oncology
Department of Obstetrics and Gynecology
Massachusetts General Hospital
Harvard Medical School
Boston, Massachusetts

Luis S. Noble
Southwest Center for Reproductive Health
and
Division of Reproductive Endocrinology
Texas Tech University Medical Center
El Paso, Texas

Carter M. Owen
Program in Reproductive and Adult Endocrinology
Eunice Kennedy Shriver National Institute of Child Health and Human Development
Bethesda, Maryland

Erika Parker New
University of South Florida Morsani College of Medicine
Tampa, Florida

John C. Petrozza
Department of Obstetrics & Gynecology
Division of Reproductive Medicine & IVF
Massachusetts General Hospital
Harvard Medical School
Boston, Massachusetts

Alexander M. Quaas
Department of Obstetrics and Gynecology
Section of Reproductive Endocrinology and Infertility
University of Oklahoma Health Sciences Center
Oklahoma City, Oklahoma

and

Reproductive Partners Fertility Center
UC San Diego Health
San Diego, California

Diego Ramirez
Texas Tech University Medical Center
El Paso, Texas

J. Alejandro Rauh-Hain
Division of Gynecologic Oncology
Department of Obstetrics and Gynecology
Massachusetts General Hospital
Boston, Massachusetts

and

Gynecologic Oncology
MD Anderson Cancer Center
Houston, Texas

Caitlin R. Sacha
Department of Obstetrics & Gynecology
Division of Reproductive Medicine & IVF
Massachusetts General Hospital
Harvard Medical School
Boston, Massachusetts

Gloria M. Salazar
Department of Radiology
Vascular Center and Interventional Radiology
Massachusetts General Hospital
Harvard Medical School
Boston, Massachusetts

May-Tal Sauerbrun-Cutler
Division of Reproductive Endocrinology and Infertility
Women & Infants Hospital of Rhode Island and
Warren Alpert Medical School of Brown University
Providence, Rhode Island

James H. Segars
Department of Gynecology and Obstetrics
Johns Hopkins University School of Medicine
Baltimore, Maryland

Emily A. Seidler
Obstetrics & Gynecology
Harvard Medical School
Boston IVF
Boston, Massachusetts

Christine C. Skiadas
Reproductive Endocrinology and Infertility
Center for Fertility and Reproductive Health
Harvard Vanguard Medical Associates/Atrius Health
Boston, Massachusetts

Matthew S. Smith
Department of Obstetrics and Gynecology
Baylor College of Medicine
and
McGovern Medical School
Houston, Texas

Jessica B. Spencer
Reproductive Endocrinology and Infertility
Emory University School of Medicine
Atlanta, Georgia

Camille Storment
Women & Children's Hospital
Reproductive Endocrinology & Infertility
Lafayette, Louisiana

John Storment
Women & Children's Hospital
Reproductive Endocrinology & Infertility
Lafayette, Louisiana

Aaron K. Styer
Vincent Center for Reproductive Biology
Vincent Department of Obstetrics and Gynecology
Massachusetts General Hospital
Boston, Massachusetts

Kathryn L. Terry
Department of Obstetrics & Gynecology
Brigham and Women's Hospital
and
Department of Epidemiology
Boston University School of Public Health
Boston, Massachusetts

Tarek Toubia
Obstetrics and Gynecology
Jennie Stuart Medical Group
Hopkinsville, Kentucky

Togas Tulandi
Department of Obstetrics and Gynecology
McGill University
Montreal, Canada

Eric Paul Wehrenberg-Klee
Department of Radiology
Vascular Center and Interventional Radiology
Massachusetts General Hospital
Harvard Medical School
Boston, Massachusetts

Lauren A. Wise
Department of Epidemiology
Boston University School of Public Health
Boston, Massachusetts

Ophelia Yin
Department of Gynecology and Obstetrics
Johns Hopkins University School of Medicine
Baltimore, Maryland

Steven L. Young
Department of Obstetrics & Gynecology
University of North Carolina School of Medicine
Chapel Hill, North Carolina

Hope Y. Yu
Department of Obstetrics and Gynecology
Women & Infants Hospital
Brown University
Providence, Rhode Island

1

The Health Care Costs of Uterine Fibroids

May-Tal Sauerbrun-Cutler and Eden R. Cardozo

Background

Approximately 588,164 women in the United States seek treatment for fibroids annually [1]. The prevalence estimates range from 4.5% to 68.6%, depending on the study population and methodology [2]. This wide range is likely due to the fact that the majority of fibroids are asymptomatic and will not be detected unless the patient becomes symptomatic. The high prevalence of uterine fibroids, along with the chronic and relapsing nature of the disease (in the absence of curative treatment such as hysterectomy) make fibroids one of the most expensive diseases to manage. Uterine fibroids are estimated to cost more annually than breast cancer, colon cancer and ovarian cancer and are almost one-fifth the estimated annual cost of diabetes in the United States (Table 1.1) [1].

Fibroids can be treated medically, surgically or alternatively through nonsurgical procedures. Generally, only hysterectomy is curative, and thus, patients who pursue other treatment modalities may require additional outpatient visits, hospitalizations, lost work time, or future procedures, and may experience future obstetric complications due to their fibroids. These direct costs (surgery, hospitalizations, outpatient visits, medications) and indirect costs (lost work time) have been quantified in studies through the use of national databases, hospital charges, insurance reimbursements and physician charges. Cardozo et al. performed a systematic review of the literature and sensitivity analysis that included obstetric complications in addition to direct and indirect costs and determined that the total annual societal cost of uterine fibroids in the United States is $5.9 billion–$34.4 billion [1]. Table 1.2, adapted from Cardozo et al., breaks down the annual estimates of costs due to uterine fibroids by direct, indirect and obstetric costs.

TABLE 1.1

Estimated Annual Cost of Various Diseases in the United States

Disease	Estimated Annual Cost
Diabetes [3]	$192,728,897,856.00
Uterine Fibroids	$34,369,314,704.00
Breast Cancer [4]	$16,057,400,853.77
Colon Cancer [4]	$14,055,718,520.64
Ovarian Cancer [4]	$5,063,759,062.27

Source: Reprinted from *Am J Obstet Gynecol*. 2012;206(3), Cardozo ER et al., The estimated annual cost of uterine leiomyomata in the United States, 211.e1–9. Copyright 2012, with permission from Elsevier.

Note: All costs are reported in 2010 dollars.

TABLE 1.2

Total Annual Estimates of Costs Due to Uterine Fibroids

	Estimate of Total Cost			
	Low	% of Total	High	% of Total
Direct Cost				
Medications, inpatient admissions, outpatient visits	$3,271,956,332	55.54%	$5,096,441,060	14.83%
Surgery	$829,213,571	14.07%	$4,312,422,131	12.55%
Indirect Cost				
Lost work	$1,552,509,693	26.35%	$17,201,602,940	50.05%
Spontaneous abortion	$983,035	0.02%	$110,698,973	0.32%
Preterm delivery	$52,056,948	0.88%	$1,468,626,480	4.27%
Cesarean delivery	$184,938,975	3.14%	$6,179,523,120	17.98%
Total Annual Estimate	$5,891,658,554	100.00%	$34,369,314,704	100.00%

Source: Reprinted from *Am J Obstet Gynecol*. 2012;206(3), Cardozo ER et al., The estimated annual cost of uterine leiomyomata in the United States, 211.e1–9. Copyright 2012, with permission from Elsevier.

Note: All costs are reported in 2010 dollars.

Direct Costs

Direct costs include surgical, medical management, inpatient admissions, outpatient visits and medication costs. Two studies report an average direct cost of $9473 [5] and $9319 [6] per patient during the year after uterine fibroid diagnosis. However, direct costs within the year in which a surgical procedure was performed are significantly higher, and estimates calculated using databases of third-party payers, payments from insurers, as well as payments from patients (deductibles and copays) range from $15,878 to $21,603 [7–10].

Surgical costs are a large driver of this cost burden. Each year, an estimated 200,000 hysterectomies and 300,000 myomectomies are performed for treatment of uterine fibroids [11,12]. Hysterectomy, myomectomy and uterine artery embolization have fairly similar cost ranges, which have been estimated between $6287 and $14,850 per patient, with

TABLE 1.3

Estimated Direct Cost of Uterine Fibroids

	Range of Women Having Each Intervention			Cost Estimates			Estimate of Total Cost		
Medical Management									
Medications, inpatient admissions, outpatient visits				$5563 [5]	–	$8665 [6]	$3,271,956,332	–	$5,096,441,060
Surgical Management									
Hysterectomy	21.00% [5]	–	52.90% [8]	$6287 [13]	–	$11,538 [8]	$776,532,518	–	$3,589,921,782
Myomectomy	1.00% [14]	–	5.93% [15]	$6805 [13]	–	$14,850 [13]	$40,027,010	–	$517,938,300
Uterine artery embolization	0.20% [14]	–	1.77% [15]	$6805 [13]	–	$12,863 [8]	$8,002,680	–	$133,916,693
Endometrial ablation	0.16% [5]	–	2.43% [15]	$4943 [8]	–	$4943 [8]	$4,651,363	–	$70,645,356
Total Direct Costs							**$4,101,169,903**	–	**$9,408,863,191**

Source: Reprinted from *Am J Obstet Gynecol.* 2012;206(3), Cardozo ER et al., The estimated annual cost of uterine leiomyomata in the United States, 211.e1–9. Copyright 2012, with permission from Elsevier.

Notes: Total women seeking treatment for fibroids was calculated by number of women aged 25–54 (63,930,821) multiplied by baseline prevalence of 0.92% = 588,164.

All costs are reported in 2010 dollars.

endometrial ablation being less costly at approximately $4943 [8,13]. Table 1.3 shows the estimated low and high costs of each surgical procedure and the percentage of women who undergo each intervention. Table 1.3 also includes the cost of medical management of uterine fibroids, which accounts for medication costs as well as inpatient hospitalizations and outpatient doctors' visits. By multiplying the range of the number of women who underwent each treatment annually by a range of published estimates of direct costs, it was estimated that the direct cost of uterine fibroids annually in the United States is between $4.1 billion and $9.4 billion [1].

It is important to remember that while surgical costs may be a substantial driver of the total health care costs of uterine fibroids, the overall lifetime cost of an individual with uterine fibroids may be lower if their fibroids are treated surgically. Table 1.3 indicates that the total annual costs of nonsurgical management of uterine fibroids are higher than that of surgical management. Carls et al. found that even though surgery cost more than expectant management in the short term, long-term cost savings were noted, and 3 years after surgery, there were significantly lower medical costs of approximately $1000 per year among hysterectomy patients compared to nonsurgical patients [8].

Indirect Costs

Most studies estimate indirect costs of uterine fibroids by examining absenteeism and disability costs based on retrospective claims analysis from third-party payers and estimated costs to employers. For example, Carls et al. calculated these costs by using 70% of daily wage multiplied by days absent from work, and estimated that missed workdays in the year after surgery cost employers more than for nonsurgical patients [8].

Estimated annual lost work time due to absenteeism and short-term disability has been calculated to be as high as $30,075 for patients who underwent hysterectomy, $25,164 for myomectomy, $18,836 for AUE, $17,385 for endometrial ablation, and $14,282 for nonsurgical treatment [1,6,8].

It should be noted that money due to lost work time, estimated to be $1.6–$17.2 billion dollars annually, is an underestimation of the indirect costs of fibroids because it measures days absent from work and not costs associated with decreased productivity at work [1]. However, the estimated cost of lost work remains substantial and contributes 26.4%–50.1% of the total annual costs attributable to uterine fibroids (Table 1.2) [1].

Obstetric Costs

Obstetric complications are also a significant contributor to the indirect health-care cost burden of uterine fibroids. Fibroids contribute to a large number of pregnancy-related complications, including spontaneous abortion, preterm delivery and cesarean delivery [1,12,16]. Coronado et al. estimated odds ratios for each obstetric outcome by comparing 2065 women with pregnancy related complications with fibroids to women who had similar complications but without fibroids [17]. Cardozo et al. used these odds ratios to calculate the proportion of each complication attributable to uterine fibroids and a prevalence of fibroids in pregnancy ranging from 0.37% to 10.7% [17,18] to determine the number of cases attributed annually to fibroids. Published costs of individual procedures and lifetime expense of a preterm infant were used to calculate the estimated annual costs of obstetric outcomes attributable to fibroids (Table 1.4) [1], which may cost up to $7.76 million annually.

Future Research

As new treatments for uterine fibroids evolve, more research is needed to understand the cost effectiveness of various treatment modalities. Furthermore, long-term follow-up in these studies is critical given the chronic nature of the disease and its high recurrence rates.

TABLE 1.4

Estimated Annual Cost of Obstetric Complications Related to Uterine Fibroids

Obstetric Outcome	Estimated Annual Number of Cases Attributed to Fibroids			Estimated Cost per Case			Estimate of Total Cost		
	Low		High						
Spontaneous abortion	421	–	12,089	$2335 [19]	–	$9157 [20]	$983,035	–	$110,698,973
Preterm delivery	906	–	25,560	$57,458 [21]	–	$57,458 [21]	$52,056,948	–	$1,468,626,480
Cesarean delivery	13,455	–	304,440	$13,745 [22]	–	$20,298 [23]	$184,938,975	–	$6,179,523,120
Combined Cost for Obstetrical Outcomes							**$237,978,958**	–	**$7,758,848,573**

Source: Reprinted from *Am J Obstet Gynecol.* 2012;206(3), Cardozo ER et al., The estimated annual cost of uterine leiomyomata in the United States, 211.e1–9. Copyright 2012, with permission from Elsevier.

Note: All costs are reported in 2010 dollars.

REFERENCES

1. Cardozo ER, Clark AD, Banks NK, Henne MB, Stegmann BJ, and Segars JH. The estimated annual cost of uterine leiomyomata in the United States. *Am J Obstet Gynecol.* 2012;206(3):211.e1–9.
2. Stewart EA, Cookson CL, Gandolfo RA, and Schulze-Rath R. Epidemiology of uterine fibroids: A systematic review. *BJOG.* 2017;124(10):1501–12.
3. Association AD. Economic costs of diabetes in the U.S. In 2007. *Diabetes Care.* 2008;31(3):596–615.
4. National Cancer Institute. *Cancer Trends Progress Report 2009/2010 Update: Costs of Cancer Care.* https://progressreport.cancer.gov/sites/default/files/archive/report2009.pdf
5. Hartmann KE, Birnbaum H, Ben-Hamadi R et al. Annual costs associated with diagnosis of uterine leiomyomata. *Obstet Gynecol.* 2006;108(4):930–7.
6. Lee DW, Ozminkowski RJ, Carls GS, Wang S, Gibson TB, and Stewart EA. The direct and indirect cost burden of clinically significant and symptomatic uterine fibroids. *J Occup Environ Med.* 2007;49(5):493–506.
7. Soliman AM, Yang H, Du EX, Kelkar SS, and Winkel C. The direct and indirect costs of uterine fibroid tumors: A systematic review of the literature between 2000 and 2013. *Am J Obstet Gynecol.* 2015;213(2):141–60.
8. Carls GS, Lee DW, Ozminkowski RJ, Wang S, Gibson TB, and Stewart E. What are the total costs of surgical treatment for uterine fibroids? *J Womens Health (Larchmt).* 2008;17(7):1119–32.
9. Epstein AJ, Groeneveld PW, Harhay MO, Yang F, and Polsky D. Impact of minimally invasive surgery on medical spending and employee absenteeism. *JAMA Surg.* 2013;148(7):641–7.
10. Dembek CJ, Pelletier EM, Isaacson KB, and Spies JB. Payer costs in patients undergoing uterine artery embolization, hysterectomy, or myomectomy for treatment of uterine fibroids. *J Vasc Interv Radiol.* 2007;18(10):1207–13.
11. Wu JM, Wechter ME, Geller EJ, Nguyen TV, and Visco AG. Hysterectomy rates in the United States, 2003. *Obstet Gynecol.* 2007;110(5):1091–5.
12. Farquhar CM and Steiner CA. Hysterectomy rates in the United States 1990–1997. *Obstet Gynecol.* 2002;99(2):229–34.
13. Mauskopf J, Flynn M, Thieda P, Spalding J, and Duchane J. The economic impact of uterine fibroids in the United States: A summary of published estimates. *J Womens Health (Larchmt).* 2005;14(8):692–703.
14. Oderda G, Asche C, Jones KP, Merrill RM, and Spalding J. Characterization of therapy and costs for patients with uterine fibroids in Utah Medicaid. *Arch Gynecol Obstet.* 2007;276(3):211–8.
15. Lee DW, Gibson TB, Carls GS, Ozminkowski RJ, Wang S, and Stewart EA. Uterine fibroid treatment patterns in a population of insured women. *Fertil Steril.* 2009;91(2):566–74.
16. Klatsky PC, Tran ND, Caughey AB, and Fujimoto VY. Fibroids and reproductive outcomes: A systematic literature review from conception to delivery. *Am J Obstet Gynecol.* 2008;198(4):357–66.
17. Coronado GD, Marshall LM, and Schwartz SM. Complications in pregnancy, labor, and delivery with uterine leiomyomas: A population-based study. *Obstet Gynecol.* 2000;95(5):764–9.
18. Laughlin SK, Baird DD, Savitz DA, Herring AH, and Hartmann KE. Prevalence of uterine leiomyomas in the first trimester of pregnancy: An ultrasound-screening study. *Obstet Gynecol.* 2009;113(3):630–5.
19. Rocconi RP, Chiang S, Richter HE, and Straughn JM. Management strategies for abnormal early pregnancy: A cost-effectiveness analysis. *J Reprod Med.* 2005;50(7):486–90.
20. Adams EK and Melvin CL. Costs of maternal conditions attributable to smoking during pregnancy. *Am J Prev Med.* 1998;15(3):212–9.
21. Behrman RE, Butler AS, Institute of Medicine (U.S.). *Preterm Birth: Causes, Consequences, and Prevention.* Washington, D.C.: National Academies Press; 2007. Committee on Understanding Premature Birth and Assuring Healthy Outcomes.
22. Healthcare T. The Healthcare Costs of Having a Baby. 2007. http://www.marchofdimes.com/downloads/The_Healthcare_Costs_of_Having_a_Baby.pdf
23. Merrill C and Steiner C. Hospitalizations Related to Childbirth, 2003: Statistical Brief #11. In: *Healthcare Cost and Utilization Project (HCUP) Statistical Briefs.* Rockville (MD): Agency for Healthcare Research and Quality (US); 2006.

2

Environmental Chemicals and Risk of Uterine Leiomyomata

Lauren A. Wise

Environmental exposures may influence risk of uterine leiomyomata (UL) via multiple mechanisms, including endocrine disruption. Endocrine-disrupting chemicals (EDCs) are naturally occurring compounds or synthetic chemicals that can alter functioning of the endocrine system by mimicking the activity of sex steroids, blocking or altering binding to hormone receptors, altering the production and breakdown of natural hormones, or modifying the function of hormone receptors. Exposure to environmental chemicals in the US population is widespread [1], with reproductive-aged women [1] and African Americans [2–5] having the highest exposure levels to several EDCs. Given the breadth of animal and human evidence indicating that sex steroid hormones (estrogens and progesterone) are involved in UL etiology [6], a link between EDCs and UL seems plausible. In the following chapter, I review the epidemiologic literature investigating risk of UL in relation to a range of environmental chemicals, starting with the most widely studied exposures (e.g., cigarette smoking) and concluding with less well-studied exposures of emerging interest.

Tobacco

Tobacco smoke constituents can inhibit aromatase [7] and shift estradiol metabolism toward less potent forms of estrogen [8,9]. Conversely, components of cigarette smoke may also exert estrogen-related effects on the uterus that could promote cell proliferation [10]. Early studies, based largely on surgical UL cases, have reported that smoking was associated with a reduced risk of UL [11–15], with risk reduction ranging from 20% to 50% lower among current or ever smokers relative to never smokers. However, more recent case-control [16,17] and prospective cohort studies [18,19] have found no such association. In the Uterine Fibroid Study (UFS), a cross-sectional ultrasound screening study, there was a positive relation of smoking with diffuse UL but not with submucosal or intramural/subserosal UL [20]. To our knowledge, there are no studies of passive smoke exposure in adulthood and UL risk. In the sole study of passive smoke exposure in early life, there was no association between *in utero* exposure to smoke (incidence rate ratio [IRR] = 1.01, 95% confidence interval [CI]: 0.94–1.09) and UL risk; passive smoke exposure from ages 0–10 was associated with a weak increase in UL risk (IRR = 1.06, 95% CI: 1.01–1.11) [21]. Because cigarette smokers are less likely than nonsmokers to seek routine medical care [19], and incidental detection of UL is common, caution should be used when interpreting the results from studies in which not all women are screened with ultrasound. Thus, detection bias is a concern in studies of smoking and UL that do not employ systematic ultrasound screening of its participants.

Diethylstilbestrol

Prenatal exposure to diethylstilbestrol (DES), a potent endocrine disruptor, has been shown to cause long-term changes in estrogen-related gene expression [22] and endogenous hormones of premenopausal women; [23] thus, a positive association with UL risk is plausible. Although an association between prenatal DES exposure and UL has been found in laboratory rodents [22,24], the epidemiologic data are conflicting, possibly because prenatal exposure to DES is difficult to assess and studies are prone to recall and reporting biases. One prospective cohort study, which used medical records to document exposure, found no association between prenatal DES exposure and UL [25]. A second prospective cohort study found a 21% increased risk of UL among women who self-reported exposure to DES in the first trimester [26]. Two cross-sectional studies [27,28], one of which was an ultrasound screening study [28], found a positive association between self-reported prenatal DES exposure and UL risk. One of these studies found that only "probable," but not "definite," prenatal DES exposure was associated with UL risk [28], suggesting that recall bias could explain these results. To minimize the influence of reporting bias, future studies should seek medical documentation of DES exposure.

Phthalates

Phthalates are a family of organic chemicals that have been used as plasticizers for polyvinylchloride plastics since the 1930s. They have been widely used in food packaging, medical devices and medications, toys and building materials, as well as cosmetics and personal-care products such as perfume, lotion and nail polish [29]. There is increasing concern that exposure to phthalates may have adverse effects on reproductive health. Studies in experimental animals suggest that phthalates possess endocrine-disrupting properties and can adversely affect reproductive function by altering steroidogenesis [30–38]. *In vitro* studies indicate that some phthalates have antiestrogenic activities [32,35,38], while others have weak estrogenic activity [39,40], lending biologic plausibility for an effect of phthalates on hormone-responsive conditions such as UL.

Exposure to phthalates is typically quantified by measuring concentrations of diester phthalate molecules in urine (or blood) that were synthesized for commercial use ("parent" molecules), or of monoester metabolites that are formed from hydrolysis or oxidation of diesters after entering living systems (Table 2.1) [41]. Monoester metabolites are rare in the environment because they arise only from biotransformation, and thus they are the preferred exposure measure. Biomonitoring studies document that more than 78% of people in the US general population have detectable amounts of phthalates in their bodies [2]. National Health and Nutrition Examination Survey (NHANES) data indicate that African Americans have significantly higher levels of some phthalate metabolites (MEP, MnBP, MiBP) than do Mexican Americans and whites [2,42,43], a disparity that has persisted over time and is present among women [44].

Five epidemiologic studies have directly evaluated UL prevalence or incidence in relation to phthalate exposure, as measured by biomarker concentrations, and have yielded inconclusive results [44–48]. All of these studies were retrospective in design (cross-sectional [44,47] or case-control [45,46,48]). (A sixth study prospectively examined use of hair relaxers as a possible proxy for phthalate exposure in relation to risk of UL, finding consistent positive associations for age at first use, frequency of use and duration of use [49].) The largest of the five "direct" studies [44], a cross-sectional nationally representative study of 1,227 women (151 UL cases), found that women with higher urinary MBP (MnBP + MiBP) concentrations were more likely to report a physician diagnosis of UL. There was little evidence of an association between UL and MEHP, MEOHP, MEP or MBzP. In the subset of women contributing data to the 2001–2004 wave of NHANES, when additional data on the oxidative phthalate metabolites were measured, the associations between phthalate metabolites of DEHP and UL were close to 1.0 [44]. Specifically, the odds ratio (OR) for MEHHP was 0.97 (highest versus the lowest three quartiles), and the associations for MEOHP and MECPP were positive but imprecise.

In a 2016 case-control study of 57 women with and without uterine leiomyoma (n = 30 and 27, respectively), the authors calculated the molar sum of DEHP metabolites: ∑3-DEHP, combining mono-(2-ethylhexyl) phthalate (MEHP), mono-(2-ethyl-5-hydroxyhexyl) phthalate (MEHHP) and mono-(2-ethyl-5-oxohexyl) phthalate; ∑4-DEHP, ∑3-DEHP plus mono-(2-ethyl-5-carboxypentyl) phthalate; and ∑5-DEHP, ∑4-DEHP plus mono-(2-(carboxylmethyl)hexyl) phthalate (2cx-MMHP) [48]). After adjustment for age, waist circumference and parity using multiple logistic regression analyses, log ∑3-DEHP (OR = 10.82, 95% CI: 1.25–93.46) and ∑4-DEHP (OR = 8.78, 95% CI: 1.03–75.29) were positively associated with UL risk.

A 2015 cross-sectional study of surgically visualized UL found no appreciable association between urinary phthalates and UL prevalence after adjusting for potential confounders [47]. An earlier case-control study reported that urinary MEHP levels were higher in UL cases than controls [46]. Another case-control study found lower serum levels of DEHP and MEHP in (prevalent) surgical cases of UL [45]. In that study, controls were shown by ultrasound to be free of UL [45], but they had undergone other hospital procedures that could have increased their levels of DEHP and MEHP [50]. In addition, that study measured serum concentrations of DEHP [44], which are subject to contamination from laboratory equipment and other external sources. Serum MEHP concentrations are also prone to contamination from DEHP present in the specimen because serum enzymes can hydrolyze DEHP to MEHP during storage [51].

A 2019 publication based on cross-sectional data from women undergoing inpatient surgery for UL (n = 57) also reported positive associations between urinary phthalate metabolites and uterine volume, but did not investigate UL incidence [148]. Associations were strongest for individual DEHP metabolites (MEHHP, MEOHP, MECPP), ∑DEHP (sum of all DEHP metabolites), and ∑AA (i.e., sum of androgenic metabolites: MBP, MiBP, MBzP, MEHP, MEHHP, MEOHP, MECPP, MEP, MHBP, MCOP, and MHiBP). Specifically, a doubling in ∑DEHP and ∑AA phthalates was associated with 33.2% (95% confidence interval 6.6–66.5) and 26.8% (95% confidence interval 2.2–57.4) increase in uterine volume, respectively [148]).

The fact that phthalates do not bioaccumulate and are rapidly excreted creates major challenges for the study of phthalates and health. Studies of UL are limited by their retrospective design, as phthalate exposure assessment may have occurred years after UL occurrence. A large interval between the etiologically relevant exposure window and the measured exposure window is a form of measurement error that may attenuate associations. Another

TABLE 2.1

Common Phthalates and their Commonly Detected Metabolites

Phthalate (Common Sources of Exposure)	Abbrev.	Metabolite(s)	Abbrev.
Dimethyl phthalate (insect repellants, plastics)	DMP	Mono-methyl phthalate	MMP
Diethyl phthalate (fragrances)	DEP	Mono-ethyl phthalate	MEP
Dibutyl phthalates (nail polish, cosmetics, pharmaceutical coatings, insecticides)	DBP	Mono-n-butyl phthalate Mono-isobutyl phthalates	MnBP MiBP
Benzylbutyl phthalate (adhesives, vinyl flooring products, sealants, car-care products)	BzBP	Mono-benzyl phthalate (includes some mono-n-butyl phthalate)	MBzP
Di-2-ethylhexyl phthalate (flexible plastics including food containers, toys, packaging film)	DEHP	Mono-2-ethylhexyl phthalate Mono-(2-ethyl-5-oxohexyl) phthalate Mono-(2-ethyl-5-hydroxyhexyl) phthalate Mono-(2-ethyl-5-carboxypentyl) phthalate	MEHP MEOHP MEHHP MECPP
Di-n-octylphthalate (flexible plastics)	DOP	Mono-3-carboxypropyl phthalate	MCPP
Di-isononyl phthalate	DiNP	Mono-carboxyoctyl phthalate	MCOP
Di-isodecyl phthalate	DiDP	Mono-carboxynonyl phthalate	MCNP

source of exposure measurement error is related to the number of measurements. Unless exposures are constant over time, measurements taken at a single point in time are less reliable indicators of typical exposures than multiple measurements. In their study of 46 women aged 35–49 who provided first morning urinary voids on 2 consecutive days, Hoppin et al. [52] reported intraclass correlation coefficients (ICCs) ranging from 0.53 to 0.80 for creatinine-corrected urinary levels of MBP, MEP, MEHP and MBzP. Other studies have observed good to excellent ICCs for urinary phthalate levels measured up to 6 weeks apart (0.33–0.66) [53,54], but ICCs were lower for longer periods of time: >3 months, ICCs in 19 men ranged from 0.28–0.52 [55]; >6 months, ICCs in 29 children were <0.30, except for MBP (0.35) and MBzP (0.62) [56]. To optimize exposure assessment, measurement of urinary phthalates at multiple time points is critical.

Bisphenol A (BPA)

BPA is one of the most common chemicals in use, with over six billion pounds produced annually for the manufacture of polycarbonate plastics and epoxy resins, which are used as dental sealants, food-can linings and other products. Biomonitoring studies have shown that 93% of the US general population have detectable amounts of BPA in their bodies [57], and BPA has been detected in the blood, urine and breast milk of most women [1,58–60]. Chemically, BPA is closely related to the potent nonsteroidal estrogen diethylstilbestrol (DES), which is known to have adverse reproductive effects [61,62] and is positively associated with UL in most [26–28,63], but not all [25], studies. In animals, BPA disrupts oocyte maturation [64–72], intraovarian steroidogenesis [73–75], development of female reproductive organs [76,77], and fertility [78]. Outbred female CD-1 mice treated with subcutaneous injections of BPA neonatally were more likely to develop UL than unexposed mice [79], and estrogen-responsive genes were repressed in BPA-exposed rats [80]. In tissue culture studies, BPA promotes myometrial cell proliferation, UL cell proliferation and uterine tumorigenesis [81,82].

BPA exposure has been associated with an increased risk of UL in most [83–85], but not all [47], previous epidemiologic studies. In a 2013 case-control study of Chinese women, mean (+/−SD) urinary BPA concentrations were significantly higher among cases (17.6 +/− 2.3 ng/mL) than controls (11.8 +/− 1.7 ng/mL) [83]. In another 2013 study of Chinese women (unknown study design and method of UL classification) [85], urinary BPA was non-significantly higher in cases (13.9 +/− 12.7 ng/mL) than controls (8.50 +/− 12.2 ng/mL). Another phenol, nonylphenol, was significantly higher in cases than controls [85], a finding that has since been replicated [86]. In a 2011 study of Chinese women, cases were divided into three groups (mild, moderate and severe) according to tumor size. Controls were shown to be free of UL based on transvaginal ultrasound examination. Higher serum BPA levels were found for "moderate/severe UL cases" relative to "mild UL cases/controls." [84] However, blood is not an optimal matrix for assessing exposure to nonpersistent chemicals such as BPA because of potential for external contamination [50]. Also, serum BPA levels are approximately an order of magnitude lower than those in urine, with serum levels for many people below the limit of detection [87].

Two replacement chemicals for BPA (bisphenol S and bisphenol F) have been introduced to the market and are now part of the latest phenols panel that can be assayed at the Centers for Disease Control and Prevention (CDC).

Polychlorinated Biphenyls (PCBs)

PCBs are ubiquitous organochlorine chemicals found in the environment that accumulate in body fat and exhibit endocrine-disrupting properties. Although PCB levels have been declining in the US because they have been banned from use [88], they are still found in most of the population [5,89,90]. Serum levels of PCBs reflect long-term exposure [88]; depending on the congener type, PCBs have half-lives of 1–10 years [90]. *In vitro* and animal models show that PCBs can bind to estrogen receptors [91–93], increase gonadotropin-releasing hormone levels, and affect production and release of luteinizing hormone from the pituitary gland [94]. PCBs are associated with greater UL risk in the Baltic gray seal (*Halichoerus grypus*) [95,96] and are hypothesized to increase UL risk in humans. In a cross-sectional analysis from the Great Lakes Study [97], UL risk was positively associated with serum levels of PCBs. Increases in risk were associated with total PCBs, estrogenic PCBs, antiestrogenic PCBs and dioxin-like PCBs, with ORs ranging from 1.6 to 1.9 per ng/g increment [97]. In a case-control study [98], significantly higher concentrations of PCBs were detected in the subcutaneous fat of UL cases compared with controls. In a 2015 cross-sectional study, PCBs measured in omental fat (PCBs 99, 138, 146, 153, 196 and 206) were associated with surgically diagnosed UL, with ORs ranging from 1.5 to 1.9 per 1-SD increment [99].

In the Study of Environment Lifestyle and Fibroids (SELF), the strength of some associations between selected predictors and PCBs varied by degree of PCB chlorination [149]. For instance, a 5-kg/m^2 higher BMI was associated with a 2.9% lower summed concentration of tri- and tetra-substituted PCBs (95% CI: 4.6%–1.2%), an 8.3% lower summed concentration of penta- and hexa-substituted PCBs (95% CI: 10.0%–6.5%), and a 12.2% lower summed concentration of hepta-, octa-, nona- and deca-substituted PCBs (95% CI: 13.8%–10.5%). Likewise, associations for age and being breastfed in infancy were stronger for higher-chlorinated PCBs. These results generally agree with previous studies on predictors of PCB body burdens. Table 2.2 shows examples of PCB groupings that are commonly used in epidemiologic research.

Finally, the Black Women's Health Study reported an increased risk of UL among women with higher consumption of marine long-chain omega-3 fatty acids and fatty fish [100], which are more likely to contain PCBs [90,101,102]. The incidence rate ratio (IRR) for the highest versus lowest quintiles of marine fatty acid intake—sum of eicosapentanoic acid, docosapentaenoic acid and docosahexaenoic acid—was 1.18 (95% CI: 1.05–1.34; $P\text{-}_{trend} = 0.005$) [100]. The IRR for highest versus lowest categories of fatty fish was 1.13 (95% CI: 1.00–1.28) [100]. Results from the SELF cohort, a prospective ultrasound study, also support an association between intake of marine long-chain omega-3 fatty acids and UL incidence: intake of docosahexaenoic acid was associated with a 49% higher incidence of UL (quartile 4 vs. 1: IRR 1.49, 95% CI: 1.04, 2.14; $P\text{-}_{trend} = 0.01$) [150]. Intakes

TABLE 2.2
Potentially Useful Groupings of Polychlorinated Biphenyls in the Study of UL

Group	PCB Congeners Included
Wolff Group 1B (weak phenobarbital inducers, persistent)	187
Wolff Group 2A (potentially antiestrogenic and immunotoxic, dioxin-like, moderately persistent)	66, 74, 105, 118, 156, 167
Wolff Group 2B (potentially antiestrogenic and immunotoxic, limited dioxin activity, persistent)	138/158, 170
Wolff Group 3 (phenobarbital, CYP1A and CYP2B inducers, biologically persistent)	99, 153, 180, 196/203, 183
Dioxin-like	105, 114, 118, 156, 157, 167, 189, 170, 180
Tri- and tetra-substituted	28, 66, 74
Penta- and hexa-substituted	99, 105, 114, 118, 138/158, 146, 153, 156, 157, 167
Hepta-, octa-, nona- and deca-substituted	170, 178, 180, 183, 187, 189, 194, 196/203, 199, 206, 209

of total marine omega-3 fatty acids were associated with a similarly-elevated UL incidence (HR 1.35, 95% CI: 0.94, 1.93; $P_{\text{-trend}} = 0.03$). It remains unclear whether the fatty acids themselves or persistent environmental pollutants (e.g., PCBs) drive the association.

Trace Elements

Several trace elements have been shown to have endocrine-disrupting properties, with the ability to interfere with the hypothalamic-pituitary-gonadal axis, and bind to and activate the estrogen receptor α. Elements with these properties include lead, mercury, cadmium, chromium, cobalt, copper, nickel and tin [103–107]. Current and former cigarette smoking were associated with higher cadmium and lead levels in uterine tissues (see Tobacco section) [108,109]. Studies of heavy metals and UL, including two *in vitro* studies of uterine tissue from women with and without UL [110,111] and two epidemiologic studies using cross-sectional designs [112,113], have been scarce and inconsistent. The following text focuses only on the elements that have been previously studied in epidemiologic studies of UL: lead, cadmium, cobalt and mercury.

Lead

Primary sources of lead exposure in humans are lead-based paint, food, drinking water, ambient air, dust and soil [114]. Data suggest that lead exposure interferes with ovarian steroid stimulation of the endometrium [107,115]. Timing of exposure may matter. In a study of rats exposed to lead acetate in drinking water *in utero*, prepubertally or postpubertally, the most severe effects were observed in the group exposed *in utero*, with disrupted estrous cycling [116]. These effects suggest direct effects of lead on the hypothalamic pituitary axis and on gonadal steroid biosynthesis.

In humans, the association between lead exposure and self-reported UL diagnosis was assessed in the NHANES, 1999–2002, a nationally representative study population of 1425 women aged 20–49 years who were premenopausal and neither pregnant nor breastfeeding [112]. Lead was measured in whole blood. In unadjusted analyses, geometric mean levels of lead were significantly higher among women with UL than those without UL, and positive associations were found between lead and the odds of UL (3rd versus 1st tertile: 1.41, 95% CI: 0.70–2.84). However, after adjusting for age, race/ethnicity, use of oral contraceptives prior to diagnosis and smoking status at diagnosis, the association was 0.82 (95% CI: 0.39–1.74) [112]. In a 2014 cross-sectional analysis of data from 473 women aged 18–44 undergoing surgery for benign gynecologic indications (ENDO study) [113], investigators analyzed 20 trace elements in whole blood and three trace elements in urine. The odds of a UL diagnosis were higher among women in the highest tertile of whole blood lead (adjusted OR = 1.31, 95% CI: 1.02–1.69) relative to the lowest tertile. However, urinary lead was not associated with UL diagnosis. Given the cross-sectional design and the lack of ultrasound screening of all participants, it cannot be determined whether increased exposure to lead contributes to UL development or whether the neoplasms themselves serve as a reservoir for lead.

Cadmium

Primary sources of cadmium exposure in humans are cigarette smoke, air pollution and contaminated food [117]. Cadmium has been shown to have estrogen-disrupting effects on reproductive development in rodents [118]. Sprague-Dawley rats exposed to cadmium 3 weeks after ovariectomy had increased uterine wet weight, promoted growth and development of the mammary glands, and induced hormone-regulated genes [119]. In the uterus, the increase in wet weight coincided with proliferation of the endometrium and induction of progesterone receptor (PgR) and complement component C3. *In utero* exposure to the metal also mimicked the effects of estrogens [119]. In a study investigating whether cadmium stimulates proliferation of estrogen-responsive human UL cells and uterine smooth muscle cells through classical interactions with ERα and ERβ, or by nongenomic mechanisms, the study found that low concentrations of cadmium indeed stimulated cell proliferation in estrogen-responsive uterine cells, but via nongenomic activation of MAPK, not through classical ER-mediated pathways [120].

In NHANES [112], a positive association was found between cadmium measured in whole blood and self-reported UL diagnosis before, but not after, adjustment for age, race/ethnicity, use of oral contraceptives prior to diagnosis and smoking status at diagnosis. In the ENDO study [113], the odds of a UL diagnosis were higher with increased whole blood cadmium (adjusted

OR = 1.44, 95% CI: 1.02–2.04). However, urinary cadmium was not associated with UL diagnosis (adjusted OR = 0.99, 95% CI: 0.77–1.29). Urinary cadmium is considered a better biomarker of exposure. Moreover, given the cross-sectional nature of the study design, it is unclear whether the positive association between cadmium and UL, if real, indicates that cadmium contributes to UL development, or that cadmium simply accumulates in UL tissue.

Cobalt

Primary sources of exposure to cobalt are soil, water, plants and animals (natural sources) and fossil fuel and waste combustion, vehicular and aircraft exhausts, processing of cobalt and cobalt-containing alloys, artificial hip and knee joints, use of cobalt chemicals and fertilizers derived from phosphate rocks (anthropogenic sources) [121]. Cobalt is an essential element and has an important role in female reproduction, but at high concentrations, it is toxic [122]. Animal studies have found an increase in the length of the estrous cycle in female mice exposed to 11.4 mg of cobalt/m^3 for 13 weeks [123], but no effects were observed in rats similarly treated for 13 weeks [124,125].

In a 2014 cross-sectional analysis of data from the ENDO study [113], the odds of a UL diagnosis were higher with increased urine cobalt (adjusted OR = 1.31, 95% CI: 1.02–1.70) [113]. Again, owing to the cross-sectional nature of the study design, it is not clear whether increased exposure to cobalt affects UL development or whether UL serve as a reservoir for cobalt accumulation.

Mercury

Humans may be exposed to mercury via fish intake, air pollution and dental amalgams [126]. Limited data are available from epidemiological studies on the relation between mercury and female reproductive function. A number of effects have been described in experimental animals exposed to mercury, including alterations in ovulation and the estrous cycle [127–130] and changes in pituitary levels of FSH and LH [131].

In NHANES [112], unadjusted geometric mean levels of whole blood mercury were significantly higher among women with UL than those without UL, and positive associations were found with self-reported UL diagnosis before and after adjusting for age, race/ethnicity, use of oral contraceptives prior to diagnosis and smoking status at diagnosis, only mercury showed a positive association with UL (3rd versus 1st tertile: 1.40, 95% CI: 0.75–2.64), albeit the association was imprecise [112]. In a 2014 cross-sectional analysis of data from the ENDO study, based on 473 women aged 18–44 undergoing surgery for benign gynecologic indications [113], neither whole blood nor urinary mercury was appreciably associated with UL.

Other EDCs

Other EDCs that have been studied in relation to UL risk include dioxin and benzophenone-type UV filters (found in sunscreens). High serum levels of dioxin measured after a chemical explosion in Seveso, Italy, were associated with reduced UL risk [132]. The inverse association may be explained by dioxin's antiestrogen effects and its ability to limit extracellular matrix production via TGF-β pathways [133]. No appreciable association was seen for five benzophenone-type chemicals in relation to UL risk in the ENDO study [47].

Analysis of Chemical Mixtures

Given that many chemicals travel together in the environment and are correlated with each other, there has been growing interest in developing novel biostatistical approaches to evaluate *mixtures* of chemicals, not merely individual chemicals. Although little consensus has been reached about which methods work best, several methods are being implemented and tested. For example, weighted quantile sum (WQS) regression can estimate the association between mixtures and health outcomes while addressing the complex correlation structure among mixture components [134,135]. By using the WQS approach, investigators can estimate a weighted sum (across chemicals) of quantiles most associated with a given health outcome and perform inference on the regression coefficient characterizing the association between the outcome and this weighted sum. WQS regression can be run using SAS statistical software. In addition, Bayesian kernel machine regression (BKMR) can be used to nonparametrically estimate and test the joint effects of multiple exposures [136–138]. Simulation studies have demonstrated the success of BKMR in estimating exposure-response functions and in identifying components of mixtures that contribute most to health outcomes [136]. Advantages of BKMR over standard multivariable regression models are that this method allows for non-linearity in relationships between exposures and outcomes, and can more fully capture uncertainty in the exposure-response function by conducting variable selection and health-effect estimation simultaneously. BKMR analyses can be run with R statistical software. Finally, random forest analysis is a novel method that produces single measures of importance for each predictor variable and takes into account interactions among variables without requiring model specification. The advantages of random forest analysis over multivariable regression models are that this approach allows for complicated interactions among constituents and does not assume a linear exposure-outcome relationship. Random forests analyses can be run using the RandomForest package in the R statistical software package [139].

Recommendations for Future Research

- Use of a prospective study design with incident cases of UL can reduce misclassification and help to clarify temporality. With retrospective studies, if levels of chemicals are influenced by having UL (e.g., by affecting metabolism of chemicals, behaviors or lifestyle factors that influence chemical levels), results could be biased. The collection of biospecimens and covariate data before the occurrence of UL can avoid reverse causation and differential misclassification of exposure and covariates.
- Studies that use ultrasound screening to detect UL incidence repeatedly over time will be able to reduce

outcome misclassification. Transvaginal ultrasound is excellent for assessing UL status and mapping size and location when there are four or fewer tumors and uterine size is <375 mL [19]. UL can go undiagnosed for years prior to symptom occurrence. Ultrasound performed in a clinic setting is considered to be the best method for detecting UL, even asymptomatic UL, because it has high sensitivity and specificity relative to histologic evidence [140]. It also is less invasive than other types of diagnostic imaging (e.g., MRI) [6]. The removal of asymptomatic subclinical UL cases from the "control" (or "non-case") group decreases attenuation of associations by misclassification of case status.

- Repeated measures of exposure are critical for nonpersistent chemicals, such as urinary phthalate metabolites and BPA, which have higher intra-individual variation due to shorter half-lives. Chemicals that are more persistent in the environment and biologically can be assessed with fewer measurements will save on costs. The analysis of mixtures of chemicals within and across chemical classes can help address the problem of correlation among chemicals and answer questions about whether or not a particular chemical or a group of chemicals is of concern health-wise.
- Collection of additional data on environmental (behavioral, psychosocial, socioeconomic) factors will allow for control of a wide range of potential confounders and exploration of factors likely to be modifiers of associations (e.g., obesity).
- Finally, the evaluation of mechanistic pathways, which is beyond the scope of epidemiologic studies, can help increase the specificity of results. For example, there is a growing body of research on epigenetics as a mechanism by which early life exposures to EDCs affect future risk of UL [141–144].

Future Research

Future studies that use prospective designs, have sufficient study size, collect data on a wide range of confounding factors, and examine classes of chemicals with large exposure variation will permit a powerful assessment of the associations between environmental chemicals and UL. An NIEHS-funded study that was launched in 2010, SELF, is well-equipped to address important research questions about the influence of environmental chemicals on UL incidence [145,146]. SELF has enrolled 1300 African American women aged 23–34 years who were free of ultrasound-detected UL at baseline (2010–2012). Comprehensive questionnaire data were collected at baseline, and participants are being followed for 5 years. Every 20 months, blood and urine are collected to allow for repeated measurement of environmental chemicals, and ultrasounds are performed by trained sonographers to detect UL. This study of African Americans, a high-risk population for EDC exposure and UL, has the potential to provide informative data on the effects of widespread pollutants on UL and seek explanations for the racial disparity in UL risk.

Conclusion

In summary, there is biological plausibility for a role of environmental chemicals, particularly EDCs, in UL pathogenesis. Exposure to environmental chemicals is widespread in the United States and, given the large numbers of chemicals that travel together in the environment, it is important to consider both their individual and combined influence on UL. Earlier reports on prenatal DES exposure indicated a possible role of EDCs on UL development, and emerging human data suggest an association between selected EDCs and UL [44–46,83–85,97–99], with recent studies showing suggestive evidence of an increased prevalence of UL among women with greater exposure to phthalates, PCBs and BPA, but much more equivocal evidence for a role of lead [113,147], cadmium [113,147], mercury [147], cobalt [113], and other trace elements. Although many of these studies support the hypothesis that exposure to higher levels of EDCs increases UL risk, some indicate biologically-plausible inverse associations (e.g., dioxin [132]), and most epidemiologic studies on EDCs and UL have been small, retrospective in design, and have relied on suboptimal measures of UL and chemical exposures (e.g., blood samples for nonpersistent EDCs). Thus, the extent to which exposure to environmental chemicals explains the Black–White disparity in UL incidence remains to be shown.

The identification of EDCs that influence UL risk could increase understanding of mechanisms for UL development. EDCs are potentially modifiable risk factors, thereby offering the opportunity for primary prevention of UL (e.g., government regulation of chemicals) should research find that they deleteriously affect UL. Given the ubiquitous nature of many EDCs (>90% exposed) and the high lifetime risk of UL among reproductive-aged women (>30%), even small associations, if real, could have an enormous public health impact. However, the evidence linking UL with EDCs is still weak, and more research is warranted in this area.

Acknowledgments

Dr. Wise acknowledges the helpful feedback of Drs. Amelia Wesselink, Jennifer Weuve, and Birgit Claus Henn on various aspects of this work.

REFERENCES

1. Centers for Disease Control and Prevention (CDC) and Department of Health and Human Services. *Fourth National Report on Human Exposure to Environmental Chemicals.* Atlanta: CDC; 2009.
2. Silva MJ, Barr DB, Reidy JA et al. Urinary levels of seven phthalate metabolites in the U.S. population from the National Health and Nutrition Examination Survey (NHANES) 1999–2000. *Environ Health Perspect.* 2004;112:331–8.
3. Axelrad DA, Goodman S, and Woodruff TJ. PCB body burdens in US women of childbearing age 2001–2002: An evaluation of alternate summary metrics of NHANES data. *Environ Res.* 2009;109:368–78.

4. Axelrad DA and Cohen J. Calculating summary statistics for population chemical biomonitoring in women of childbearing age with adjustment for age-specific natality. *Environ Res.* 2011;111:149–55.
5. Sjodin A, Jones RS, Caudill SP, Wong LY, Turner WE, and Calafat AM. Polybrominated diphenyl ethers, polychlorinated biphenyls, and persistent pesticides in serum from the national health and nutrition examination survey: 2003–2008. *Environ Sci Technol.* 2014;48:753–60.
6. Wise LA and Laughlin-Tommaso SK. Uterine Leiomyomata. In: Goldman MB, Troisi R, and Rexrode KM (eds). *Women and Health.* 2nd ed. San Diego, CA: Academic Press, 2013, pp. 285–306.
7. Barbieri RL, McShane PM, and Ryan KJ. Constituents of cigarette smoke inhibit human granulosa cell aromatase. *Fertil Steril.* 1986;46:232–6.
8. Michnovicz JJ, Hershcopf RJ, Nagunuma H, Bradlow HL, and Fishman J. Increased 2-hydroxylation of estradiol as a possible mechanism for the anti-estrogenic effect of cigarette smoking. *N Engl J Med.* 1986;315:1305–9.
9. Bradlow L. Variations in estrogen metabolism. In: Snow R and Hall P, (eds). *Steroid Contraceptives and Women's Response.* New York: Plenum Press, 1994, pp. 171–8.
10. Ohtake F, Takeyama K, Matsumoto T et al. Modulation of oestrogen receptor signalling by association with the activated dioxin receptor. *Nature.* 2003;423:545–50.
11. Ross RK, Pike MC, Vessey MP, Bull D, Yeates D, and Casagrande JT. Risk factors for uterine fibroids: Reduced risk associated with oral contraceptives. *Br Med J Clin Res Ed.* 1986;293:359–62.
12. Lumbiganon P, Rugpao S, Phandhu-fung S, Laopaiboon M, Vudhikamraksa N, and Werawatakul Y. Protective effect of depot-medroxyprogesterone acetate on surgically treated uterine leiomyomas: A multicentre case-control study. *Br J Obstet Gynaecol.* 1996;103:909–14.
13. Romieu I, Walker AM, and Jick S. Determinants of uterine fibroids. *Post Mark Surveill.* 1991;5:119–33.
14. Parazzini F, Negri E, La Vecchia C et al. Uterine myomas and smoking. Results from an Italian study. *J Reprod Med.* 1996;41:316–20.
15. Templeman C, Marshall SF, Clarke CA et al. Risk factors for surgically removed fibroids in a large cohort of teachers. *Fertil Steril.* 2009;92:1436–46.
16. Faerstein E, Szklo M, and Rosenshein N. Risk factors for uterine leiomyoma: A practice-based case-control study. I. African-American heritage, reproductive history, body size, and smoking. *Am J Epidemiol.* 2001;153:1–10.
17. Chen CR, Buck GM, Courey NG, Perez KM, and Wactawski-Wende J. Risk factors for uterine fibroids among women undergoing tubal sterilization. *Am J Epidemiol.* 2001;153:20–6.
18. Marshall LM, Spiegelman D, Manson JE et al. Risk of uterine leiomyomata among premenopausal women in relation to body size and cigarette smoking. *Epidemiology.* 1998;9:511–7.
19. Wise LA, Palmer JR, Harlow BL et al. Risk of uterine leiomyomata in relation to tobacco, alcohol and caffeine consumption in the Black Women's Health Study. *Hum Reprod.* 2004;19:1746–54.
20. Dragomir AD, Schroeder JC, Connolly A et al. Potential risk factors associated with subtypes of uterine leiomyomata. *Reprod Sci.* 2010;17:1029–35.
21. Wise LA, Radin RG, Palmer JR, and Rosenberg L. Association of intrauterine and early life factors with uterine leiomyomata in black women. *Ann Epidemiol.* 2012;22:847–54.
22. Greathouse KL, Cook JD, Lin K et al. Identification of uterine leiomyoma genes developmentally reprogrammed by neonatal exposure to diethylstilbestrol. *Reprod Sci.* 2008;15:765–78.
23. Wise LA, Troisi R, Hatch EE, Titus LJ, Rothman KJ, and Harlow BL. Prenatal diethylstilbestrol exposure and reproductive hormones in premenopausal women. *J Dev Orig Health Dis.* 2015;6:208–16.
24. Newbold R. Cellular and molecular effects of developmental exposure to diethylstilbestrol: Implications for other environmental estrogens. *Environ Health Perspect.* 1995;103:83–7.
25. Wise LA, Palmer JR, Rowlings K et al. Risk of benign gynecologic tumors in relation to prenatal diethylstilbestrol exposure. *Obstet Gynecol.* 2005;105:167–73.
26. Mahalingaiah S, Hart JE, Wise LA, Terry KL, Boynton-Jarrett R, and Missmer SA. Prenatal diethylstilbestrol exposure and risk of uterine leiomyomata in the Nurses' Health Study II. *Am J Epidemiol.* 2013;179:186–91.
27. D'Aloisio AA, Baird DD, DeRoo LA, and Sandler DP. Association of intrauterine and early-life exposures with diagnosis of uterine leiomyomata by 35 years of age in the Sister Study. *Environ Health Perspect.* 2010;118:375–81.
28. Baird DD and Newbold R. Prenatal diethylstilbestrol (DES) exposure is associated with uterine leiomyoma development. *Reprod Toxicol.* 2005;20:81–4.
29. Blount BC, Silva MJ, Caudill SP et al. Levels of seven urinary phthalate metabolites in a human reference population. *Environ Health Perspect.* 2000;108:979–82.
30. Agarwal DK, Lawrence WH, and Autian J. Antifertility and mutagenic effects in mice from parenteral administration of di-2-ethylhexyl phthalate (DEHP). *J Toxicol Environ Health.* 1985;16:71–84.
31. Agarwal DK, Lawrence WH, Turner JE, and Autian J. Effects of parenteral di-(2-ethylhexyl)phthalate (DEHP) on gonadal biochemistry, pathology, and reproductive performance of mice. *J Toxicol Environ Health.* 1989;26:39–59.
32. Lamb JC, Chapin RE, Teague J, Lawton AD, and Reel JR. Reproductive effects of four phthalic acid esters in the mouse. *Toxicol Appl Pharmacol.* 1987;88:255–69.
33. Berman E and Laskey JW. Altered steroidogenesis in whole-ovary and adrenal culture in cycling rats. *Reprod Toxicol.* 1993;7:349–58.
34. Laskey JW and Berman E. Steroidogenic assessment using ovary culture in cycling rats: Effects of bis(2-diethylhexyl)phthalate on ovarian steroid production. *Reprod Toxicol.* 1993;7:25–33.
35. Davis BJ, Maronpot RR, and Heindel JJ. Di-(2-ethylhexyl) phthalate suppresses estradiol and ovulation in cycling rats. *Toxicol Appl Pharmacol.* 1994;128:216–23.
36. Arcadi FA, Costa C, Imperatore C et al. Oral toxicity of bis(2-ethylhexyl) phthalate during pregnancy and suckling in the Long-Evans rat. *Food Chem Toxicol.* 1998;36:963–70.
37. Lovekamp TN and Davis BJ. Mono-(2-ethylhexyl) phthalate suppresses aromatase transcript levels and estradiol production in cultured rat granulosa cells. *Toxicol Appl Pharmacol.* 2001;172:217–24.
38. Davis BJ, Weaver R, Gaines LJ, and Heindel JJ. Mono-(2-ethylhexyl) phthalate suppresses estradiol production independent of FSH-cAMP stimulation in rat granulosa cells. *Toxicol Appl Pharmacol.* 1994;128:224–8.

39. Picard K, Lhuguenot J-C, Lavier-Canivenc M-C, and Chagnon M-C. Estrogenic activity and metabolism of *n*-butyl benzyl phthalate *in vitro*: Identification of the active molecule(s). *Toxicol Appl Pharmacol.* 2001;172:108–18.
40. Harris CA, Henttu P, Parker MG, and Sumpter JP. The estrogenic activity of phthalate esters *in vitro. Environ Health Perspect.* 1997;105:802–11.
41. Hauser R and Calafat AM. Phthalates and human health. *Occup Environ Med.* 2005;62:806–18.
42. Centers for Disease Control and Prevention. *Fourth Report on Human Exposure to Environmental Chemicals, Updated Tables*, (September 2013). Atlanta, GA: U.S. Department of Health and Human Services, Centers for Disease Control and Prevention; 2013. http://www.cdc.gov/exposurereport/
43. Centers for Disease Control and Prevention. *Fourth Report on Human Exposure to Environmental Chemicals.* Atlanta, GA: U.S. Department of Health and Human Services, Centers for Disease Control and Prevention; 2009. http://www.cdc.gov/exposurereport/
44. Weuve J, Hauser R, Calafat AM, Missmer SA, and Wise LA. Association of exposure to phthalates with endometriosis and uterine leiomyomata: Findings from NHANES, 1999–2004. *Environ Health Perspect.* 2010;118:825–32.
45. Luisi S, Latini G, de Felice C et al. Low serum concentrations of di-(2-ethylhexyl)phthalate in women with uterine fibromatosis. *Gynecol Endocrinol.* 2006;22:92–5.
46. Huang PC, Tsai EM, Li WF et al. Association between phthalate exposure and glutathione *S*-transferase M1 polymorphism in adenomyosis, leiomyoma and endometriosis. *Hum Reprod.* 2010;25:986–94.
47. Pollack AZ, Buck Louis GM, Chen Z et al. Bisphenol A, benzophenone-type ultraviolet filters, and phthalates in relation to uterine leiomyoma. *Environ Res.* 2015;137:101–7.
48. Kim YA, Kho Y, Chun KC et al. Increased urinary phthalate levels in women with uterine leiomyoma: A case-control study. *Int J Environ Res Public Health.* 2016;13.
49. Wise LA, Palmer JR, Reich D, Cozier YC, and Rosenberg L. Hair relaxer use and risk of uterine leiomyomata in African-American women. *Am J Epidemiol.* 2012;175:432–40.
50. Calafat AM, Koch HM, Swan SH et al. Misuse of blood serum to assess exposure to bisphenol A and phthalates. *Breast Cancer Res.* 2013;15:403.
51. Kato K, Silva MJ, Brock JW et al. Quantitative detection of nine phthalate metabolites in human serum using reversed-phase high-performance liquid chromatography-electrospray ionization-tandem mass spectrometry. *J Anal Toxicol.* 2003;27:284–9.
52. Hoppin JA, Brock JW, Davis BJ, and Baird DD. Reproducibility of urinary phthalate metabolites in first morning urine samples. *Environ Health Perspect.* 2002;110:515–8.
53. Adibi JJ, Whyatt RM, Williams PL et al. Characterization of phthalate exposure among pregnant women assessed by repeat air and urine samples. *Environ Health Perspect.* 2008;116:467–73.
54. Baird DD, Saldana TM, Nepomnaschy PA et al. Within-person variability in urinary phthalate metabolite concentrations: Measurements from specimens after long-term frozen storage. *J Expo Sci Environ Epidemiol.* 2010;20:169–75.
55. Hauser R, Meeker JD, Park S, Silva MJ, and Calafat AM. Temporal variability of urinary phthalate metabolite levels in men of reproductive age. *Environ Health Perspect.* 2004;112:1734–40.
56. Teitelbaum SL, Britton JA, Calafat AM et al. Temporal variability in urinary concentrations of phthalate metabolites, phytoestrogens and phenols among minority children in the United States. *Environ Res.* 2008;106:257–69.
57. Calafat AM, Ye X, Wong LY, Reidy JA, and Needham LL. Exposure of the U.S. population to bisphenol A and 4-tertiary-octylphenol: 2003–2004. *Environ Health Perspect.* 2008;116:39–44.
58. Lee YJ, Ryu HY, Kim HK et al. Maternal and fetal exposure to bisphenol A in Korea. *Reprod Toxicol.* 2008;25:413–9.
59. Tsutsumi O. Assessment of human contamination of estrogenic endocrine-disrupting chemicals and their risk for human reproduction. *J Steroid Biochem Mol Biol.* 2005; 93:325–30.
60. Mok-Lin E, Ehrlich S, Williams PL et al. Urinary bisphenol A concentrations and ovarian response among women undergoing IVF. *Int J Androl.* 2010;33:385–93.
61. Giusti RM, Iwamoto K, and Hatch EE. Diethylstilbestrol revisited: A review of the long-term health effects. *Ann Intern Med.* 1995;122:778–88.
62. Hoover RN, Hyer M, Pfeiffer RM et al. Adverse health outcomes in women exposed in utero to diethylstilbestrol. *N Engl J Med.* 2011;365:1304–14.
63. D'Aloisio AA, Baird DD, DeRoo LA, and Sandler DP. Early-life exposures and early onset uterine Leiomyomata in black women in the Sister Study. *Environ Health Perspect.* 2012;120:406–12.
64. Hunt PA, Koehler KE, Susiarjo M et al. Bisphenol a exposure causes meiotic aneuploidy in the female mouse. *Curr Biol.* 2003;13:546–53.
65. Can A, Semiz O, and Cinar O. Bisphenol-A induces cell cycle delay and alters centrosome and spindle microtubular organization in oocytes during meiosis. *Mol Hum Reprod.* 2005;11:389–96.
66. Mohri T and Yoshida S. Estrogen and bisphenol A disrupt spontaneous [Ca(2+)](i) oscillations in mouse oocytes. *Biochem Biophys Res Commun.* 2005;326:166–73.
67. Mlynarcikova A, Kolena J, Fickova M, and Scsukova S. Alterations in steroid hormone production by porcine ovarian granulosa cells caused by bisphenol A and bisphenol A dimethacrylate. *Mol Cell Endocrinol.* 2005;244:57–62.
68. Mlynarcikova A, Fickova M, and Scsukova S. The effects of selected phenol and phthalate derivatives on steroid hormone production by cultured porcine granulosa cells. *Altern Lab Anim.* 2007;35:71–7.
69. Hunt PA, Lawson C, Gieske M et al. Bisphenol A alters early oogenesis and follicle formation in the fetal ovary of the rhesus monkey. *Proc Natl Acad Sci U S A.* 2012; 109:17525–30.
70. Eichenlaub-Ritter U, Vogt E, Cukurcam S, Sun F, Pacchierotti F, and Parry J. Exposure of mouse oocytes to bisphenol A causes meiotic arrest but not aneuploidy. *Mutat Res.* 2008;651:82–92.
71. Lenie S, Cortvrindt R, Eichenlaub-Ritter U, and Smitz J. Continuous exposure to bisphenol A during *in vitro* follicular development induces meiotic abnormalities. *Mutat Res.* 2008;651:71–81.
72. Mlynarcikova A, Nagyova E, Fickova M, and Scsukova S. Effects of selected endocrine disruptors on meiotic maturation, cumulus expansion, synthesis of hyaluronan and progesterone by porcine oocyte-cumulus complexes. *Toxicol In Vitro.* 2009;23:371–7.

73. Xi W, Lee CK, Yeung WS et al. Effect of perinatal and postnatal bisphenol A exposure to the regulatory circuits at the hypothalamus-pituitary-gonadal axis of CD-1 mice. *Reprod Toxicol.* 2011;31:409–17.
74. Akingbemi BT, Sottas CM, Koulova AI, Klinefelter GR, and Hardy MP. Inhibition of testicular steroidogenesis by the xenoestrogen bisphenol A is associated with reduced pituitary luteinizing hormone secretion and decreased steroidogenic enzyme gene expression in rat Leydig cells. *Endocrinology.* 2004;145:592–603.
75. Lenie S and Smitz J. Steroidogenesis-disrupting compounds can be effectively studied for major fertility-related endpoints using *in vitro* cultured mouse follicles. *Toxicol Lett.* 2009;185:143–52.
76. Kato H, Ota T, Furuhashi T, Ohta Y, and Iguchi T. Changes in reproductive organs of female rats treated with bisphenol A during the neonatal period. *Reprod Toxicol.* 2003;17:283–8.
77. Hiyama M, Choi EK, Wakitani S et al. Bisphenol-A (BPA) affects reproductive formation across generations in mice. *J Vet Med Sci.* 2011;73:1211–5.
78. Cabaton NJ, Wadia PR, Rubin BS et al. Perinatal exposure to environmentally relevant levels of bisphenol A decreases fertility and fecundity in CD-1 mice. *Environ Health Perspect.* 2011;119:547–52.
79. Newbold RR, Jefferson WN, and Padilla-Banks E. Long-term adverse effects of neonatal exposure to bisphenol A on the murine female reproductive tract. *Reprod Toxicol.* 2007;24:253–8.
80. Greathouse KL, Bredfeldt T, Everitt JI et al. Environmental estrogens differentially engage the histone methyltransferase EZH2 to increase risk of uterine tumorigenesis. *Mol Cancer Res.* 2012;10:546–57.
81. Wang KH, Kao AP, Chang CC, Lin TC, and Kuo TC. Bisphenol A at environmentally relevant doses induces cyclooxygenase-2 expression and promotes invasion of human mesenchymal stem cells derived from uterine myoma tissue. *Taiwan J Obstet Gynecol.* 2013;52:246–52.
82. Shen Y, Ren ML, Feng X, Cai YL, Gao YX, and Xu Q. An evidence *in vitro* for the influence of bisphenol A on uterine leiomyoma. *Eur J Obstet Gynecol Reprod Biol.* 2014;178:80–3.
83. Shen Y, Xu Q, Ren M, Feng X, Cai Y, and Gao Y. Measurement of phenolic environmental estrogens in women with uterine leiomyoma. *PLOS ONE.* 2013;8:e79838.
84. Han MS, Byun JC, Park JE, Kim JY, Chung JY, and Kim JM. Bisphenol-A concentrations from leiomyoma patients by LC/MS. *Toxicol Res.* 2011;27:49–52.
85. Zhou F, Zhang L, Liu A et al. Measurement of phenolic environmental estrogens in human urine samples by HPLC-MS/MS and primary discussion the possible linkage with uterine leiomyoma. *J Chromatogr B Analyt Technol Biomed Life Sci.* 2013;938:80–5.
86. Shen Y, Ren ML, Feng X, Gao YX, Xu Q, and Cai YL. Does nonylphenol promote the growth of uterine fibroids? *Eur J Obstet Gynecol Reprod Biol.* 2014;178:134–7.
87. Teeguarden JG, Calafat AM, Ye X et al. Twenty-four hour human urine and serum profiles of bisphenol a during high-dietary exposure. *Toxicol Sci.* 2011;123:48–57.
88. Hagmar L, Wallin E, Vessby B, Jonsson BA, Bergman A, and Rylander L. Intra-individual variations and time trends 1991–2001 in human serum levels of PCB, DDE and hexachlorobenzene. *Chemosphere.* 2006;64:1507–13.
89. Longnecker MP, Rogan WJ, and Lucier G. The human health effects of DDT (dichlorodiphenyltrichloroethane) and PCBS (polychlorinated biphenyls) and an overview of organochlorines in public health. *Annu Rev Public Health.* 1997;18:211–44.
90. Xue J, Liu SV, Zartarian VG, Geller AM, and Schultz BD. Analysis of NHANES measured blood PCBs in the general US population and application of SHEDS model to identify key exposure factors. *J Expo Sci Environ Epidemiol.* 2014;24:615–21.
91. Korach KS, Sarver P, Chae K, McLachlan JA, and McKinney JD. Estrogen receptor-binding activity of polychlorinated hydroxybiphenyls: Conformationally restricted structural probes. *Mol Pharmacol.* 1988;33:120–6.
92. Hodges LC, Bergerson JS, Hunter DS, and Walker CL. Estrogenic effects of organochlorine pesticides on uterine leiomyoma cells *in vitro*. *Toxicol Sci.* 2000;54:355–64.
93. Hodges LC, Hunter DS, Bergerson JS, Fuchs-Young R, and Walker CL. An *in vivo/in vitro* model to assess endocrine disrupting activity of xenoestrogens in uterine leiomyoma. *Ann N Y Acad Sci.* 2001;948:100–11.
94. Jansen HT, Cooke PS, Porcelli J, Liu TC, and Hansen LG. Estrogenic and antiestrogenic actions of PCBs in the female rat: *In vitro* and *in vivo* studies. *Reprod Toxicol.* 1993;7:237–48.
95. Backlin BM, Eriksson L, and Olovsson M. Histology of uterine leiomyoma and occurrence in relation to reproductive activity in the Baltic gray seal (*Halichoerus grypus*). *Vet Pathol.* 2003;40:175–80.
96. Bredhult C, Backlin BM, Bignert A, and Olovsson M. Study of the relation between the incidence of uterine leiomyomas and the concentrations of PCB and DDT in Baltic gray seals. *Reprod Toxicol.* 2008;25:247–55.
97. Lambertino A, Turyk M, Anderson H, Freels S, and Persky V. Uterine leiomyomata in a cohort of Great Lakes sport fish consumers. *Environ Res.* 2011;111:565–72.
98. Qin Y, Leung C, Leung A, Wu S, Zheng J, and Wong M. Persistent organic pollutants and heavy metals in adipose tissues of patients with uterine leiomyomas and the association of these pollutants with seafood diet, BMI, and age. *Environmental Science and Pollution Research.* 2010;17:229–40.
99. Trabert B, Chen Z, Kannan K et al. Persistent organic pollutants (POPs) and fibroids: Results from the ENDO study. *J Expo Sci Environ Epidemiol.* 2015;25:278–85.
100. Wise LA, Radin RG, Kumanyika SK, Ruiz-Narvaez EA, Palmer JR, and Rosenberg L. A prospective study of dietary fat and risk of uterine leiomyomata. *Am J Clin Nutr.* 2014;99:1105–16.
101. McGraw JE and Waller DP. Fish ingestion and congener specific polychlorinated biphenyl and p,p'-dichlorodiphenyldichloroethylene serum concentrations in a great lakes cohort of pregnant African American women. *Environ Int.* 2009;35:557–65.
102. Mozaffarian D and Rimm EB. Fish intake, contaminants, and human health: Evaluating the risks and the benefits. *JAMA.* 2006;296:1885–99.
103. Stoica A, Katzenellenbogen BS, and Martin MB. Activation of estrogen receptor-alpha by the heavy metal cadmium. *Mol Endocrinol.* 2000;14:545–53.
104. Fechner P, Damdimopoulou P, and Gauglitz G. Biosensors paving the way to understanding the interaction between cadmium and the estrogen receptor alpha. *PLOS ONE.* 2011;6:e23048.

105. Martin MB, Reiter R, Pham T et al. Estrogen-like activity of metals in MCF-7 breast cancer cells. *Endocrinology.* 2003;144:2425–36.
106. Nasiadek M, Swiatkowska E, Nowinska A, Krawczyk T, Wilczynski JR, and Sapota A. The effect of cadmium on steroid hormones and their receptors in women with uterine myomas. *Arch Environ Contam Toxicol.* 2011;60:734–41.
107. Wide M and Wide L. Estradiol receptor activity in uteri of pregnant mice given lead before implantation. *Fertil Steril.* 1980;34:503–8.
108. Rzymski P, Niedzielski P, Rzymski P, Tomczyk K, Kozak L, and Poniedzialek B. Metal accumulation in the human uterus varies by pathology and smoking status. *Fertil Steril.* 2016;105:1511–8 e3.
109. Rzymski P, Rzymski P, Tomczyk K et al. Metal status in human endometrium: Relation to cigarette smoking and histological lesions. *Environ Res.* 2014;132:328–33.
110. Nasiadek M, Krawczyk T, and Sapota A. Tissue levels of cadmium and trace elements in patients with myoma and uterine cancer. *Hum Exp Toxicol.* 2005;24:623–30.
111. Cunzhi H, Jiexian J, Xianwen Z, Jingang G, Shumin Z, and Lili D. Serum and tissue levels of six trace elements and copper/zinc ratio in patients with cervical cancer and uterine myoma. *Biol Trace Elem Res.* 2003;94:113–22.
112. Jackson LW, Zullo MD, and Goldberg JM. The association between heavy metals, endometriosis and uterine myomas among premenopausal women: National Health and Nutrition Examination Survey 1999–2002. *Hum Reprod.* 2008;23:679–87.
113. Johnstone EB, Louis GM, Parsons PJ et al. Increased urinary cobalt and whole blood concentrations of cadmium and lead in women with uterine leiomyomata: Findings from the ENDO Study. *Reprod Toxicol.* 2014;49:27–32.
114. Abadin H, Ashizawa A, Stevens YW et al. *Toxicological Profile for Lead.* Atlanta (GA); 2007.
115. Wide M. In: *Reproductive and Developmental Toxicity of Metals.* Clarkson TW, Nordberg GF, Sager PR (eds). New York: Plenum Press, 1983, pp. 343–56.
116. Ronis MJ, Badger TM, Shema SJ, Roberson PK, and Shaikh F. Reproductive toxicity and growth effects in rats exposed to lead at different periods during development. *Toxicol Appl Pharmacol.* 1996;136:361–71.
117. Faroon O, Ashizawa A, Wright S et al. *Toxicological Profile for Cadmium.* Atlanta (GA); 2012.
118. Wang HJ, Liu ZP, Jia XD, Chen H, and Tan YJ. Endocrine disruption of cadmium in rats using the OECD enhanced TG 407 test system. *Biomed Environ Sci.* 2014;27:950–9.
119. Johnson MD, Kenney N, Stoica A et al. Cadmium mimics the *in vivo* effects of estrogen in the uterus and mammary gland. *Nat Med.* 2003;9:1081–4.
120. Gao X, Yu L, Moore AB, Kissling GE, Waalkes MP, and Dixon D. Cadmium and proliferation in human uterine leiomyoma cells: Evidence of a role for EGFR/MAPK pathways but not classical estrogen receptor pathways. *Environ Health Perspect.* 2015;123:331–6.
121. Crinnion WJ. The CDC fourth national report on human exposure to environmental chemicals: What it tells us about our toxic burden and how it assist environmental medicine physicians. *Altern Med Rev.* 2010;15:101–9.
122. Simonsen LO, Harbak H, and Bennekou P. Cobalt metabolism and toxicology—a brief update. *Sci Total Environ.* 2012;432:210–5.
123. Bucher JR, Elwell MR, Thompson MB, Chou BJ, Renne R, and Ragan HA. Inhalation toxicity studies of cobalt sulfate in F344/N rats and B6C3F1 mice. *Fundam Appl Toxicol.* 1990;15:357–72.
124. Bucher JR, Hailey JR, Roycroft JR et al. Inhalation toxicity and carcinogenicity studies of cobalt sulfate. *Toxicol Sci.* 1999;49:56–67.
125. NTP. Toxicity studies of cobalt sulphate heptahydrate (CAS No. 10026–24–1) in F344/N rats and B6C3F1 mice (inhalation studies). Research Triangle Park: United States Department of Health and Human Services, National Institutes of Health, National Toxicology Program (NIH Publication No. 91-3124), 1991.
126. Risher JF, De Rosa CT, Jones DE, and Murray HE. Summary report for the expert panel review of the toxicological profile for mercury. *Toxicol Ind Health.* 1999;15:483–516.
127. Burbacher TM, Shen DD, Liberato N, Grant KS, Cernichiari E, and Clarkson T. Comparison of blood and brain mercury levels in infant monkeys exposed to methylmercury or vaccines containing thimerosal. *Environ Health Perspect.* 2005;113:1015–21.
128. Stadnicka A. Localization of mercury in the rat ovary after oral administration of mercuric chloride. *Acta Histochem.* 1980;67:227–33.
129. Lamperti AA and Printz RH. Localization, accumulation, and toxic effects of mercuric chloride on the reproductive axis of the female hamster. *Biol Reprod.* 1974;11:180–6.
130. Khan AT, Atkinson A, Graham TC, Thompson SJ, Ali S, and Shireen KF. Effects of inorganic mercury on reproductive performance of mice. *Food Chem Toxicol.* 2004;42:571–7.
131. Lamperti A and Niewenhuis R. The effects of mercury on the structure and function of the hypothalamo-pituitary axis in the hamster. *Cell Tissue Res.* 1976;170:315–24.
132. Eskenazi B, Warner M, Samuels S et al. Serum dioxin concentrations and risk of uterine leiomyoma in the Seveso Women's Health Study. *Am J Epidemiol.* 2007;166:79–87.
133. Gomez-Duran A, Carvajal-Gonzalez JM, Mulero-Navarro S, Santiago-Josefat B, Puga A, and Fernandez-Salguero PM. Fitting a xenobiotic receptor into cell homeostasis: How the dioxin receptor interacts with TGFbeta signaling. *Biochem Pharmacol.* 2009;77:700–12.
134. Czarnota J, Gennings C, and Wheeler DC. Assessment of weighted quantile sum regression for modeling chemical mixtures and cancer risk. *Cancer Inform.* 2015;14:159–71.
135. Gennings C, Carrico C, Factor-Litvak P, Krigbaum N, Cirillo PM, and Cohn BA. A cohort study evaluation of maternal PCB exposure related to time to pregnancy in daughters. *Environ Health.* 2013;12:66.
136. Bobb JF, Valeri L, Claus Henn B et al. Bayesian kernel machine regression for estimating the health effects of multi-pollutant mixtures. *Biostatistics.* 2015;16:493–508.
137. Liu D, Lin X, and Ghosh D. Semiparametric regression of multidimensional genetic pathway data: Least-squares kernel machines and linear mixed models. *Biometrics.* 2007;63:1079–88.
138. Liu D, Ghosh D, and Lin X. Estimation and testing for the effect of a genetic pathway on a disease outcome using logistic kernel machine regression via logistic mixed models. *BMC Bioinformatics.* 2008;9:292.
139. Liaw A and Wiener M. Classification and regression by random forest. *R News.* 2002;2(3):18–22. http://CRAN.R-project.org/doc/Rnews/

140. Dueholm M, Lundorf E, Hansen ES, Ledertoug S, and Olesen F. Accuracy of magnetic resonance imaging and transvaginal ultrasonography in the diagnosis, mapping, and measurement of uterine myomas. *Am J Obstet Gynecol.* 2002;186:409–15.
141. Katz TA, Yang Q, Trevino LS, Walker CL, and Al-Hendy A. Endocrine-disrupting chemicals and uterine fibroids. *Fertil Steril.* 2016;106:967–77.
142. Mas A, Stone L, O'Connor PM et al. Developmental exposure to endocrine disruptors expands murine myometrial stem cell compartment as a prerequisite to leiomyoma tumorigenesis. *Stem Cells.* 2017;35:666–78.
143. Prusinski Fernung LE, Yang Q, Sakamuro D, Kumari A, Mas A, and Al-Hendy A. Endocrine disruptor exposure during development increases incidence of uterine fibroids by altering DNA repair in myometrial stem cells. *Biol Reprod.* 2018;99:735–48.
144. Prusinski L, Al-Hendy A, and Yang Q. Developmental exposure to endocrine disrupting chemicals alters the epigenome: Identification of reprogrammed targets. *Gynecol Obstet Res.* 2016;3:1–6.
145. Baird DD, Harmon QE, Upson K et al. A prospective, ultrasound-based study to evaluate risk factors for uterine fibroid incidence and growth: Methods and results of recruitment. *J Womens Health (Larchmt).* 2015;24:907–15.
146. Wise LA. Study of Environment Lifestyle and Fibroids (SELF): Advancing the field of fibroid epidemiology. *J Womens Health (Larchmt).* 2015;24:862–4.
147. Jackson LW, Howards PP, Wactawski-Wende J, and Schisterman EF. The association between cadmium, lead and mercury blood levels and reproductive hormones among healthy, premenopausal women. *Hum Reprod.* 2011;26:2887–95.
148. Zota AR, Geller RJ, Calafat AM, Marfori CQ, Baccarelli AA, and Moawad GN. Phthalates exposure and uterine fibroid burden among women undergoing surgical treatment for fibroids: A preliminary study. *Fertil Steril.* 2019; 111(1):112–21.
149. Wesselink AK, Bethea TN, McClean M, Weuve J, Williams PL, Hauser R, Sjödin A, Brasky TM, Baird DD, and Wise LA. Predictors of plasma polychlorinated biphenyl concentrations among reproductive-aged black women. *Int J Hyg Environ Health.* 2019;222(7):1001–1010.
150. Brasky TM, Bethea TN, Wesselink AK, Wegienka GR, Baird DD, and Wise LA. Dietary fat intake and risk of uterine leiomyomata: A prospective ultrasound study. *Am J Epidemiol*, in press.

3

Dietary Factors and Uterine Fibroids

Holly R. Harris, Stacey A. Missmer, and Kathryn L. Terry

Dietary factors may play a role in fibroid etiology due to their potential to modify endogenous hormones as well as their inflammatory effects; however, few studies have examined diet and UL risk, and few clear dietary associations have been established. Characteristics of the peer-reviewed studies that have examined dietary factors and uterine fibroids though June 2016 are provided in Table 3.1, and the observed associations are summarized in Table 3.2.

Fruits and Vegetables

Fruits and vegetables contain vitamins, minerals, antioxidants and phytochemicals that may decrease fibroid risk. One of the most consistent associations between diet and fibroid risk has been with fruit and vegetable consumption (Table 3.3). The prospective Black Women's Health Study (BWHS) cohort and case-control studies in China and Italy all reported decreased risk of fibroids with fruit and vegetable intake [1–4]. Specifically, the BWHS reported a statistically significant decreased risk with total fruits and vegetables combined, with a stronger association for fruits than vegetables, which appeared to be driven by a significant inverse association with citrus fruits [2]. He et al. also reported a significant inverse association with total fruit and vegetable intake [1], while Shen et al. reported significant inverse associations for broccoli, cabbage, Chinese cabbage, tomatoes and apples [4], and Chiaffarino et al. reported a significant inverse association with fresh fruit and green vegetable consumption [3]. Animal data have suggested that lycopene, a carotenoid with strong antioxidant properties, decreases fibroid risk [5]. However, in both case-control and cohort studies, lycopene, other carotenoids, vitamins C and E, folate and fiber did not explain the decreased risk observed with fruits and vegetables [2,6,7]. The BWHS observed an inverse association with dietary vitamin A and fibroids risk that appeared to be driven by preformed vitamin A, not pro-vitamin A carotenoids [2]. In contrast, a cross-sectional study in the National Health and Nutrition Examination Survey examined serum micronutrient levels and reported higher serum vitamin A concentrations among women with fibroids compared to those without, but no serum difference was observed for other carotenoids or micronutrients [8].

Dietary Fat

Trans fat intake influences circulating levels of IL-6, IL-1β, TNF-α and other inflammatory markers [9–11], and markers including IL-6, IL-1 and TNF-α have been reported to influence the secretion of enzymes that digest endometrial extracellular matrices [12]. In contrast, dietary intake and plasma levels of omega-3 fatty acids have been inversely associated with inflammatory cytokines, including IL-6, TNF-α and TNF-α receptors [13,14]. Omega-6 fatty acids have also been hypothesized to reduce fibroid risk through their anti-inflammatory properties. However, few studies have examined the associations between dietary fats and fibroid risk [3,7,15]. The BWHS examined the association between dietary fats and fibroid risk, reporting statistically significant increased risks of fibroids with intake of specific long-chain omega-3 fatty acids but no significant associations with total fat or other fat subtypes [15]. However, no associations between dietary fats and fibroids were observed in a cross-sectional study of Japanese women enrolled through a health check-up program [7] or in an Italian case-control study that examined butter, margarine and oil intake [12].

Dairy Foods

Dairy foods also contain multiple components that may protect against fibroids through their anti-tumorigenic and anti-inflammatory effects [16,17], as well as through influences on circulating estrogens [18]. In mouse models, a milk diet has been demonstrated to reduce markers of oxidative and inflammatory stress, including tumor necrosis factor alpha and IL-6 [17]. In addition, milk consumption has also been shown to increase circulating insulin-like growth factor-I (IGF-I) levels [19–21], and IGF-I has been shown to promote fibroid cell proliferation in culture [22,23]. Baird et al. has reported a suggestive inverse association between high circulating IGF-I levels and fibroid prevalence [24]. The BWHS has examined the association between dairy intake and fibroids, reporting a reduced risk of fibroids with increasing consumption, with similar associations observed for low-fat and high-fat dairy foods [16]. In contrast, case-control studies in China and Italy reported no significant associations with dairy foods [1], milk or cheese [3]. Wise et al. also examined vitamins, minerals and fatty acids commonly found in dairy foods but, after adjustment for total dairy intake, did not observe significant associations with any of these dietary factors [16].

Vitamin D

Although human levels of vitamin D are primarily derived from sun exposure, vitamin D is naturally occurring in some

TABLE 3.1
Summary of Previous Observational Studies on Dietary Factors and Fibroid Risk

Author/Year	Study Name/Type	Number of Fibroid Cases and Controls or Total Study Population	Dietary or Biomarker Assessment Method	Exposure(s) Evaluated	Exposure Categorization	Adjustment Variables
Questionnaire-Based Dietary Assessment						
Shen 2016 [4]	Hospital-based case-control study, Nanjing, China	600 fibroid cases; 600 controls	Questionnaire	Green tea, honey, coffee, green onions, vitamin D, garlic, strawberries, grapes, cranberries, blueberries, walnuts, pomegranate, broccoli, cabbage, cauliflower, Chinese cabbage, turnip, tomatoes, watermelon, pawpaw, lemon, onions, apples	Frequent, occasional, no consumption	Age, education
Wise 2014 [15]	Prospective cohort 2001–2009, Black Women's Health Study	2695 incident fibroid cases; 12,044 participants at start of follow-up	85-item food frequency questionnaire (FFQ)	Total fat, saturated fat, monounsaturated fat, polyunsaturated fat, omega-6 fatty acid intake, omega-3 fatty acid intake, ratio of omega-6 to omega-3 fatty acids, trans fats, all fish/seafood, dark-meat fish, other fish/seafood	Quintiles of intake for fats; Quartiles of intake for fish/seafood	Age, questionnaire cycle, energy intake, age at menarche, parity, age at first birth, years since last birth, ever use of oral contraceptives, age at first oral contraceptive use, alcohol, smoking, body mass index (BMI), education, occupation, income, marital status, US region of residence
He 2013 [1]	Hospital-based case-control study, Beijing, China	73 fibroid cases; 210 controls	Short-form FFQ	Cereals, soy, meat, fish, dairy food, eggs, vegetables and fruits, desserts, fried food, salty food	High (more than 3 days/week), intermediate (1–2 days/week), low (never/less than 1 day/week) consumption	Age, gravidity, parity
Wise 2011 [2]	Prospective cohort 1997–2009, Black Women's Health Study	6627 incident fibroid cases; 22,583 participants at start of follow-up	68-item FFQ (1995) and 85-item FFQ (2001)	Total fruits and vegetables, vegetables (total, cruciferous, green leafy, yellow–orange), fruit (total, citrus, cantaloupe, apples, pears and bananas, orange and grapefruit juice), vitamin A (total, dietary, pro-vitamin A, preformed retinol), vitamin C (total, dietary), vitamin E (total, dietary), folate (total, dietary), carotenoids (lycopene, alpha-carotene, beta-carotene, carotene, beta-cryptoxanthin, lutein/zeaxanthin), fiber (total, insoluble, soluble)	Various categories of intake for foods (i.e., <1/day, 1/d, 2–3/d, 4+/day); Quintiles of intake for nutrients	Age, time period, energy intake, parity, age at first birth, years since last birth, ever use of oral contraceptives, age at first oral contraceptive use, BMI, smoking, current alcohol intake, multivitamin use, education, income, marital status, US region of residence

(Continued)

TABLE 3.1 (*Continued*)

Summary of Previous Observational Studies on Dietary Factors and Fibroid Risk

Author/Year	Study Name/Type	Number of Fibroid Cases and Controls or Total Study Population	Dietary or Biomarker Assessment Method	Exposure(s) Evaluated	Exposure Categorization	Adjustment Variables
Wise 2010 [16]	Prospective cohort 1997–2007, Black Women's Health Study	5871 incident fibroid cases; 22,120 participants at start of follow-up	68-item FFQ (1995) and 85-item FFQ (2001)	Dairy foods (total, high-fat, low-fat, milk, high-fat milk, low-fat milk, cheese, ice cream, yogurt, butter), soy (total soy foods, soy milk, tofu, soy/veggie burgers), calcium, phosphorus, calcium-to-phosphorus ratio, dietary vitamin D, butyric acid intake	Various categories of intake for foods (i.e., <1/day, 1/d, 2/d, 3/d, 4+/day); Quintiles of intake for nutrients	Age, time period, energy intake, age at menarche, parity, age at first birth, years since last birth, ever use of oral contraceptives, age at first oral contraceptive use, vigorous exercise, BMI, smoking, alcohol intake, diabetes, education, occupation, income, marital status, geographic region
Radin 2010 [31]	Prospective cohort 1997–2007, Black Women's Health Study	5800 incident fibroid cases; 22,861 participants at start of follow-up	68-item FFQ (1995) and 85-item FFQ (2001)	Glycemic load, glycemic index	Quintiles	Age, questionnaire cycle, energy intake, servings of dairy foods, age at menarche, current use of hormonal contraception, BMI, diabetes, current alcohol consumption, smoking, vigorous physical activity, current US region of residence, marital status, household income, occupation, education, parity, age at first birth, years since last birth
Nagata 2009 [7]	Hospital based case-control study, Gifu, Japan	54 fibroid cases; 231 controls	169-item FFQ	Total energy, fat (total, SFA, MUFA, PUFA), dietary fiber, soya isoflavones, alcohol (total, beer/light beer, other types of liquor)	Tertiles	Age, BMI, smoking, number of live births, age at menarche
Terry 2008 [6]	Prospective cohort 1991–2001, Nurses' Health Study II	6302 incident fibroid cases; 82,512 participants at start of follow-up	130-item FFQ (assessed in 1991, 1995 and 1999)	Lycopene, alpha-carotene, beta-carotene, beta-cryptoxanthin, lutein/zeaxanthin	Quintiles	Age, age at menarche, infertility, marital status, ancestry, age at first oral contraceptive use, parity, age at first birth, time since last birth, BMI, diastolic blood pressure, antihypertensive therapy, calories

(*Continued*)

TABLE 3.1 (*Continued*)

Summary of Previous Observational Studies on Dietary Factors and Fibroid Risk

Author/Year	Study Name/Type	Number of Fibroid Cases and Controls or Total Study Population	Dietary or Biomarker Assessment Method	Exposure(s) Evaluated	Exposure Categorization	Adjustment Variables
Wise 2004 [30]	Prospective cohort 1997–2001, Black Women's Health Study	2177 incident fibroid cases; 22,885 participants at start of follow-up	68-item FFQ	Alcohol consumption status, current alcohol consumption, years of alcohol consumption, type of alcohol (beer, wine, liquor), coffee (caffeinated, decaffeinated), tea, soft drinks, caffeine	Various categories of intake (i.e., cups/day: almost never, <1, 1, 2, 3, 3 or more)	Age, time period, age at menarche, age at first birth, years since last birth, use of oral contraceptives, education, smoking, current alcohol consumption, BMI
Chiaffarino 1999 [3]	Hospital-based case-control study, Milan, Italy	843 fibroid cases; 1,557 controls	Questionnaire	Milk, beef and other red meat, liver, carrots, green vegetables, fresh fruit, eggs, ham, fish, cheese, whole-grain foods, butter, margarine, oil, coffee, tea, alcohol	High, intermediate, low	Age, education, marital status, parity, BMI, smoking, calendar year at interview
Biomarker-Based Exposure Assessment						
Baird 2013 [25]	Health plan-based cross-sectional study, National Institute for Environmental Health Sciences Uterine Fibroid Study	674 participants with fibroids; 362 participants without fibroids	Plasma levels using radioimmunoassay	25-hydroxyvitamin D	Linear term and 5-ng/mL categories	Age, age at menarche, full-term pregnancies after age 24 years, BMI, physical activity, ethnicity
Paffoni 2013 [27]	Infertility clinic-based case-control study, Milan, Italy	128 fibroid cases; 256 controls	Serum levels using radioimmunoassay	25-hydroxyvitamin D_3	Continuous (ng/mL) and categorical (<10 ng/mL, 10–19.9 ng/mL, 20+ ng/mL)	BMI, parity, ethnicity
Sabry 2013 [26]	Outpatient clinic-based cross-sectional study, Sohag, Egypt	104 participants with fibroids; 50 participants without fibroid	Serum levels using radioimmunoassay	25-hydroxyvitamin D_3	Continuous (ng/mL)	Stratification by ethnicity
Martin 2011 [8]	Population-based cross-sectional study, 2003–2004 National Health and Nutrition Examination Survey	68 participants with fibroids; 819 participants without fibroids	Serum blood levels	Beta-carotene, vitamin A, vitamin B_6, vitamin B_{12}, vitamin C, vitamin E, folate	Tertiles	Age, race, BMI, education, parity, oral contraceptive use, age at first birth, age at last birth
Atkinson 2006 [29]	Health plan-based case-control study, Washington, US	170 fibroid cases; 173 controls	Urinary excretion of phytoestrogens measured using gas chromatography-mass spectrometry	Isoflavones and lignans	Continuous (nmol/mg Cr^x) and quartiles	Age, BMI, race, family history of uterine fibroids, mean lignin or isoflavone excretion

TABLE 3.2

Summary of Associations between Selected Dietary Factors and Uterine Fibroids

Dietary Factor	Summary of Association(s)	References
Fruits and vegetables	Consistently decreased risk	[1–4]
Carotenoids	No associations	[2,6]
Fats	No associations overall, suggestion of increased risk with specific long chain omega-3 fatty acids	[3,7,15]
Dairy	Inconsistent	[1,3,16]
Dietary vitamin D	No associations	[4,16]
Plasma vitamin D	Consistently decreased risk	[25–27]
Fish	Inconsistent	[1,3,15,28]
Soy	No associations	[1,7,16]
Meat	Inconsistent	[1,3]
Alcohol	Suggestion of increased risk among beer drinkers	[3,7,30]

foods such as fatty fish, liver and eggs, while other foods, such as milk or orange juice, are fortified with vitamin D. Dietary vitamin D was not associated with fibroid risk in the BWHS or a China-based case-control study [4,16]. However, given that only a small portion of vitamin D comes from diet, plasma levels may be a more accurate indicator of an individual's vitamin D level, and three cross-sectional studies have reported a reduced risk of fibroids among women with higher levels of plasma vitamin D [25–27].

Fish

Four studies conducted in three different geographic regions have examined fish intake. While fish can be rich in polyunsaturated fats, it also can be a source of toxin exposure—particularly persistent organic pollutants (POPs) and other phytoestrogenic compounds. A case-control study from China reported no association between fish consumption and fibroid risk [1], while an Italian case-control study reported a protective effect of fish consumption on fibroid risk [3]. In the US, the BWHS observed the suggestion of an increased risk with consumption of dark-meat fish [15]. In the midwestern US, consumption of sport fish, which are known to be high in a number of POPs, was marginally associated with increased fibroid risk [28]. The varied types of fish consumed in different countries, assorted preparation methods and differing POP burdens across studies make the interpretation of these results challenging.

Soy

Soy intake has been examined in populations with high and low intakes of soy products with no clear association. In a case-control study in Japan, no significant association was observed between soy isoflavones and fibroid risk [7]. Soy intake was also not associated with fibroid risk in a case-control study in China or in the BWHS in the US [1,16].

Meat

Only two studies have examined meat intake in relation to fibroid risk, with inconsistent results. Chiaffario et al. observed a significant increased risk of fibroids with higher beef and other red meat consumption [3] while He et al. observed no association between meat intake and fibroid risk [1].

Alcohol

Alcohol consumption has been associated with an increased risk of fibroids in two of three studies that have examined this

TABLE 3.3

Main Results from Studies Evaluating the association(s) between Fruit and Vegetable Intake and Uterine Fibroids

Author/Year	Selected Exposure(s)	Multivariable Hazard Ratio (HR) or Odds Ratio (OR) and 95% Confidence Intervals (CI)	Serving Categories
Shen 2016 [4]	Broccoli	OR = 0.55; 95% CI = 0.32–0.96	Continuous servings
	Cabbage	OR = 0.45; 95% CI = 0.21–0.95	
	Chinese cabbage	OR = 0.31; 95% CI = 0.10–0.95	
	Tomato	OR = 0.45; 95% CI = 0.24–0.85	
	Apple	OR = 0.41; 95% CI = 0.21–0.81	
He 2013 [1]	Vegetables and fruits	OR = 0.4; 95% CI = 0.2–0.9	High vs. low consumption (reference)
Wise 2011 [2]	Total fruits and vegetables	HR = 0.90; 95% CI = 0.82–0.98	≥4 servings/day vs. <1/day (reference)
	Total vegetables	HR = 0.97; 95% CI = 0.89–1.05	≥2 servings/day vs. <4/week (reference)
	Cruciferous	HR = 0.97; 95% CI = 0.89–1.06	≥6 servings/week vs. <1/week (reference)
	Green leafy	HR = 0.93; 95% CI = 0.85–1.01	≥6 servings/week vs. <1/week (reference)
	Yellow-orange	HR = 1.00; 95% CI = 0.92–1.09	≥6 servings/week vs. <1/week (reference)
	Total fruits	HR = 0.89; 95% CI = 0.81–0.98	≥2 servings/day vs. <2/week (reference)
	Citrus	HR = 0.92; 95% CI = 0.86–1.00	≥3 servings/week vs. <1/month (reference)
	Cantaloupe	HR = 0.95; 95% CI = 0.86–1.04	≥3 servings/week vs. <1/month (reference)
	Apples, pears and bananas	HR = 0.98; 95% CI = 0.89–1.08	≥3 servings/week vs. <1/month (reference)
	Orange and grapefruit juice	HR = 1.02; 95% CI = 0.93–1.12	≥1 serving/day vs. <1/month (reference)
Chiaffarino 1999 [3]	Green vegetables	OR = 0.5; 95% CI = 0.4–0.6	Third vs. first tertile (reference)

association. The BWHS reported significantly higher risks of fibroids among women who were current drinkers and those who had consumed alcohol for a longer period of time. This association was strongest for beer consumption [30]. Nagata et al. also observed an increased risk of fibroids with increasing alcohol consumption that was strongest among beer drinkers [7]. An Italian case-control study observed no association between alcohol intake and fibroids; however, wine was the alcohol consumed by 90% of women included in this study, with only a small proportion consuming beer [3].

In summary, few studies have examined the associations between dietary factors and fibroid risk and the majority of these studies have been cross-sectional in design—severely reducing the ability to draw temporal cause and effect conclusions. To date, consistent associations between diet and fibroid risks are limited to two consistent discoveries: a reduced risk with higher fruit and vegetable intake (although the primary food contributors remain to be determined) and increased risk with lower vitamin D levels (although the impact of sun versus food sources remains unclear). Much more research is needed to clarify the role of other dietary factors in relation to fibroid risk. Given the prevalence of fibroids and the effects on women's lives, understanding the impact of this modifiable group of risk or preventive factors would have a large clinical and public health impact.

REFERENCES

1. He Y, Zeng Q, Dong S, Qin L, Li G, and Wang P. Associations between uterine fibroids and lifestyles including diet, physical activity and stress: A case-control study in China. *Asia Pac J Clin Nutr.* 2013;22(1):109–17.
2. Wise LA, Radin RG, Palmer JR, Kumanyika SK, Boggs DA, and Rosenberg L. Intake of fruit, vegetables, and carotenoids in relation to risk of uterine leiomyomata. *Am J Clin Nutr.* 2011;94(6):1620–31.
3. Chiaffarino F, Parazzini F, La Vecchia C, Chatenoud L, Di Cintio E, and Marsico S. Diet and uterine myomas. *Obstet Gynecol.* 1999;94(3):395–8.
4. Shen Y, Wu Y, Lu Q, and Ren M. Vegetarian diet and reduced uterine fibroids risk: A case-control study in Nanjing, China. *J Obstet Gynaecol Res.* 2016;42(1):87–94.
5. Sahin K, Ozercan R, Onderci M et al. Lycopene supplementation prevents the development of spontaneous smooth muscle tumors of the oviduct in Japanese quail. *Nutr Cancer.* 2004;50(2):181–9.
6. Terry KL, Missmer SA, Hankinson SE, Willett WC, and De Vivo I. Lycopene and other carotenoid intake in relation to risk of uterine leiomyomata. *Am J Obstet Gynecol.* 2008;198(1):37.el–e8.
7. Nagata C, Nakamura K, Oba S, Hayashi M, Takeda N, and Yasuda K. Association of intakes of fat, dietary fibre, soya isoflavones and alcohol with uterine fibroids in Japanese women. *Br J Nutr.* 2009;101(10):1427–31.
8. Martin C, Huber L, Thompson M, and Racine E. Serum micronutrient concentrations and risk of uterine fibroids. *J Womens Health (Larchmt).* 2011;20(6):915–21.
9. Baer DJ, Judd JT, Clevidence BA, and Tracy RP. Dietary fatty acids affect plasma markers of inflammation in healthy men fed controlled diets: A randomized crossover study. *Am J Clin Nutr.* 2004;79(6):969–73.
10. Mozaffarian D, Pischon T, Hankinson SE et al. Dietary intake of trans fatty acids and systemic inflammation in women. *Am J Clin Nutr.* 2004;79(4):606–12.
11. Mozaffarian D, Rimm EB, King IB, Lawler RL, McDonald GB, and Levy WC. Trans fatty acids and systemic inflammation in heart failure. *Am J Clin Nutr.* 2004;80(6):1521–5.
12. Bischof P. Endocrine, paracrine, and autocrine regulation of trophoblastic metalloproteinases. *Early Pregnancy.* 2001;5(1):30–1.
13. Ferrucci L, Cherubini A, Bandinelli S et al. Relationship of plasma polyunsaturated fatty acids to circulating inflammatory markers. *J Clin Endocrinol Metab.* 2006;91(2):439–46.
14. Pischon T, Hankinson SE, Hotamisligil GS, Rifai N, Willett WC, and Rimm EB. Habitual dietary intake of n-3 and n-6 fatty acids in relation to inflammatory markers among US men and women. *Circulation.* 2003;108(2):155–60.
15. Wise LA, Radin RG, Kumanyika SK, Ruiz-Narváez EA, Palmer JR, and Rosenberg L. Prospective study of dietary fat and risk of uterine leiomyomata. *Am J Clin Nutr.* 2014;99(5):1105–16.
16. Wise LA, Radin RG, Palmer JR, Kumanyika SK, and Rosenberg L. A prospective study of dairy intake and risk of uterine leiomyomata. *Am J Epidemiol.* 2010;171(2):221–32.
17. Zemel MB and Sun X. Dietary calcium and dairy products modulate oxidative and inflammatory stress in mice and humans. *J Nutr.* 2008;138(6):1047–52.
18. Wolford ST and Argoudelis CJ. Measurement of estrogens in cow's milk, human milk, and dairy products. *J Dairy Sci.* 1979;62(9):1458–63.
19. Giovannucci E, Pollak M, Liu Y et al. Nutritional predictors of insulin-like growth factor I and their relationships to cancer in men. *Cancer Epidemiol Biomarkers Prev.* 2003; 12(2):84–9.
20. Heaney RP, McCarron DA, Dawson-Hughes B et al. Dietary changes favorably affect bone remodeling in older adults. *J Am Diet Assoc.* 1999;99(10):1228–33.
21. Holmes MD, Pollak MN, Willett WC, and Hankinson SE. Dietary correlates of plasma insulin-like growth factor i and insulin-like growth factor binding protein 3 concentrations. *Cancer Epidemiol Biomarkers Prev.* 2002;11(9):852–61.
22. Strawn EY, Novy MJ, Burry KA, and Bethea CL. Insulin-like growth factor I promotes leiomyoma cell growth *in vitro*. *Am J Obstet Gynecol.* 1995;172(6):1837–44.
23. van der Ven L, Van Buul-Offers S, Gloudemans T et al. Modulation of insulin-like growth factor (IGF) action by IGF-binding proteins in normal, benign, and malignant smooth muscle tissues. *J Clin Endocrinol Metab.* 1996;81(10):3629–35.
24. Baird D, Travlos G, Wilson R et al. Uterine leiomyomata in relation to insulin-like growth factor-I, insulin, and diabetes. *Epidemiology.* 2009;20(4):604–10.
25. Baird D, Hill M, Schnectman J, and Hollis B. Vitamin D and the risk of uterine fibroids. *Epidemiology.* 2013;24(3):447–53.
26. Sabry M, Halder S, Allah A, Roshdy E, Rajaratnam V, and Al-Hendy A. Serum vitamin D3 level inversely correlates with uterine fibroid volume in different ethnic groups: A cross-sectional observational study. *Int J Womens Health.* 2013;5:93–100.
27. Paffoni A, Somigliana E, Viganò P et al. Vitamin D status in women with uterine leiomyomas. *J Clin Endocrinol Metab.* 2013;98(8):E1374–E8.

28. Lambertino A, Turyk M, Anderson H, Freels S, and Persky V. Uterine leiomyomata in a cohort of Great Lakes sport fish consumers. *Environ Res.* 2011;111(4):565–72.
29. Atkinson C, Lampe JW, Scholes D, Chen C, Wähälä K, and Schwartz SM. Lignan and isoflavone excretion in relation to uterine fibroids: A case-control study of young to middle-aged women in the United States. *Am J Clin Nutr.* 2006;84(3):587–93.
30. Wise L, Palmer J, Harlow B et al. Risk of uterine leiomyomata in relation to tobacco, alcohol and caffeine consumption in the Black Women's Health Study. *Human Reproduction.* 2004;19(8):1746–54.
31. Radin RG, Palmer JR, Rosenberg L, Kumanyika SK, and Wise LA. Dietary glycemic index and load in relation to risk of uterine leiomyomata in the Black Women's Health Study. *Am J Clin Nutr.* 2010;91(5):1281–8.

4

Types of Fibroids

Christine C. Skiadas

Fibroids are the most common pelvic tumor found in women [1], and their existence has been recognized in some of the earliest anatomical descriptions of the uterus, from writings dating back to the first century [2]. The presence of fibroids detected in hysterectomy specimens indicate that there are many fibroids that go clinically unnoticed [3], and if ultrasound is employed for diagnosis, the cumulative incidence by age 50 can be greater than 80% [4].

For some women, fibroids have significant clinical implications. Symptomatic fibroids typically present with abnormal uterine bleeding, pelvic pressure or increasing abdominal girth. Fibroids can also be detected as part of an evaluation for infertility or recurrent pregnancy loss; however, the extent to which fibroids are symptomatic varies widely among women [5,6].

The clinical impact of fibroids depends on a host of factors, including location, number, size and consistency; therefore, understanding these different elements is critical. In addition, histologic and pathologic features of fibroids, such as degeneration or calcification, may also cause significant variability in presentation. Furthermore, although the vast majority of uterine smooth muscle tumors are benign, there are certain subsets that have developed genetic features or mutations ranging from uncertain malignant potential to leiomyosarcoma. This chapter seeks to address the main types of fibroids and to provide an overview of the variability of fibroids.

Anatomic Location

Although often diagnosed on physical exam and palpation of the uterus, improved imaging modalities, and minimally invasive diagnostic techniques (including transvaginal ultrasound, saline sonohysterography and office hysteroscopy) have allowed for noninvasive methods for diagnosis, as well as further characterization of fibroids prior to management decisions. Similarly, the diagnosis of fibroids must be excluded from other gynecologic conditions that may present with common symptoms [7]. One of the most important defining characteristics of a uterine fibroid is its anatomic location within the uterus.

Fibroids have traditionally been categorized anatomically in relationship to the endometrial cavity, largely owing to the fact that proximity to the endometrium is clinically significant in terms of the symptom of abnormal bleeding and also the strong clinical implications for future pregnancy outcomes as well as management options. The first numerical classification system was defined for submucosal fibroids and was based on the extension into the endometrial cavity. Wamsteker et al. [8] attempted to identify the subset of fibroids that could be completely cured with hysteroscopic resection and devised a classification system based on hysteroscopic evaluation and the visualized angle of the fibroid's attachment to the myometrial wall when directly observed hysteroscopically [8]. Intracavitary fibroids were classified as type 0, and submucosal fibroids with a myometrial component were defined as type 1 if >50% of the fibroid was within the endometrial cavity or type 2 if <50% of the fibroid was within the cavity.

An extension of this classification system was developed as part of a comprehensive evaluation of causes of abnormal uterine bleeding by the Federation International de Gynecologie et d'Obstetrique (FIGO) and published in 2011 [9]. The main causes of abnormal uterine bleeding were identified to be either structural (polyp, adenomyosis, leiomyoma, malignancy and hyperplasia) or nonstructural (coagulopathy, ovulatory dysfunction, endometrial, iatrogenic and not yet classified), resulting in the development of the pneumonic PALM-COEIN [10]. One of the goals of developing this classification system was to allow for a clear diagnosis of the cause abnormal bleeding, but also to facilitate definitions for research and to tailor clinical management.

Although the broader category of presence of a leiomyoma alone may be useful for defining an etiology for abnormal bleeding, further subgroups were classified within the subcategory of "leiomyoma." The FIGO working group expanded upon the original hysteroscopic classification of submucosal fibroids to a 0–8 numerical score defining the location of the fibroid, ranging from type 0 (completely intracavitary) to type 8 (no anatomical connection to the uterus) (see Figures 4.1–4.4, [11,12]). Intramural fibroids are described as type 3 fibroids, which touch the endometrium, and type 4 fibroids, which are completely intramural without endometrial contact. Subserosal fibroids are classified as types 5–7, with fibroids <50% subserosal being a type 5, >50% subserosal type 6, and a type 7 fibroid, which is pedunculated on the external surface of the uterus in a subserosal manner [9]. Furthermore, this system allows for classification of transmural fibroids, those that extend from endometrium to the serosa as two numbers (i.e., 2–5), with the first number indicating the relationship to the endometrium and the second number defining the serosal relationship. A final category of type 8 leiomyomata is reserved for fibroids that do not relate to the myometrium at all, including cervical fibroids, broad ligament fibroids and other parasitic lesions [9].

Polyp	
Adenomyosis	
Leiomyoma	→ Submucosal / Other
Malignancy & hyperplasia	

Coagulopathy
Ovulatory dysfunction
Endometrial
Iatrogenic
Not yet classified

Leiomyoma subclassification system

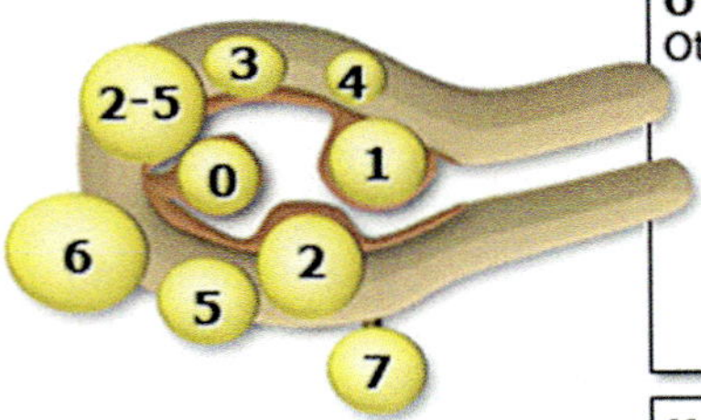

SM - Submucosal	0	Pedunculated intracavitary
	1	<50 percent intramural
	2	≥50 percent intramural
O - Other	3	Contacts endometrium; 100 percent intramural
	4	Intramural
	5	Subserosal ≥50 percent intramural
	6	Subserosal <50 percent intramural
	7	Subserosal pedunculated
	8	Other (specify, e.g., cervical, parasitic)

Hybrid leiomyomas (impact both endometrium and serosa)	Two numbers are listed separated by a hyphen. By convention, the first refers to the relationship with the endometrium while the second refers to the relationship to the serosa. One example is below.	
	2-5	Submucosal and subserosal, each with less than half the diameter in the endometrial and peritoneal cavities, respectively.

FIGURE 4.1 FIGO classification system for abnormal uterine bleeding with the leiomyoma subclassification system highlighted. Submucosal fibroids (type 0–2) range from those completely intracavitary (type 0) to those with >50% of the fibroid within the cavity (type 1) and <50% within the cavity (type 2). Intramural fibroids include type 3 lesions (those that abut the endometrium) and type 4 lesions (completely within the myometrium). Subserosal fibroids range from those fibroids where >50% is intramural, but extends to the serosa (type 5) to type 6 (<50% intramural) and type 7, which represents fibroids that are pedunculated and attached to the uterus via a stalk. Fibroids that are transmural (i.e., extending from endometrium to serosal surface are denoted with two numbers, with the endometrial relationship denoted first (i.e., 2–5). Type 8 fibroids are those with no direct myometrial attachment and include cervical fibroids, broad ligament fibroids, round ligament fibroids and parasitic fibroids. (Reproduced with permission from Munro MG, Critchley HO, Fraser IS, Group FMDW. *Fertil Steril*. 2011;95(7):2204–8, 8.e1–3.)

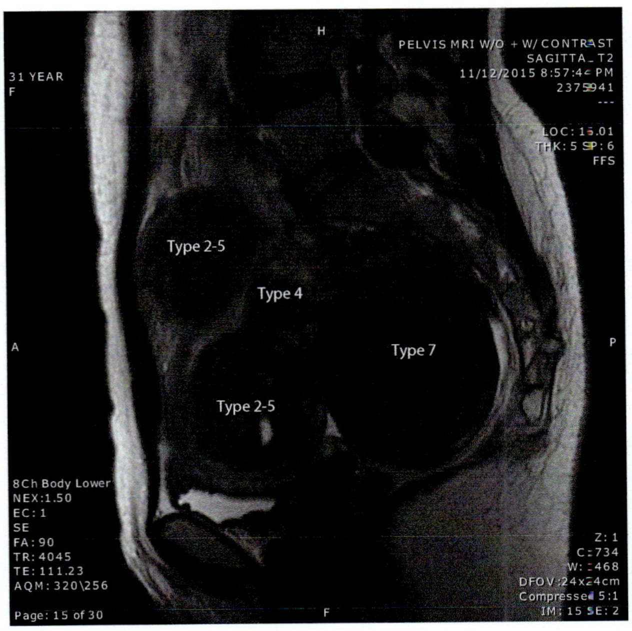

FIGURE 4.2 Sagittal images of pelvic MRI demonstrating different fibroid types within a patient.

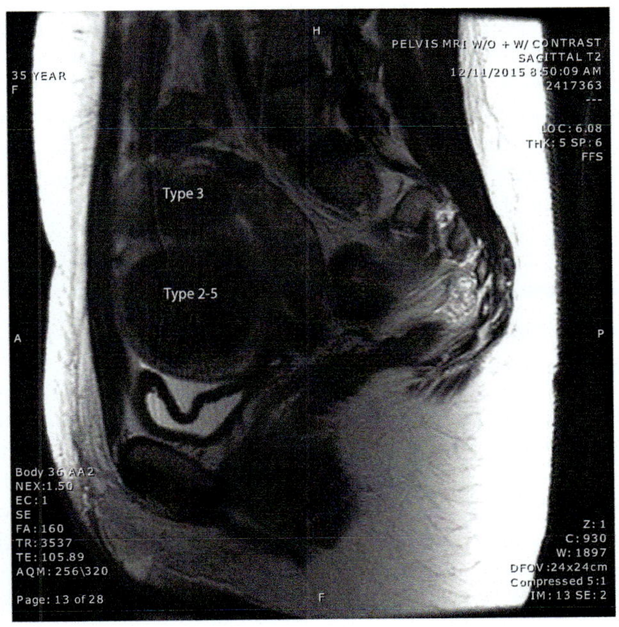

FIGURE 4.3 Sagittal images of pelvic MRI demonstrating different fibroid types within a patient.

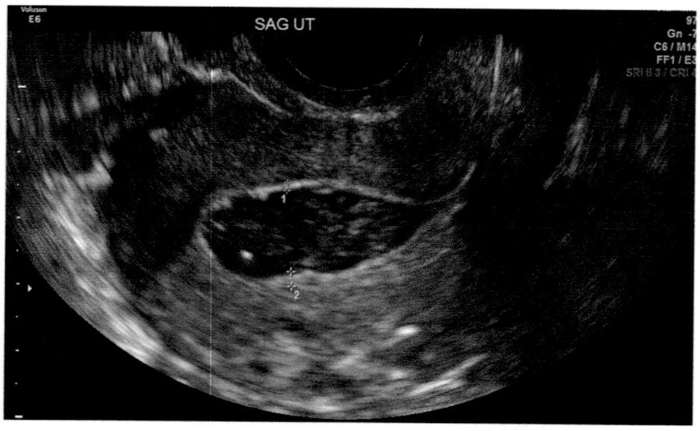

FIGURE 4.4 Saline sonohysterogram of the same patient whose MRI is displayed in Figure 4.1 three months postoperative from robotic-assisted laparoscopic myomectomy.

Unusual Locations

Although the vast majority of fibroids occur within the corpus of the uterus, they can arise throughout the Mullerian tract, including the Mullerian remnants [13] of a patient with Mullerian agenesis, the round ligament [14,15] and the Fallopian tube [16]. Leiomyoma can arise in the broad ligament and represents the most common type of broad ligament growth [17]. Submucosal fibroids can prolapse through the cervical os and present as a vaginal mass [18,19].

Fibroids can also develop as an extension of the cervical stroma, which can significantly distort normal pelvic anatomy, and occasionally can present with obstructive symptoms [20] and create further challenges in terms of surgical approach and management and have also been reported as growing in a cervical stump remaining after supracervical hysterectomy [21]. Parasitic lesions typically refer to myomatous tissue that has become detached from the uterus and subsequently established a blood supply in a different location. Parasitic fibroids have been reported since the 1950s [22]. Recently, the introduction of minimally invasive surgical techniques and morcellation devices for removal of fibroids has led to further recognition of this condition; however, the incidence remains small, representing less than 1% of fibroids [23].

Number and Size of Fibroids and Diagnostic Imaging

Although some patients may present with a solitary fibroid, many patients have multiple fibroids of different types, with may act to compound symptoms [1]. Although bimanual exam or abdominal physical exam can be used to diagnose fibroids, there is poor correlation between bimanual exam and the extent of fibroids when evaluated by imaging [24].

Ultrasound was first developed for use in gynecology in the late 1950s [25] and, over the subsequent decades, has markedly evolved. Development of transvaginal ultrasound allowed for improved visualization of the endometrium and pelvic organs [26], as well as the ability to identify the size and location of individual fibroids, which has led to increased diagnosis of fibroids prior to development of symptoms. In a study by Donna Day Baird et al., where randomly selected members of an urban health plan were screened with ultrasound, the estimated cumulative incidence of fibroid tumors by the age of 50 was more than 80% for black women and nearly 70% for white women [4]. Interestingly, 51% of the premenopausal women with no previous diagnosis of fibroids showed ultrasound evidence of fibroid tumors [4]. In another study of younger asymptomatic women (ages 18–30), fibroids were identified on ultrasound in 26% of black women and 7% of white women [27].

Number and size of fibroids tend to work synergistically to cause symptoms—with increasing clinical significance with larger and more numerous fibroids [5]. In the ultrasound study by Baird et al., ultrasound measurements of women with a previous diagnosis of fibroids tended to have larger fibroids than those with newly detected fibroids [4], and another study showed that at initial ultrasound diagnosis, more than 60% of women were found to have multiple fibroids [28]. The number of fibroids at time of diagnosis has also been linked with racial differences, with one study reporting black women to have a significantly higher risk of having multiple focal fibroids (73% versus 45%) in comparison to white women [4]. The reasons why some women develop multiple fibroids and some develop solitary fibroids are still being uncovered, but may relate to genetic differences as well as hormonal environment. For example, some studies have demonstrated differential expression of the receptors for estrogen [29] and progesterone [30] between women with solitary versus multiple fibroids.

Fibroid Growth

The growth of fibroids can be unpredictable and can also demonstrate significant variability among individual patients, including noted growth differences between black and white women [31], as well as among individual fibroids [5,28]. Flake et al. has proposed that growth may begin with a predominantly proliferative phase in the initial development of the fibroid, and later evolution may manifest in terms of collagen deposition [32]. These proposed developmental phases are outlined in Table 4.1. Although the pathogenesis of initial fibroid growth remains unknown, there has been described a "2-hit" hypothesis whereby a myometrial cell undergoes a genetic mutation and then the surrounding hormonal environment and paracrine factors from the surrounding myometrial cells induce subsequent growth and development of the resulting fibroid [33].

Fibroid growth tends also to correlate with hormonal status, with essentially no reports of uterine fibroids prepubertally and increasing incidence over the reproductive lifespan. Although classic teaching was that fibroids tend to grow in pregnancy, ultrasound studies have demonstrated that although 22%–32% of fibroids grow in pregnancy [34,35], 78% showed no increase in size [34]. Postmenopause, there is relief of symptoms of bleeding associated with fibroids with the cessation of menstruation, and most women experience some shrinkage of fibroids. Fibroid growth rate has been raised as a concern for the possible detection of leiomyosarcoma, although this has not been reported in

TABLE 4.1

Proposed Developmental Phases of Fibroids

Phase	Estimate Collagen Content	Functional Status
Phase 1	No, or insignificant, collagen matrix	Proliferation of myocytes
Phase 2	<10% collagen	Proliferation of myocytes and synthesis of collagen
Phase 3	10%–50% collagen	Proliferation, synthesis of collagen, and early senescence in late Phase 3
Phase 4	>50% collagen	Involution

Source: Reproduced with permission from Flake GL et al. *Obstet Gynecol Int.* 2013;2013:528376.

all studies. In one study in which patients were identified to have rapidly growing fibroids, the incidence of uterine sarcoma was no different when compared to patients not experiencing rapid growth [36].

Fibroids are hormonally responsive to estrogen and progesterone, and estrogen and progesterone receptors have been shown to be expressed in both fibroid and normal myometrial tissue [37–39]; however, owing to the great variability in clinical presentation, the exact role in pathogenesis that is played by estrogen and progesterone is unclear. Therefore, counseling of patients in regard to the ability to predict future fibroid growth remains a clinical challenge and growth patterns will be further discussed in Chapter 6. The mainstay of medical treatment options for fibroids include manipulation of hormones in some way to either affect bleeding pattern or attempt to induce shrinkage of fibroids. A comprehensive discussion of the medical management of fibroids is undertaken in Chapters 10–14.

Degeneration and Histologic Features

Occasionally, fibroids can outgrow their blood supply, resulting in the general term "fibroid degeneration." Fibroids without degeneration classically appear as firm, white, whorled, solid round lesions, whereas fibroids that have undergone degeneration may have a cystic center, or a softening of the interior portion of the fibroid. Degenerated fibroids can appear atypical on imaging studies or at the time of surgery, with central necrosis. Pathologically, degeneration can be classified as hyaline degeneration, the most common form, although other forms of degeneration include cystic, hydropic, myxomatous, fatty, red, necrotic and calcific [40]. Calcified fibroids are thought to represent a long-term consequence of fibroid degeneration and can either appear as a complete calcification within the myometrium or, more commonly, a calcified rim around the fibroid. Rarer types of leiomyomata include diffuse leiomyomatosis, which presents with innumerable nodules within the myometrium as well as dissecting leiomyomatosis, leiomyoma with vascular invasion and intravenous leiomyomatosis [40].

Even fibroids that appear grossly as "typical fibroids" can demonstrate heterogeneity in terms of mitotic activity, collagenous component, cellularity and fibrotic stroma [32]. Pathologically, the mitotic count has also been implicated in identifying fibroids on the spectrum of completely benign tumors to those of uncertain malignant potential and frank sarcoma [32]. Mitotic activity (greater than 10 or more mitoses per 10 high-power fields) has been one of the hallmarks of the diagnosis of leiomyosarcoma. In addition, cytologic atypia and tumor cell necrosis also play a role in diagnostic evaluation [18], and a further discussion of sarcomas will occur in Chapter 23. Smooth muscle tumors that have some features that are concerning for malignancy, but did not meet all diagnostic criteria, fall into the category of smooth muscle tumors of uncertain malignant potential [41].

Conclusion

Fibroids are one of the most common benign gynecologic conditions affecting women. Improved diagnostic techniques have led to a significant increase in early diagnosis and have allowed for further preoperative evaluation to classify and describe the types of fibroids within an individual patient, including number, size and anatomic location. Improved characterization has led to individual tailoring of treatment options based on symptomatic presentation, as well as desired fertility. Hopefully, with further improvements in identification of the different types of fibroids (perhaps on a molecular and genetic level), treatment options will continue to become less invasive and more targeted to specific patients.

REFERENCES

1. Buttram VC and Reiter RC. Uterine leiomyomata: Etiology, symptomatology, and management. *Fertil Steril.* 1981;36(4):433–45.
2. Speroff L and Fritz MA. *Clinical Gynecologic Endocrinology and Infertility.* 7th ed. Philadelphia: Lippincott Williams & Wilkins; 2005. 1334 pp.
3. Cramer SF and Patel A. The frequency of uterine leiomyomas. *Am J Clin Pathol.* 1990;94(4):435–8.
4. Baird DD, Dunson DB, Hill MC, Cousins D, and Schectman JM. High cumulative incidence of uterine leiomyoma in black and white women: Ultrasound evidence. *Am J Obstet Gynecol.* 2003;188(1):100–7.
5. DeWaay DJ, Syrop CH, Nygaard IE, Davis WA, and Van Voorhis BJ. Natural history of uterine polyps and leiomyomata. *Obstet Gynecol.* 2002;100(1):3–7.
6. Stewart EA. Uterine fibroids. *N Engl J Med.* 2015;372(17):1646–55.
7. McLucas B. Diagnosis, imaging and anatomical classification of uterine fibroids. *Best Pract Res Clin Obstet Gynaecol.* 2008;22(4):627–42.
8. Wamsteker K, Emanuel MH, and de Kruif JH. Transcervical hysteroscopic resection of submucous fibroids for abnormal uterine bleeding: Results regarding the degree of intramural extension. *Obstet Gynecol.* 1993;82(5):736–40.
9. Munro MG, Critchley HO, Broder MS, Fraser IS, Disorders FWGoM. FIGO classification system (PALM-COEIN) for causes of abnormal uterine bleeding in nongravid women of reproductive age. *Int J Gynaecol Obstet.* 2011;113(1):3–13.
10. Munro MG, Critchley HO, and Fraser IS. The FIGO classification of causes of abnormal uterine bleeding: Malcolm G. Munro, Hilary O.D. Crithcley, Ian S. Fraser, for the FIGO Working Group on Menstrual Disorders. *Int J Gynaecol Obstet.* 2011;113(1):1–2.

11. Munro MG. *Abnormal Uterine Bleeding*. Cambridge: New York: Cambridge University Press; 2010. 251 pp.
12. Munro MG, Critchley HO, Fraser IS, Group FMDW. The FIGO classification of causes of abnormal uterine bleeding in the reproductive years. *Fertil Steril*. 2011;95(7):2204–8, 8.e1–3.
13. Narayanan R, Mariappan S, Paulraj S, and Shankar B. Imaging of leiomyomas arising from Müllerian remnants in a case of Mayer-Rokitansky-Küster-Hauser syndrome. *BMJ Case Rep*. 2015;2015.
14. Kirkham JC, Nero CJ, Tambouret RH, and Yoon SS. Leiomyoma and leiomyosarcoma arising from the round ligament of the uterus. *J Am Coll Surg*. 2008;207(3):452.
15. Vignali M, Bertulessi C, Spreafico C, and Busacca M. A large symptomatic leiomyoma of the round ligament. *J Minim Invasive Gynecol*. 2006;13(5):375–6.
16. Wen KC, Yang CC, and Wang PH. Primary fallopian tube leiomyoma managed by laparoscopy. *J Minim Invasive Gynecol*. 2005;12(3):193.
17. Heller DS. Lesions of the broad ligament: A review. *J Minim Invasive Gynecol*. 2015;22(7):1163–8.
18. Toledo G and Oliva E. Smooth muscle tumors of the uterus: A practical approach. *Arch Pathol Lab Med*. 2008;132(4):595–605.
19. Matytsina-Quinlan L and Matytsina L. Submucosal uterine fibroid prolapsed into vagina in a symptomatic patient with IUS. *BMJ Case Rep*. 2014;2014:bcr2014203877. doi:10.1136/bcr-2014-203877
20. Mihmanli V, Cetinkaya N, Kilickaya A, Kilinc A, and Kose D. Giant cervical myoma associated with urinary incontinence and hydroureteronephrosis. *Clin Exp Obstet Gynecol*. 2015;42(5):690–1.
21. Chu CM, Acholonu UC, Jr., Chang-Jackson SC, and Nezhat FR. Leiomyoma recurrent at the cervical stump: Report of two cases. *J Minim Invasive Gynecol*. 2012;19(1):131–3.
22. Brody S. Parasitic fibroid. *Am J Obstet Gynecol*. 1953;65(6): 1354–6.
23. Van der Meulen JF, Pijnenborg JM, Boomsma CM, Verberg MF, Geomini PM, and Bongers MY. Parasitic myoma after laparoscopic morcellation: A systematic review of the literature. *BJOG*. 2016;123(1):69–75.
24. Stoelinga B, Huirne J, Heymans MW, Reekers JA, Ankum WM, and Hehenkamp WJ. The estimated volume of the fibroid uterus: A comparison of ultrasound and bimanual examination versus volume at MRI or hysterectomy. *Eur J Obstet Gynecol Reprod Biol*. 2015;184:89–96.
25. Donald I, Macvicar J, and Brown T. Investigation of abdominal masses by pulsed ultrasound. *Lancet*. 1958;1(7032):1188–95.
26. Mendelson EB, Bohm-Velez M, Joseph N, and Neiman HL. Gynecologic imaging: Comparison of transabdominal and transvaginal sonography. *Radiology*. 1988;166(2):321–4.
27. Marsh EE, Ekpo GE, Cardozo ER, Brocks M, Dune T, and Cohen LS. Racial differences in fibroid prevalence and ultrasound findings in asymptomatic young women (18–30 years old): A pilot study. *Fertil Steril*. 2013;99(7):1951–7.
28. Mavrelos D, Ben-Nagi J, Holland T, Hoo W, Naftalin J, and Jurkovic D. The natural history of fibroids. *Ultrasound Obstet Gynecol*. 2010;35(2):238–42.
29. Shao R, Fang L, Xing R, Xiong Y, and Wang Z. Differential expression of estrogen receptor α and β isoforms in multiple and solitary leiomyomas. *Biochem Biophys Res Commun*. 2015;468(1–2):136–42.
30. Tsigkou A, Reis FM, Lee MH et al. Increased progesterone receptor expression in uterine leiomyoma: Correlation with age, number of leiomyomas, and clinical symptoms. *Fertil Steril*. 2015;104(1):170–5.e1.
31. Peddada SD, Laughlin SK, Miner K et al. Growth of uterine leiomyomata among premenopausal black and white women. *Proc Natl Acad Sci U S A*. 2008;105(50):19887–92.
32. Flake GP, Moore AB, Sutton D et al. The natural history of uterine leiomyomas: Light and electron microscopic studies of fibroid phases, interstitial ischemia, inanosis, and reclamation. *Obstet Gynecol Int*. 2013;2013:528376.
33. Bulun SE. Uterine fibroids. *N Engl J Med*. 2013;369(14):1344–55.
34. Aharoni A, Reiter A, Golan D, Paltiely Y, and Sharf M. Patterns of growth of uterine leiomyomas during pregnancy. A prospective longitudinal study. *Br J Obstet Gynaecol*. 1988;95(5):510–3.
35. Rosati P, Exacoustòs C, and Mancuso S. Longitudinal evaluation of uterine myoma growth during pregnancy. A sonographic study. *J Ultrasound Med*. 1992;11(10):511–5.
36. Parker WH, Fu YS, and Berek JS. Uterine sarcoma in patients operated on for presumed leiomyoma and rapidly growing leiomyoma. *Obstet Gynecol*. 1994;83(3):414–8.
37. Moravek MB and Bulun SE. Endocrinology of uterine fibroids: Steroid hormones, stem cells, and genetic contribution. *Curr Opin Obstet Gynecol*. 2015;27(4):276–83.
38. Pedeutour F, Quade BJ, Weremowicz S, Dal Cin P, Ali S, and Morton CC. Localization and expression of the human estrogen receptor beta gene in uterine leiomyomata. *Genes Chromosomes Cancer*. 1998;23(4):361–6.
39. Andersen J and Barbieri RL. Abnormal gene expression in uterine leiomyomas. *J Soc Gynecol Investig*. 1995;2(5):663–72.
40. Clement PB and Young RH. *Atlas of Gynecologic Surgical Pathology*. 3rd ed. London: Saunders/Elsevier; 2014. 568 pp.
41. D'Angelo E and Prat J. Uterine sarcomas: A review. *Gynecol Oncol*. 2010;116(1):131–9.

5

Genetics of Uterine Leiomyomata

C. Scott Gallagher and Cynthia C. Morton

Clonality

Early isoenzymatic studies of *G6PD* (glucose-6-phosphate dehydrogenase) of UL in women heterozygous for A and B isotypes were fundamental in establishing the paradigm of monoclonality in neoplasms [1–3]. Subsequent molecular investigations employing methylation-sensitive restriction-enzyme assays in women with polymorphisms in the X-linked genes *PGK* (phosphoglycerol kinase) and *AR* (androgen receptor) further substantiated the monoclonal origin of UL [2,4,5]. Identification of unique, tumor-specific somatic point mutations in *MED12* (mediator complex subunit 12) by whole-exome sequencing (WES) of individual neoplasms supported the theory of monoclonality [6].

Recently, however, whole-genome sequencing (WGS) of independent tumor nodules obtained from the same uterus uncovered identical patterns of chromosomal rearrangements and copy-number alterations that were complex in nature [7,8]. Review of clinical histories indicated only two of five patients with clonally related tumors had prior myomectomies, suggesting genetically identical UL might arise non-iatrogenically in a single uterus [7,8]. On the one hand, observations of spatially distinct tumors with overlapping complex genomic abnormalities challenge the historical perspective that all UL are monoclonal. Alternatively, in women who have not had surgical or morcellation-based interventions, multiple genetically identical neoplasms may instead reflect a naturally occurring, local dispersion of tumorlets.

Somatic and Germline Alterations

Somatic Chromosome Rearrangements

Karyotypic abnormalities are detected in ~40% of UL and are predominantly simple in nature, affecting one to a few chromosomes [2,9–19]. Comparative expression analyses of UL with either t(12;14)(q14-q15;q23-q24) or various deletions of the long arm of chromosome 7 have revealed transcriptional signatures specific to each cytogenetic subgroup [20,21]. These diverse gene expression profiles provide evidence that underlying cellular pathologies of individual tumors may be driven by distinct biological mechanisms.

The t(12;14)(q14-q15;q23-q24) is observed in nearly 20% of all cytogenetically abnormal UL and is associated with larger-sized neoplasms than karyotypically normal tumors [2,14,18,19,22–30]. Breakpoints on chromosome 12 span a large genomic region 5′ and 3′ of *HMGA2* (high mobility group AT-hook 2) [31,32], which encodes a DNA architectural factor that regulates transcription [33,34]. Generally, balanced translocations result in dysregulated expression of the transcript (a gain or loss of function) or fusion genes (production of chimeric protein with novel function), as illustrated in Figure 5.1 [35–37]. Expression of *HMGA2* is elevated in UL with t(12;14) compared to karyotypically normal UL and myometrium, suggesting the rearrangement has a gain-of-function effect on *HMGA2* [38,39]. Truncation of *HMGA2* with deletion of the 3′-UTR removes a site of transcription inhibition mediated by the microRNA *let-7* [40,41]. Overexpression in both cases suggests *HMGA2* harbors potential for dysregulated growth in UL, which is also supported by the observation of trisomy 12 in UL [9,13,18]. Interestingly, in a male with a pericentric inversion of chromosome 12 that results in constitutional truncation of *HMGA2*, extreme somatic overgrowth and multiple lipomas (another common mesenchymal tumor with documented frequent chromosomal rearrangements in *HMGA2* [40,41]) were reported [31,42,43]. A number of additional "UL genes" have been implicated through chromosomal studies: *HMGA1* at 6p21.3 [2,13,18,26,44,45], *CUX1* at 7q22.1 [7,46], *KAT6B* at 10q22 [47], *RAD51L1* at 14q23-q24 [18,37,48] and both *COL4A5* and *COL4A6* at Xq22.3 [7].

Somatic Mutations

WES of 18 UL revealed somatic heterozygous mutations specific to exons 1 and 2 of *MED12* (mediator complex subunit 12), as demonstrated in Figure 5.2a [6]. Follow-up targeted sequencing analyses in multiple populations have consistently reported between approximately 50% and 90% of UL to harbor *MED12* mutations specific to this highly conserved region [6,49–53]. While uterine-specific *Med12* knockout in mice does not result in UL development, introduction of the most frequent *Med12* mutation (c.131G>A) into either the conditional *Med12*-knockout or wild-type background results in UL-like tumors [54]. WGS analysis in UL with *MED12* mutations revealed widespread, complex chromosomal abnormalities, leading to the hypothesis that *MED12* mutations may result in genomic instability [7]. Examination of *HMGA2* expression in leiomyomata with and without mutations in *MED12* revealed overexpression of *HMGA2* and *MED12* mutations are mutually exclusive, suggesting the two genes participate in different pathways in UL tumorigenesis [6–8,55,56].

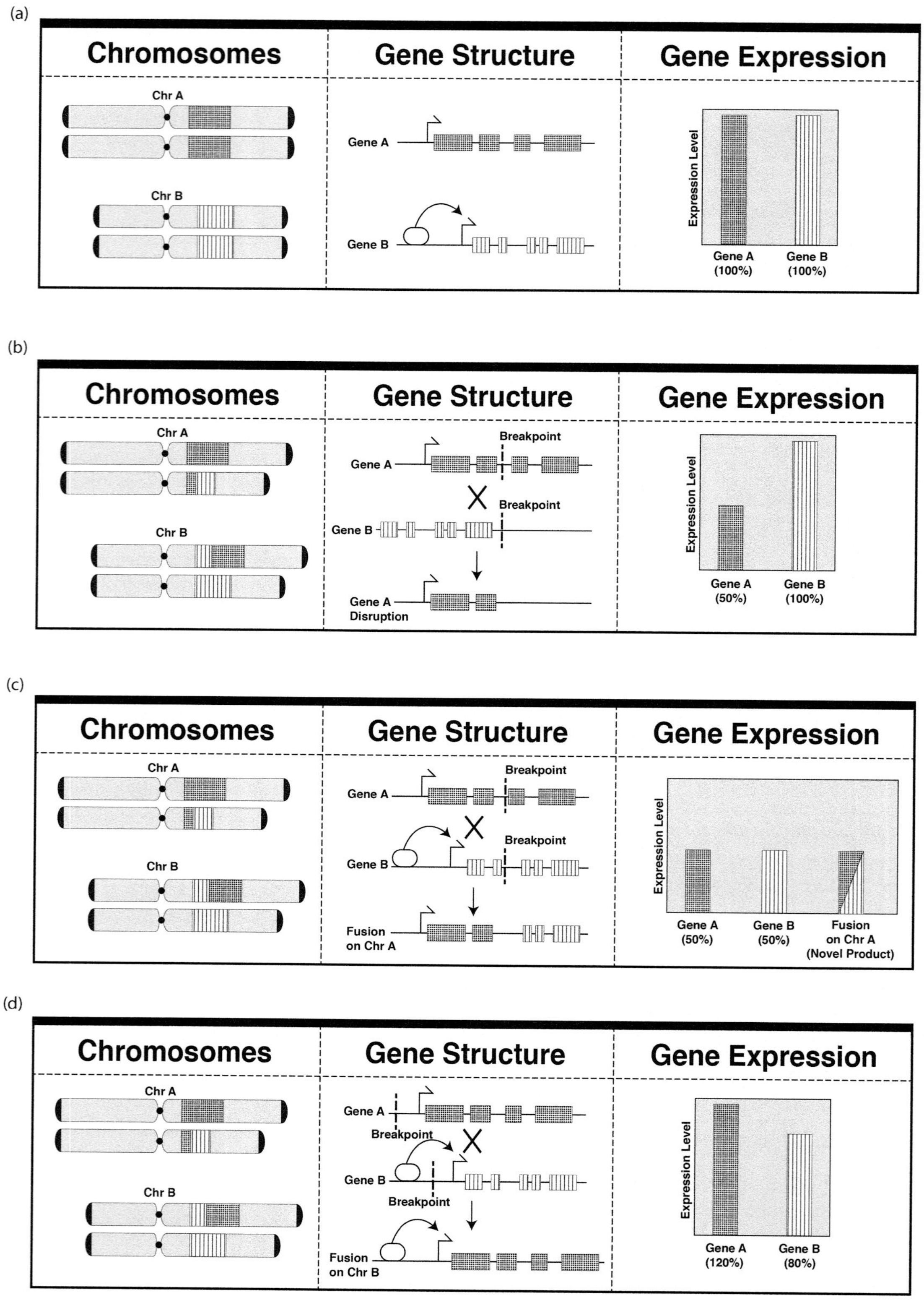

FIGURE 5.1 Possible effects of chromosomal rearrangements on genes and their expression. (a) In wild-type cells, the chromosomes are structurally normal with an intact, normal gene structure, and gene expression is at normal levels. (b) Rearrangement displaces the 3′ region of Gene A, causing gene disruption and decreased overall expression. When the allelic copy of Gene A has an inactivating mutation, is imprinted or is located on the inactivated X chromosome, disruption may result in complete loss of Gene A expression. (c) Intragenic rearrangement may result in a fusion gene. The rectangle shaded with both patterns in the "Gene Expression" column indicates expression of the novel, fusion gene product. (d) Rearrangement upstream of the coding regions can introduce foreign *cis*-regulatory elements that enhance the basal level of Gene A transcription. Shaded rectangles correspond to the individual genes on the chromosomes and in the gene structure, while clear circles represent *cis*-regulatory elements, such as enhancers. Shaded rectangles in gene expression correspond to the level of expression of each gene.

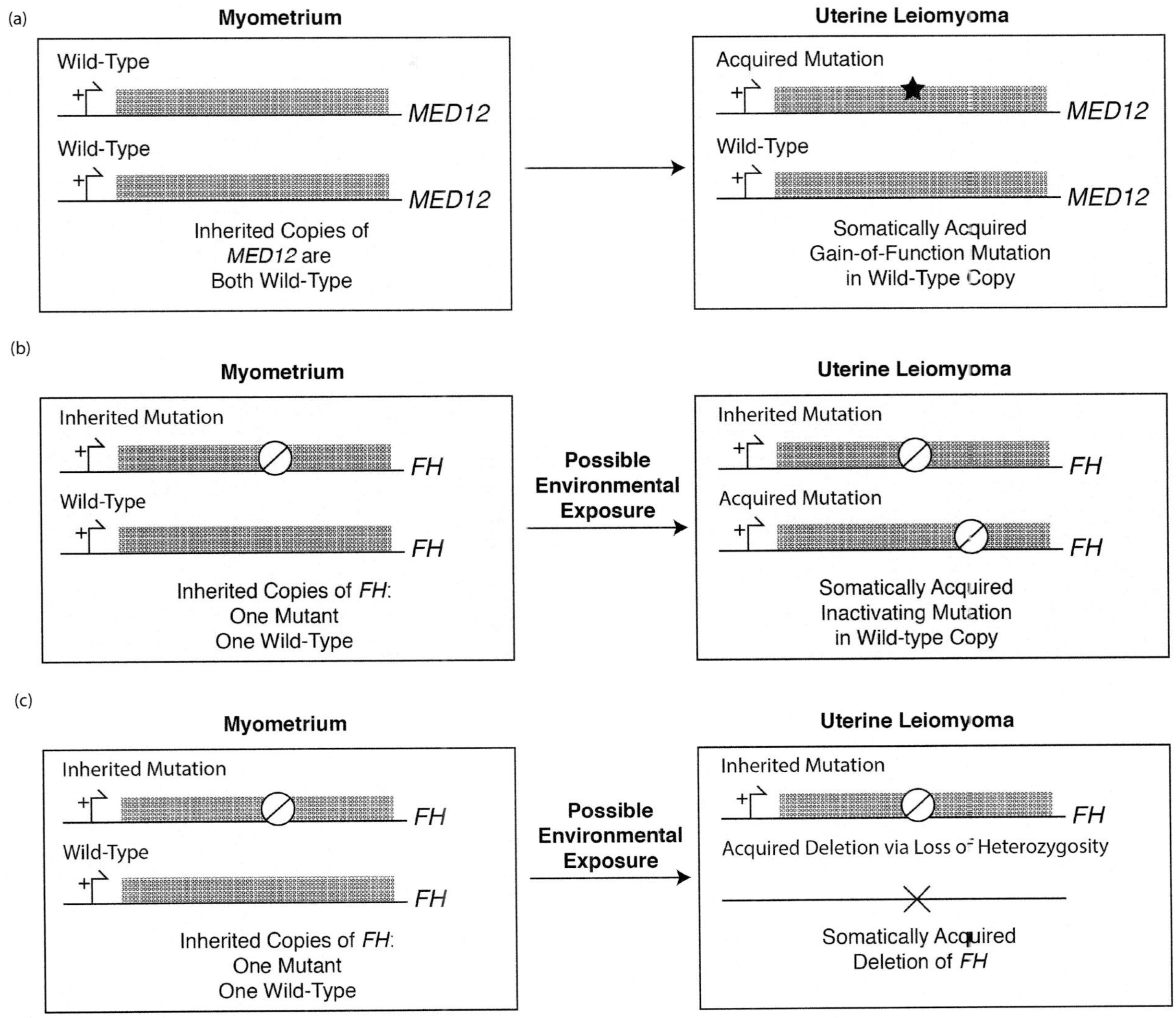

FIGURE 5.2 Genetic mechanisms of transformation of myometrium to benign uterine leiomyoma in familial and non-familial cases. (a) Both inherited copies of *MED12* are wild type and encode functional protein. A single "hit" in one *MED12* allele is observed in approximately 70% of karyotypically normal UL, resulting in dysregulation of the MED12 protein. (b and c) In HLRCC, individuals inherit an inactivated copy of the tumor suppressor *FH*, which is insufficient for development of UL. In accordance with Knudson's two-hit hypothesis for cancer, transformation of myometrial tissue into UL is consistent with acquiring somatic inactivation of the functional wild-type copy through mutation (b) or loss of heterozygosity (c).

Genomic Instability

Genomic instability is a common observation in UL. Whether or not cytogenetic abnormalities direct tumor transformation remains unclear, especially as they have been considered secondary events from clonality studies [2]. Alternatively, UL may result from driver mutations that induce dysregulation of chromosomal stability, as appears to be the case with *MED12* mutations in mice [54]. WGS analysis in UL has revealed widespread, complex chromosomal abnormalities that involve greater than three chromosomal abnormalities [7,57].

Chromosomal rearrangement is hypothesized to alter gene activity by recombining regions of the genome (Figure 5.1). Breakage and repair may be nonviable in many cases, but, at a low frequency, they can create gene fusions encoding novel chimeric proteins and dysregulate gene expression by introducing foreign regulatory elements or removing native ones. Resolution of chromosomal damage can generate cells with survival or growth advantages and result in benign transformation of a myometrial cell [7,57]. Alternatively, chromosomal instability may mostly be inert, with dysregulated growth resulting from primary mutations elsewhere in the genome [6].

Rare Familial Uterine Leiomyomata

Loss-of-function heterozygous mutations in *FH* (fumarate hydratase) at 1q43 are etiologic in a rare autosomal dominant tumor predisposition syndrome known as hereditary leiomyomatosis and renal cell carcinoma (HLRCC) [58–62]. Individuals with *FH* mutations may develop cutaneous leiomyomas of the erector piliform muscles, earlier-onset UL, uterine leiomyosarcoma and renal cell carcinoma [58,60,63,64]. As shown in Figure 5.2b, somatic inactivation of the wild-type copy of *FH* either through loss of heterozygosity or mutation is frequently observed in HLRCC-associated neoplasms and is consistent with Knudson's two-hit hypothesis, suggesting *FH* is a *bona fide* tumor suppressor gene [59,65–67]. In cells deficient in *FH*, both fumarate and succinate accumulate and inhibit the hypoxia-inducible factor prolyl hydroxylase, which in turn results in overexpression of the transcription factor HIF-1α (hypoxia-inducible factor 1α) and a "pseudo-hypoxic" state [68–71]. Of note, a single functional copy of *FH* is sufficient for maintaining normal metabolic activity [72]. In HLRCC, patients heterozygous for a missense or nonsense *FH* mutation, *MED12* mutations and somatic biallelic inactivation of *FH* appear to be mutually exclusive, suggesting a distinct molecular mechanism involving oxidative phosphorylation through mitochondrial complex 2, leading to UL in HLRCC [52,61,66–68,72,73]. Albeit an infrequent event, biallelic inactivation of *FH* has also been reported in sporadic cases of UL [74–76].

Alport syndrome with diffuse leiomyomatosis (AS-DL) is an X-linked-dominant, hereditary nephropathy associated with development of leiomyomata in the esophagus, tracheobronchial tree and genital tract [77–79]. Disease phenotypes observed in both AS and AS-DL are a consequence of abnormal basement membranes resulting from improper assembly of collagen IV protomers [80,81]. *COL4A5* (collagen type IV alpha 5) and *COL4A6* (collagen type IV alpha 6) reside in a head-to-head orientation on the X chromosome, and AS-DL is associated specifically with deletions spanning from the 5′ region of *COL4A5* into the 5′ region of *COL4A6* [78,79,82–84]. Of note, null mutations in the 5′ end of *COL4A5* that do not extend into *COL4A6* are sufficient to cause AS but insufficient to cause AS-DL [78,85]. WGS of isolated cases of UL without AS-DL have detected somatic deletions and rearrangements in the *COL4A5-COL4A6* locus, further supporting a role for the two collagen type IV alpha chains in development and growth of UL [7,53].

Common Constitutional Variants

Various observations indicate a genetic basis for UL liability. Women with first-degree affected relatives are at greater risk for developing UL than women with no immediate family history, suggesting common heritable factors influence burden for developing UL [86–91]. Concordance rates of hospitalization for UL are significantly greater in monozygotic twins compared to dizygotic twins at rates consistent with their degree of genetic relationship [92,93]. Lastly, black women have a comparatively higher prevalence and greater disease morbidity than age-matched white women [94,95]. Significant racial differences in disease rates persist after adjustment for confounding variables, suggesting population-specific, common genetic variants influence susceptibility to UL, as illustrated in Figure 5.3 [94–100].

Admixture-based analysis of the ancestral genetic content of 2453 cases and 2102 controls of African American women revealed a significant decrease in the mean percentage of European ancestry in cases versus controls (20.00% versus 21.63%; $p < 0.0001$). The association of ancestral genomic content and case-control status in African American women further suggests germline factors influence racial discrepancies in prevalence and symptomatology. Interestingly, an age-adjusted, admixture-based analysis in the same cohort revealed an even greater difference in the mean percentage of European ancestry in women who were diagnosed at an age younger than 35 years: 18.40% in cases versus 21.63% in controls ($p < 0.00001$ [101]). Observation of an even more pronounced association in younger cases is consistent with genetic factors influencing greater UL morbidity in black women [91,94–101].

High frequency in the general population and phenotypic heterogeneity of UL support a polygenic model [91]. Genome-wide association studies (GWASs) apply case-control methods to identify common genetic variants, or single nucleotide polymorphisms (SNPs), that are significantly associated with a specific disease or phenotype [102–104]. The initial UL GWAS was performed in a Japanese cohort of 5073 clinically diagnosed cases of UL and 4673 controls with no history of the disease. Significant associations ($p < 5.00 \times 10^{-8}$) were observed at SNPs located in three loci: 10q24.33 ($p = 8.65 \times 10^{-14}$; odds ratio [OR] = 1.47, 95% confidence interval [CI] = 1.23–1.75), 11p15.1 ($p = 3.82 \times 10^{-12}$; OR = 1.39; 95% CI = 1.17–1.64) and 22q13.1 ($p = 2.79 \times 10^{-12}$; OR = 1.23; 95% CI = 1.11–1.37) [105].

Genome-wide linkage analysis in 261 self-reported white UL sister-pair families identified seven linkage regions with an LOD (logarithm of the odds) score greater than 2.0 [106]. Significant linkage regions were observed in 10p11 (LOD = 4.15) and 3p21

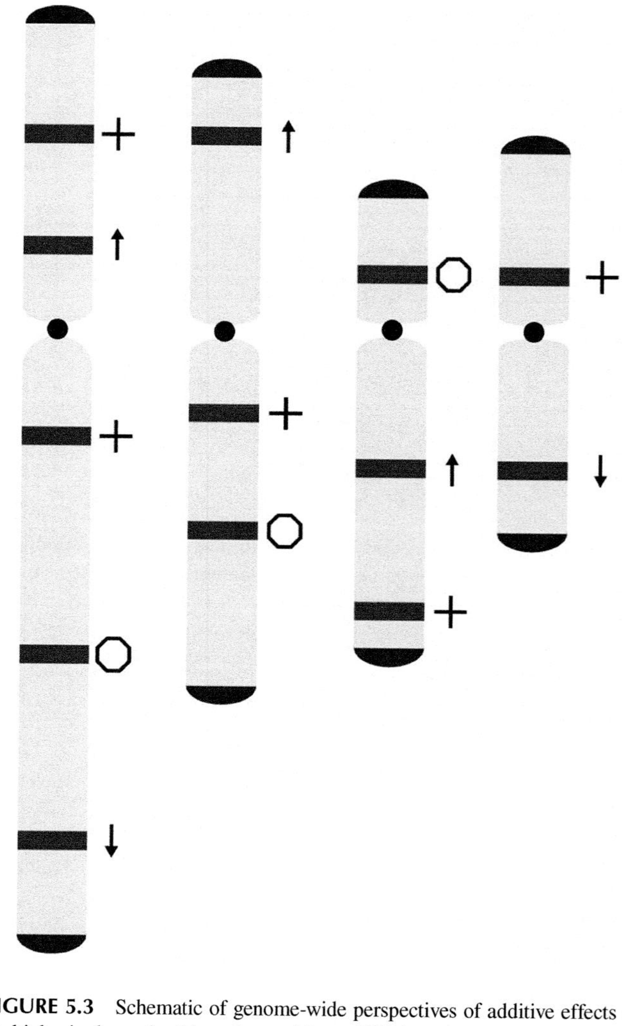

FIGURE 5.3 Schematic of genome-wide perspectives of additive effects of multiple single nucleotide polymorphisms (SNPs) on neoplasms. Genes that influence tumor phenotype are illustrated as dark bands across the chromosomes. Individual effects of each variant are summed to influence transformation of myometrial tissue to uterine leiomyomata, as well as possible subsequent rare transformation of leiomyoma to leiomyosarcoma. Effects of each variant are marked as either positively influencing tumorigenic transformation (+), inhibiting transformation (○), promoting malignant transformation (↑) or protecting against malignancy (↓). Though only one chromosome of each of the four representative pairs is shown, the cell is presumed to be diploid.

(LOD = 3.73), and five additional linkage regions with LOD scores >2 were detected in 2q37, 5p13, 11p15, 12q14 and 17q25. Two of these linkage blocks, located in 11p15.5 and 12q14, have further genomic evidence to support their association with UL predisposition [106]: 11p15.5 was reported as one of the three significant loci in the Japanese cohort, and *HMGA2* resides within the region of linkage at 12q14 [33,105,106].

Meta-analysis across two independent cohorts of white women, the Women's Genome Health Study (WGHS; n = 746 cases, 4487 controls) and the Queensland Institute of Medical Research (QIMR; n = 484 cases, 610 controls), identified one SNP at 17q25.3 as having genome-wide significant association with UL ($p = 3.05 \times 10^{-8}$; OR = 1.30; 95% CI = 1.18–1.43). The candidate SNP resides under the previously mentioned linkage peak on the long arm of chromosome 17 and in a block of linkage disequilibrium (LD) in 17q25.3, which contains *FASN* (fatty acid synthase). Tissue microarray immunohistochemistry analysis revealed a three-fold elevation in FAS protein levels in UL when compared to patient-matched myometrial tissue [106]. *FASN* transcript and protein levels have also been reported to be upregulated in many cancer types and are involved in promoting tumor cell growth [107,108]. Aside from a small-scale study that replicated the association in 11p15.1 [109,110], results from the Japanese GWAS, the genome-wide linkage analysis, and the GWAS meta-analysis have yet to be reproduced rigorously, but such a study is now underway in the FibroGENE Consortium [111]. Replication of association is necessary to ensure that variants identified through GWAS are not erroneously detected owing to hidden substructure in the population—a phenomenon known as the "winner's curse" [91,102,112].

Interactions between Germline and Somatic Mutations

Recently, genomic screening of pediatric cancer patients has uncovered an enrichment of mutations in cancer predisposition genes compared with individuals with no reported history of cancer. The early onset of pediatric cancer argues in favor of a model in which a patient's risk may be predominantly genetic in nature, and such findings may inform our understanding of the heritability and biology of UL. WES and WGS of 1120 cancer patients less than 20 years of age identified germline mutations associated with an increased risk of developing childhood cancer in 8.5% (n = 95), of whom only 40% (n = 23) had a family history of cancer. Four participants were mosaics for mutations in cancer-predisposition genes, indicating that at least a subset of mutations occurs post-implantation [113]. Constitutional genetic mutations may therefore be important factors that predispose individuals to neoplasms at a frequency greater than previously recognized, including both those segregating in families and those arising *de novo*. In the latter cases, detection of constitutional genetic mutations may be of greater value than family medical history in evaluating a patient's risk. For further thought, both forms of constitutional genetic mutations lend support to an argument for implementation of genomic sequencing in newborn screening to optimize health and management of disease [114–118].

As described herein, inherited genomic variants, as well as constitutional and acquired genetic mutations, are associated with the biology of UL. Exactly how they may interact with one another remains to be determined. Shown in Figure 5.4,

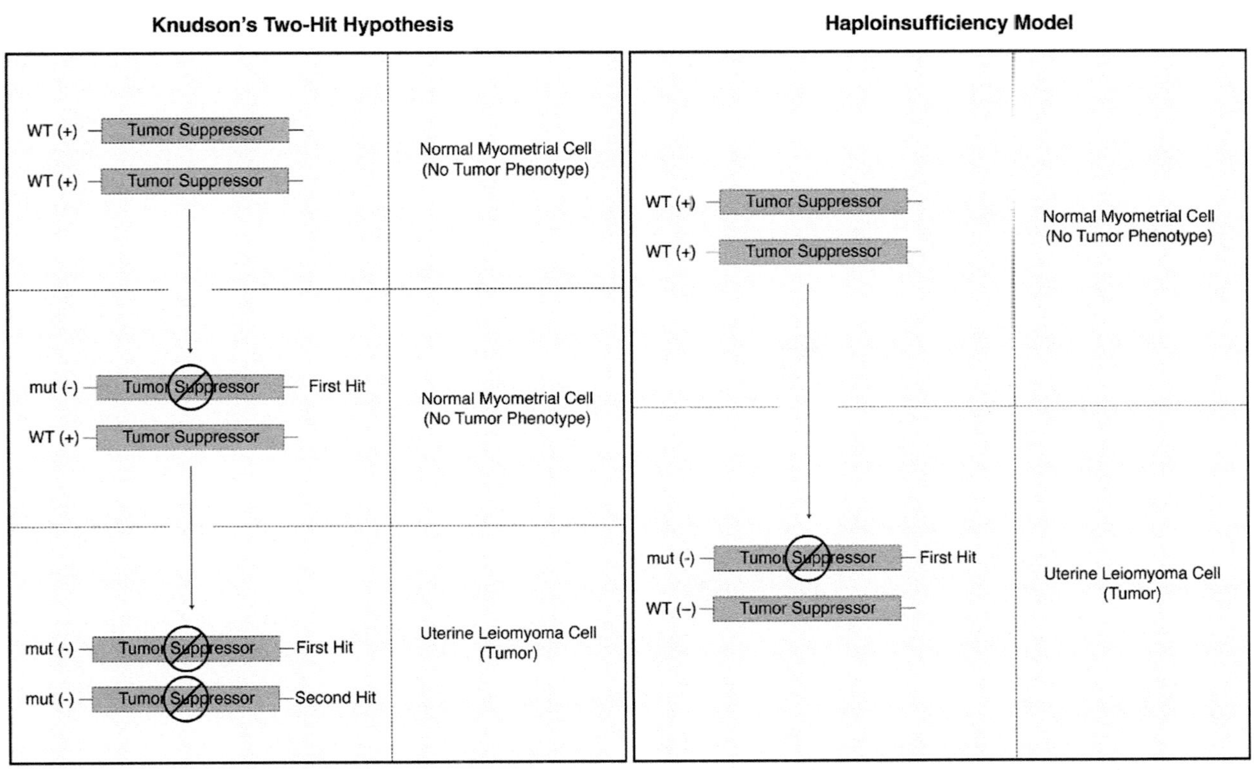

FIGURE 5.4 Comparison of genetic models of benign transformation by loss-of-function mutations occurring in tumor suppressor genes. Knudson's two-hit hypothesis model is shown on the left and illustrates how two mutations are required to develop a tumor. On the right, the haploid insufficiency model demonstrates how a single loss-of-function mutation in certain tumor suppressor genes is sufficient to produce a tumor.

Knudson's classical two-hit hypothesis, in which an individual inherits a mutant allele and subsequently acquires a second mutation, or "hit," in the wild-type allele, may explain both the late onset of UL and its well-demonstrated association with exposure to steroid hormones at puberty. This model can be applied to the rare familial cases of HLRCC and AS-DL and mutations in *FH* and *COL4A5-COL4A6*, respectively [65]. Alternatively, synergistic combinations of heterozygous loss-of-function mutations in tumor suppressor genes may be sufficient to drive tumorigenesis in the relevant biological context [119]. Under the former model, constitutional and acquired mutations act consecutively and additively in the pathobiology of UL. Under the latter, acquired point mutations and chromosomal abnormalities may be facilitators to advanced pathogenesis. In light of the exceptionally high frequency of UL and the comparatively very low frequency of uterine leiomyosarcoma, evaluating whether the observed somatic changes are harbingers of carcinogenesis or protection against malignant transformation will be valuable in gaining an understanding of the role of acquired genomic instability in UL [95,98,120].

Acknowledgments

We thank Zehra Ordulu, MD, for her edits and review of the manuscript, and for support of the research by the NIH/NICHD (HD060530 to C.C.M.).

REFERENCES

1. Townsend DE, Sparkes RS, Baluda MC, and McClelland G. Unicellular histogenesis of uterine leiomyomas as determined by electrophoresis by glucose-6-phosphate dehydrogenase. *Am J Obstet Gynecol.* 1970;107(8):1168–73.
2. Ligon AH and Morton CC. Genetics of uterine leiomyomata. *Genes Chromosomes Cancer.* 2000;28(3):235–45.
3. Linder D and Gartler SM. Glucose-6-phosphate dehydrogenase mosaicism: Utilization as a cell marker in the study of leiomyomas. *Science.* 1965;150(3692):67–9.
4. Mashal RD, Fejzo ML, Friedman AJ et al. Analysis of androgen receptor DNA reveals the independent clonal origins of uterine leiomyomata and the secondary nature of cytogenetic aberrations in the development of leiomyomata. *Genes Chromosomes Cancer.* 1994;11(1):1–6.
5. Hashimoto K, Azuma C, Kamiura S et al. Clonal determination of uterine leiomyomas by analyzing differential inactivation of the X-chromosome-linked phosphoglycerokinase gene. *Gynecol Obstet Invest.* 1995;40(3):204–8.
6. Makinen N, Mehine M, Tolvanen J et al. MED12, the mediator complex subunit 12 gene, is mutated at high frequency in uterine leiomyomas. *Science.* 2011;334(6053):252–5.
7. Mehine M, Kaasinen E, Makinen N et al. Characterization of uterine leiomyomas by whole-genome sequencing. *N Engl J Med.* 2013;369(1):43–53.
8. Mehine M, Heinonen HR, Sarvilinna N et al. Clonally related uterine leiomyomas are common and display branched tumor evolution. *Hum Mol Genet.* 2015;24(15):4407–16.
9. Nibert M and Heim S. Uterine leiomyoma cytogenetics. *Genes Chromosomes Cancer.* 1990;2(1):3–13.
10. Rein MS, Friedman AJ, Barbieri RL, Pavelka K, Fletcher JA, and Morton CC. Cytogenetic abnormalities in uterine leiomyomata. *Obstet Gynecol.* 1991;77(6):923–6.
11. Hodge JC and Morton CC. Genetic heterogeneity among uterine leiomyomata: Insights into malignant progression. *Hum Mol Genet.* 2007;16 Spec No 1:R7–13. doi: 10.1093/hmg/ddm043
12. Sandberg AA and Bridge JA. *The Cytogenetics of Bone and Soft Tissue Tumors.* Austin: R.G. Landes, 1994. 469 pp.
13. Kiechle-Schwarz M, Sreekantaiah C, Berger CS et al. Nonrandom cytogenetic changes in leiomyomas of the female genitourinary tract. A report of 35 cases. *Cancer Genet Cytogenet.* 1991;53(1):125–36.
14. Meloni AM, Surti U, Contento AM, Davare J, and Sandberg AA. Uterine leiomyomas: Cytogenetic and histologic profile. *Obstet Gynecol.* 1992;80(2):209–17.
15. Mrozek K, Gibas Z, and Limon J. Specific chromosome aberrations in human soft-tissue tumors and their diagnostic significance. *Pol Tyg Le.* 1995;50(36–39):85–9.
16. Pandis N, Heim S, Bardi G et al. Chromosome analysis of 96 uterine leiomyomas. *Cancer Genet Cytogenet.* 1991;55(1):11–8.
17. Quade BJ. Pathology, cytogenetics and molecular biology of uterine leiomyomas and other smooth muscle lesions. *Curr Opin Obstet Gynecol.* 1995;7(1):35–42.
18. Sandberg AA. Updates on the cytogenetics and molecular genetics of bone and soft tissue tumors: Leiomyoma. *Cancer Genet Cytogenet.* 2005;158(1):1–26.
19. Gross KL and Morton CC. Genetics and the development of fibroids. *Clin Obstet Gynecol.* 2001;44(2):335–49.
20. Hodge JC, Kim TM, Dreyfuss JM et al. Expression profiling of uterine leiomyomata cytogenetic subgroups reveals distinct signatures in matched myometrium: Transcriptional profiling of the t(12;14) and evidence in support of predisposing genetic heterogeneity. *Hum Mol Genet.* 2012;21(10):2312–29.
21. Hodge JC, Park PJ, Dreyfuss JM et al. Identifying the molecular signature of the interstitial deletion 7q subgroup of uterine leiomyomata using a paired analysis. *Genes Chromosomes Cancer.* 2009;48(10):865–85.
22. Turc-Carel C, Dal Cin P, Boghosian L, Terk-Zakarian J, and Sandberg AA. Consistent breakpoints in region 14q22-q24 in uterine leiomyoma. *Cancer Genet Cytogenet.* 1988;32(1):25–31.
23. Heim S, Nilbert M, Vanni R et al. A specific translocation, t(12;14)(q14-15;q23-24), characterizes a subgroup of uterine leiomyomas. *Cancer Genet Cytogenet.* 1988;32(1):13–7.
24. Vanni R, Nieddu M, Paoli R, and Lecca U. Uterine leiomyoma cytogenetics. I. Rearrangements of chromosome 12. *Cancer Genet Cytogenet.* 1989;37(1):49–54.
25. Fan SX, Sreekantaiah C, Berger CS, Medchill M, Pedron S, and Sandberg AA. Cytogenetic findings in nine leiomyomas of the uterus. *Cancer Genet Cytogenet.* 1990;47(2):179–89.
26. Mark J, Havel G, Grepp C, Dahlenfors R, and Wedell B. Chromosomal patterns in human benign uterine leiomyomas. *Cancer Genet Cytogenet.* 1990;44(1):1–13.
27. Hennig Y, Deichert U, Bonk U, Thode B, Bartnitzke S, and Bullerdiek J. Chromosomal translocations affecting 12q14-15 but not deletions of the long arm of chromosome 7 associated with a growth advantage of uterine smooth muscle cells. *Mol Hum Reprod.* 1999;5(12):1150–4.
28. Brosens I, Deprest J, Dal Cin P, and Van den Berghe H. Clinical significance of cytogenetic abnormalities in uterine myomas. *Fertil Steril.* 1998;69(2):232–5.

29. Rein MS, Powell WL, Walters FC et al. Cytogenetic abnormalities in uterine myomas are associated with myoma size. *Mol Hum Reprod.* 1998;4(1):83–6.
30. Kataoka S, Yamada H, Hoshi N et al. Cytogenetic analysis of uterine leiomyoma: The size, histopathology and GnRHa-response in relation to chromosome karyotype. *Eur J Obstet Gynecol Reprod Biol.* 2003;110(1):58–62.
31. Fejzo MS, Yoon SJ, Montgomery KT et al. Identification of a YAC spanning the translocation breakpoints in uterine leiomyomata, pulmonary chondroid hamartoma, and lipoma: Physical mapping of the 12q14-q15 breakpoint region in uterine leiomyomata. *Genomics.* 1995;26(2):265–71.
32. Ashar HR, Fejzo MS, Tkachenko A et al. Disruption of the architectural factor HMGI-C: DNA-binding AT hook motifs fused in lipomas to distinct transcriptional regulatory domains. *Cell.* 1995;82(1):57–65.
33. Schoenmakers EF, Mols R, Wanschura S et al. Identification, molecular cloning, and characterization of the chromosome 12 breakpoint cluster region of uterine leiomyomas. *Genes Chromosomes Cancer.* 1994;11(2):106–18.
34. Fusco A and Fedele M. Roles of HMGA proteins in cancer. *Nat Rev Cancer.* 2007;7(12):899–910.
35. Schoenmakers EF, Wanschura S, Mols R, Bullerdiek J, Van den Berghe H, and Van de Ven WJ. Recurrent rearrangements in the high mobility group protein gene, *HMGI-C*, in benign mesenchymal tumours. *Nat Genet.* 1995;10(4):436–44.
36. Rogalla P, Drechsler K, Frey G et al. *HMGI-C* expression patterns in human tissues. Implications for the genesis of frequent mesenchymal tumors. *Am J Pathol.* 1996;149(3):775–9.
37. Schoenmakers EF, Huysmans C, and Van de Ven WJ. Allelic knockout of novel splice variants of human recombination repair gene *RAD51B* in t(12;14) uterine leiomyomas. *Cancer Res.* 1999;59(1):19–23.
38. Ingraham SE, Lynch RA, Surti U et al. Identification and characterization of novel human transcripts embedded within HMGA2 in t(12;14)(q15;q24.1) uterine leiomyoma. *Mutat Res.* 2006;602(1–2):43–53.
39. Gattas GJ, Quade BJ, Nowak RA, and Morton CC. *HMGIC* expression in human adult and fetal tissues and in uterine leiomyomata. *Genes Chromosomes Cancer.* 1999;25(4):316–22.
40. Lee YS and Dutta A. The tumor suppressor microRNA let-7 represses the *HMGA2* oncogene. *Genes Dev.* 2007; 21(9):1025–30.
41. Mayr C, Hemann MT, and Bartel DP. Disrupting the pairing between *let-7* and *Hmga2* enhances oncogenic transformation. *Science.* 2007;315(5818):1576–9.
42. Ligon AH, Moore SD, Parisi MA et al. Constitutional rearrangement of the architectural factor *HMGA2*: A novel human phenotype including overgrowth and lipomas. *Am J Hum Genet.* 2005;76(2):340–8.
43. Sreekantaiah C, Leong SP, Karakousis CP et al. Cytogenetic profile of 109 lipomas. *Cancer Res.* 1991;51(1):422–33.
44. Kazmierczak B, Bol S, Wanschura S, Bartnitzke S, and Bullerdiek J. PAC clone containing the *HMGI(Y)* gene spans the breakpoint of a 6p21 translocation in a uterine leiomyoma cell line. *Genes Chromosomes Cancer.* 1996;17(3):191–3.
45. Williams AJ, Powell WL, Collins T, and Morton CC. *HMGI(Y)* expression in human uterine leiomyomata. Involvement of another high-mobility group architectural factor in a benign neoplasm. *Am J Pathol.* 1997;150(3):911–8.
46. Schoenmakers EF, Bunt J, Hermers L et al. Identification of *CUX1* as the recurrent chromosomal band 7q22 target gene in human uterine leiomyoma. *Genes Chromosomes Cancer.* 2013;52(1):11–23.
47. Moore SD, Herrick SR, Ince TA et al. Uterine leiomyomata with t(10;17) disrupt the histone acetyltransferase MORF. *Cancer Res.* 2004;64(16):5570–7.
48. Ingraham SE, Lynch RA, Kathiresan S, Buckler AJ, and Menon AG. *hREC2*, a *RAD51*-like gene, is disrupted by t(12;14) (q15;q24.1) in a uterine leiomyoma. *Cancer Genet Cytogenet.* 1999;115(1):56–61.
49. Makinen N, Heinonen HR, Moore S, Tomlinson IP, van der Spuy ZM, and Aaltonen LA. *MED12* exon 2 mutations are common in uterine leiomyomas from South African patients. *Oncotarget.* 2011;2(12):966–9.
50. McGuire MM, Yatsenko A, Hoffner L, Jones M, Surti U, and Rajkovic A. Whole exome sequencing in a random sample of North American women with leiomyomas identifies *MED12* mutations in majority of uterine leiomyomas. *PLOS ONE.* 2012;7(3):e33251.
51. Je EM, Kim MR, Min KO, Yoo NJ, and Lee SH. Mutational analysis of *MED12* exon 2 in uterine leiomyoma and other common tumors. *Int J Cancer.* 2012;131(6):E1044–7.
52. Kampjarvi K, Park MJ, Mehine M et al. Mutations in exon 1 highlight the role of *MED12* in uterine leiomyomas. *Hum Mutat.* 2014;35(9):1136–41.
53. Mehine M, Makinen N, Heinonen HR, Aaltonen LA, and Vahteristo P. Genomics of uterine leiomyomas: Insights from high-throughput sequencing. *Fertil Steril.* 2014;102(3):621–9.
54. Mittal P, Shin YH, Yatsenko SA, Castro CA, Surti U, and Rajkovic A. *Med12* gain-of-function mutation causes leiomyomas and genomic instability. *J Clin Invest.* 2015;125(8):3280–4.
55. Bertsch E, Qiang W, Zhang Q et al. *MED12* and *HMGA2* mutations: Two independent genetic events in uterine leiomyoma and leiomyosarcoma. *Mod Pathol.* 2014;27(8):1144–53.
56. Markowski DN, Bartnitzke S, Loning T, Drieschner N, Helmke BM, and Bullerdiek J. *MED12* mutations in uterine fibroids–their relationship to cytogenetic subgroups. *Int J Cancer.* 2012;131(7):1528–36.
57. Forment JV, Kaidi A, and Jackson SP. Chromothripsis and cancer: Causes and consequences of chromosome shattering. *Nat Rev Cancer.* 2012;12(10):653–70.
58. Reed WB, Walker R, and Horowitz R. Cutaneous leiomyomata with uterine leiomyomata. *Acta Derm Venereol.* 1973;53(5):409–16.
59. Tomlinson IP, Alam NA, Rowan AJ et al. Germline mutations in *FH* predispose to dominantly inherited uterine fibroids, skin leiomyomata and papillary renal cell cancer. *Nat Genet.* 2002;30(4):406–10.
60. Launonen V, Vierimaa O, Kiuru M et al. Inherited susceptibility to uterine leiomyomas and renal cell cancer. *Proc Natl Acad Sci U S A.* 2001;98(6):3387–92.
61. Alam NA, Rowan AJ, Wortham NC et al. Genetic and functional analyses of *FH* mutations in multiple cutaneous and uterine leiomyomatosis, hereditary leiomyomatosis and renal cancer, and fumarate hydratase deficiency. *Hum Mol Genet.* 2003;12(11):1241–52.
62. Kiuru M, Launonen V, Hietala M et al. Familial cutaneous leiomyomatosis is a two-hit condition associated with renal cell cancer of characteristic histopathology. *Am J Pathol.* 2001;159(3):825–9.

63. Merino MJ, Torres-Cabala C, Pinto P, and Linehan WM. The morphologic spectrum of kidney tumors in hereditary leiomyomatosis and renal cell carcinoma (HLRCC) syndrome. *Am J Surg Pathol.* 2007;31(10):1578–85.
64. Thyresson HN and Su WP. Familial cutaneous leiomyomatosis. *J Am Acad Dermatol.* 1981;4(4):430–4.
65. Knudson AG, Jr. Mutation and cancer: Statistical study of retinoblastoma. *Proc Natl Acad Sci U S A.* 1971;68(4):820–3.
66. Gaude E and Frezza C. Defects in mitochondrial metabolism and cancer. *Cancer Metab.* 2014;2:10.
67. King A, Selak MA, and Gottlieb E. Succinate dehydrogenase and fumarate hydratase: Linking mitochondrial dysfunction and cancer. *Oncogene.* 2006;25(34):4675–82.
68. Bayley JP, Launonen V, and Tomlinson IP. The *FH* mutation database: An online database of fumarate hydratase mutations involved in the MCUL (HLRCC) tumor syndrome and congenital fumarase deficiency. *BMC Med Genet.* 2008;9:20.
69. Selak MA, Armour SM, MacKenzie ED et al. Succinate links TCA cycle dysfunction to oncogenesis by inhibiting HIF-alpha prolyl hydroxylase. *Cancer Cell.* 2005;7(1):77–85.
70. Pollard PJ, Briere JJ, Alam NA et al. Accumulation of Krebs cycle intermediates and over-expression of HIF1alpha in tumours which result from germline FH and SDH mutations. *Hum Mol Genet.* 2005;14(15):2231–9.
71. Isaacs JS, Jung YJ, Mole DR et al. HIF overexpression correlates with biallelic loss of fumarate hydratase in renal cancer: Novel role of fumarate in regulation of HIF stability. *Cancer Cell.* 2005;8(2):143–53.
72. Kampjarvi K, Makinen N, Mehine M et al. *MED12* mutations and *FH* inactivation are mutually exclusive in uterine leiomyomas. *Br J Cancer.* 2016;114(12):1405–11.
73. Alam NA, Olpin S, Rowan A et al. Missense mutations in fumarate hydratase in multiple cutaneous and uterine leiomyomatosis and renal cell cancer. *J Mol Diagn.* 2005; 7(4):437–43.
74. Kiuru M, Lehtonen R, Arola J et al. Few *FH* mutations in sporadic counterparts of tumor types observed in hereditary leiomyomatosis and renal cell cancer families. *Cancer Res.* 2002;62(16):4554–7.
75. Lehtonen R, Kiuru M, Vanharanta S et al. Biallelic inactivation of fumarate hydratase (*FH*) occurs in nonsyndromic uterine leiomyomas but is rare in other tumors. *Am J Pathol.* 2004;164(1):17–22.
76. Harrison WJ, Andrici J, Maclean F et al. Fumarate hydratase-deficient uterine leiomyomas occur in both the syndromic and sporadic settings. *Am J Surg Pathol.* 2016;40(5):599–607.
77. Kashtan CE and Michael AF. Alport syndrome: From bedside to genome to bedside. *Am J Kidney Dis.* 1993;22(5):627–40.
78. Miner JH. Alport syndrome with diffuse leiomyomatosis. When and when not? *Am J Pathol.* 1999;154(6):1633–5.
79. Mothes H, Heidet L, Arrondel C et al. Alport syndrome associated with diffuse leiomyomatosis: *COL4A5-COL4A6* deletion associated with a mild form of Alport nephropathy. *Nephrol Dial Transplant.* 2002;17(1):70–4.
80. Hudson BG, Reeders ST, and Tryggvason K. Type IV collagen: Structure, gene organization, and role in human diseases. Molecular basis of Goodpasture and Alport syndromes and diffuse leiomyomatosis. *J Biol Chem.* 1993;268(35):26033–6.
81. Antignac C. Molecular genetics of basement membranes: The paradigm of Alport syndrome. *Kidney Int Suppl.* 1995;49:S29–33.
82. Zhou J, Mochizuki T, Smeets H et al. Deletion of the paired alpha 5(IV) and alpha 6(IV) collagen genes in inherited smooth muscle tumors. *Science.* 1993;261(5125):1167–9.
83. Heidet L, Dahan K, Zhou J et al. Deletions of both alpha 5(IV) and alpha 6(IV) collagen genes in Alport syndrome and in Alport syndrome associated with smooth muscle tumours. *Hum Mol Genet.* 1995;4(1):99–108.
84. Heidet L, Cohen-Solal L, Boye E et al. Novel *COL4A5/COL4A6* deletions and further characterization of the diffuse leiomyomatosis-Alport syndrome (DL-AS) locus define the DL critical region. *Cytogenet Cell Genet.* 1997;78(3–4):240–6.
85. Barker DF, Hostikka SL, Zhou J et al. Identification of mutations in the *COL4A5* collagen gene in Alport syndrome. *Science.* 1990;248(4960):1224–7.
86. Vikhlyaeva EM, Khodzhaeva ZS, and Fantschenko ND. Familial predisposition to uterine leiomyomas. *Int J Gynaecol Obstet.* 1995;51(2):127–31.
87. Sato F, Mori M, Nishi M, Kudo R, and Miyake H. Familial aggregation of uterine myomas in Japanese women. *J Epidemiol.* 2002;12(3):249–53.
88. Kurbanova M, Koroleva AG, and Sergeev AS. Genetic-epidemiologic analysis of uterine myoma: Assessment of repeated risk. *Genetika.* 1989;25(10):1896–8.
89. Kurbanova M, Koroleva AG, and Sergeev AS. Genetic analysis of the predisposition to uterine myoma. Prevalence and morbidity. *Genetika.* 1989;25(6):1122–4.
90. Van Voorhis BJ, Romitti PA, and Jones MP. Family history as a risk factor for development of uterine leiomyomas. Results of a pilot study. *J Reprod Med.* 2002;47(8):663–9.
91. Gallagher CS and Morton CC. Genetic association studies in uterine fibroids: Risk alleles presage the path to personalized therapies. *Semin Reprod Med.* 2016;34(4):235–41.
92. Treloar SA, Martin NG, Dennerstein L, Raphael B, and Heath AC. Pathways to hysterectomy: Insights from longitudinal twin research. *Am J Obstet Gynecol.* 1992;167(1):82–8.
93. Luoto R, Kaprio J, Rutanen EM, Taipale P, Perola M, and Koskenvuo M. Heritability and risk factors of uterine fibroids—the Finnish Twin Cohort study. *Maturitas.* 2000; 37(1):15–26.
94. Marshall LM, Spiegelman D, Barbieri RL et al. Variation in the incidence of uterine leiomyoma among premenopausal women by age and race. *Obstet Gynecol.* 1997;90(6):967–73.
95. Baird DD, Dunson DB, Hill MC, Cousins D, and Schectman JM. High cumulative incidence of uterine leiomyoma in black and white women: Ultrasound evidence. *Am J Obstet Gynecol.* 2003;188(1):100–7.
96. Kjerulff K, Langenberg P, and Guzinski G. The socioeconomic correlates of hysterectomies in the United States. *Am J Public Health.* 1993;83(1):106–8.
97. Kjerulff KH, Langenberg P, Seidman JD, Stolley PD, and Guzinski GM. Uterine leiomyomas. Racial differences in severity, symptoms and age at diagnosis. *J Reprod Med.* 1996;41(7):483–90.
98. Buttram VC, Jr. and Reiter RC. Uterine leiomyomata: Etiology, symptomatology, and management. *Fertil Steril.* 1981;36(4):433–45.
99. Stewart EA. Uterine fibroids. *Lancet.* 2001;357(9252):293–8.
100. Schwartz SM, Marshall LM, and Baird DD. Epidemiologic contributions to understanding the etiology of uterine leiomyomata. *Environ Health Perspect.* 2000;108(Suppl 5):821–7.

101. Wise LA, Ruiz-Narvaez EA, Palmer JR et al. African ancestry and genetic risk for uterine leiomyomata. *Am J Epidemiol.* 2012;176(12):1159–68.
102. Bush WS and Moore JH. Chapter 11: Genome-wide association studies. *PLoS Comput Biol.* 2012;8(12):e1002822.
103. Reich DE and Lander ES. On the allelic spectrum of human disease. *Trends Genet.* 2001;17(9):502–10.
104. Hindorff LA, Sethupathy P, Junkins HA et al. Potential etiologic and functional implications of genome-wide association loci for human diseases and traits. *Proc Natl Acad Sci USA.* 2009;106(23):9362–7.
105. Cha PC, Takahashi A, Hosono N et al. A genome-wide association study identifies three loci associated with susceptibility to uterine fibroids. *Nat Genet.* 2011;43(5):447–50.
106. Eggert SL, Huyck KL, Somasundaram P et al. Genome-wide linkage and association analyses implicate FASN in predisposition to Uterine Leiomyomata. *Am J Hum Genet.* 2012;91(4):621–8.
107. Rossi S, Graner E, Febbo P et al. Fatty acid synthase expression defines distinct molecular signatures in prostate cancer. *Mol Cancer Res.* 2003;1(10):707–15.
108. Ogino S, Nosho K, Meyerhardt JA et al. Cohort study of fatty acid synthase expression and patient survival in colon cancer. *J Clin Oncol.* 2008;26(35):5713–20.
109. Edwards TL, Michels KA, Hartmann KE, and Velez Edwards DR. *BET1L* and *TNRC6B* associate with uterine fibroid risk among European Americans. *Hum Genet.* 2013;132(8):943–53.
110. Edwards TL, Hartmann KE, and Velez Edwards DR. Variants in *BET1L* and *TNRC6B* associate with increasing fibroid volume and fibroid type among European Americans. *Hum Genet.* 2013;132(12):1361–9.
111. Gallagher CS, Velez-Edwards DR, Cantor RM et al. Identification of 10 novel uterine leiomyomata susceptibility loci by genome-wide association analysis in population-based conventional and direct-to-consumer cohorts. *(Abstract/Program #885/T). Presented at the 65th Annual Meeting of the American Society of Human Genetics*, October 8, 2015, Baltimore, MD.
112. Zollner S and Pritchard JK. Overcoming the winner's curse: Estimating penetrance parameters from case-control data. *Am J Hum Genet.* 2007;80(4):605–15.
113. Zhang J, Walsh MF, Wu G et al. Germline mutations in predisposition genes in pediatric cancer. *N Engl J Med.* 2015;373(24):2336–46.
114. Baker H. Genetic mutations in paediatric cancer. *Lancet Oncol.* 2016;17(1):e8.
115. D'Orazio JA. Inherited cancer syndromes in children and young adults. *J Pediatr Hematol Oncol.* 2010;32(3):195–228.
116. Krepischi AC, Capelli LP, Silva AG et al. Large germline copy number variations as predisposing factor in childhood neoplasms. *Future Oncol.* 2014;10(9):1627–33.
117. Maris JM. Defining why cancer develops in children. *N Engl J Med.* 2015;373(24):2373–5.
118. Shen J and Morton CC. Next generation newborn hearing screening. In: *Genetics of Deafness.* Vona B, Haaf T (eds). Monogr Hum Genet. 2016;20:30–9.
119. Solimini NL, Xu Q, Mermel CH et al. Recurrent hemizygous deletions in cancers may optimize proliferative potential. *Science.* 2012;337(6090):104–9.
120. Brooks SE, Zhan M, Cote T, and Baquet CR. Surveillance, epidemiology, and end results analysis of 2677 cases of uterine sarcoma 1989–1999. *Gynecol Oncol.* 2004;93(1):204–8.

6

Growth Patterns and Endometrial Changes

Jovana Kaludjerovic

Introduction

Uterine fibroids (UFs), also known as uterine leiomyomas, are benign mesenchymal tumors that form in the myometrium of up to 80% of women by the age of 50 [1]. In a non-gravid uterus, fibroids can undergo both growth and regression [2], and can have a substantial impact on women's quality of life. Many women with UF experience heavy menstrual bleeding, dysmenorrhea, pregnancy complications and infertility [3,4]. The symptom severity is often positively correlated with tumor size and location. So, it was traditionally believed that fibroids are inert masses [5]. However, advances in pathophysiology have highlighted that fibroids can influence endometrial function at a molecular level and that their effects can extend beyond the local endometrial environment [5,6]. This chapter provides a summary of UF growth patterns and endometrial changes.

There are three broad categories of fibroids: submucosal, subserosal and intramural. Submucosal fibroids lie directly under the endometrium and can extend into the uterine cavity. Subserosal fibroids project to the outside of the uterus and intramural fibroids grow within the muscular uterine wall. Regardless of their size or location, fibroids are hormonally responsive tumors that can disrupt normal uterine tissue by altering endometrial gene expression through paracrine interactions and, in turn, cause excessive uterine bleeding or defective implantation [7]. The submucosal fibroids are the most disruptive to endometrial integrity, implantation and the capacity of the myometrium to contract and stop menstrual bleeding from the endometrial blood vessels. Thus, submucosal fibroids are most often associated with excessive or irregular bleeding, infertility and recurrent pregnancy loss.

Cellular Composition and Development of Uterine Fibroids

It is accepted that fibroids are monoclonal tumors that arise from a single myocyte, but the initiating event for the neoplastic transformation of a myocyte has not been elucidated [8,9]. There are three cell populations in UFs: fully differentiated smooth muscle cells, a population with intermediate characteristics and fibroid stem cells [5,10]. It is believed that a genetic hit to a myometrial stem cell—such as trisomy of chromosome 12, deletion in 7q, point mutations in the mediator complex subunit 12 (*MED12*) or chromosomal rearrangement involving the high-mobility group AT-hook2 (*HMGA2*)—gives rise to a fibroid stem cell [11–15]. The fibroid stem cell, like the myometrial stem cell, has minimal to no estrogen receptor (ER) and progesterone receptor (PR) expression [16], yet, it is critical for steroid-hormone-dependent fibroid growth and expansion. This was first demonstrated in a mouse xenograph model [7]. In this model, tumors composed of fibroid stem cells and myometrial cells grew into significantly larger tumors and had faster growth rates, under the influence of estrogen and progesterone, than tumors composed of only differentiated fibroid and myometrial cells. Most notably, fibroid stem cells could only induce tumor growth or proliferation in the presence of differentiated fibroid or myometrial cells. These findings highlighted that fibroid stem cells rely on paracrine signaling from surrounding mature fibroid and myometrial cells to facilitate estrogen and progesterone action. In addition, the growth of fibroid xenografts depended on the combination of estrogen and progesterone and could not be induced with either treatment alone.

Steroid-Induced Regulation of Uterine Fibroid Growth and Development

During a normal menstrual cycle, the ovary produces estrogen and progesterone under the influence of the hypothalamus as part of the hypothalamic-pituitary-ovarian axis. The cyclic rise in estrogen and progesterone play a critical role in UF growth and proliferation. The healthy myometrial tissue expresses ERs and PRs [17,18]. But mature fibroid cells overexpress ERs, PRs and the aromatase enzyme, which causes *in situ* synthesis of estrogen to increase and contribute to estrogen-induced signaling [18–20]. Once bound to its receptor, estrogen derived locally or centrally translocates to the nucleus, where it binds to an estrogen response element in the promoter region of the response genes. This triggers the recruitment of co-regulatory proteins including chromatin-remodeling complexes, co-activators and co-repressors, that upregulate signaling pathways and stimulate production of cytokines resulting in fibroid growth.

There are two types of ERs: ERα and ERβ. UFs express both receptors, but the abundance of ERα relative to ERβ is significantly higher in UFs than the myometrium, allowing ERα in UFs to bind to the estrogen response element as a homodimer, as well as a heterodimer with ERβ [18]. Recent evidence suggests that a high ERα-to-ERβ ratio rather than the level of ERα alone is what has a more profound effect on UF growth and proliferation. But, much remains unknown about the exact roles of these receptors in UFs.

Traditionally, estrogen was viewed as a primary mitogenic factor in the uterus. However, Ishikawa et al [7] showed that the primary roles of estrogen and ERα in fibroid growth are permissive in that they enable tissue to respond to progesterone by inducing the expression of PRs, including PR-A and PR-B. In line with this, it has been observed that mitotic activity in UFs is the highest during the luteal/secretory phase of the menstrual cycle, when progesterone is dominant [21,22]. In postmenopausal women, fibroid proliferation is significantly higher with combined estrogen and progestin therapy than estrogen alone [21]. In addition, estrogen and progesterone induce secretion of a growth permissive extracellular matrix (ECM) by stimulating production of collagen, proteoglycans and fibronectin [23]. The ECM traps a number of growth factors, keeping them in close proximity to the fibroid, where they further stimulate cell proliferation and growth, leading to cellular hypertrophy [24–26]. So, tumor growth is often characterized by slow proliferation with concurrent deposition of abundant ECM, usually in a steroid-hormone-dependent manner.

Wnt/β-Catenin Regulation of Uterine Fibroid Growth and Development

An important mechanism involved in UF growth is the Wnt/β-catenin pathway [5,27]. In this pathway, secreted Wnt proteins bind to frizzled family cell surface receptors and cause activated β-catenin to translocate to the nucleus and induce expression of specific target genes, including cell proliferation genes like *c-Myc*, *WISP1* and the cyclin D1 gene [28]. Interestingly, overexpression of constitutively activated β-catenin in uterine mesenchyme during embryonic development and adulthood gave rise to UF-like tumors in mice with 100% penetrance [29]. The occurrence was more common in multiparous mice, suggesting that steroid hormones may interact with activated β-catenin to accelerate tumorigenesis. Moreover, activation of the Wnt/β-catenin pathways led to increased levels of TGF-β, which has been shown to exert paracrine effects on endometrial stromal cells and epithelial cells [6,30], as well as regulate cell proliferation and deposition of ECM [29].

As previously noted, *MED12* mutations in myometrial stem cells can give rise to fibroid stem cells [5,31]. Fibroids with *MED12* mutations express significantly higher levels of Wnt4 [32]. Since estrogen rapidly induces Wnt4 expression in an ER-dependent and -independent manner [32,33], it is thought that mutated *MED12* and estrogen cooperate in activating transcriptional targets of the Wnt pathway including β-catenin. *MED12* knockdown in human fibroid cells leads to decreased cell proliferation via downregulation of the Wnt4/β-catenin signaling pathway [34]. In mice, deletion of β-catenin in uterine mesenchyme reduced uterine size and caused a cell fate change that replaces smooth muscle cells with adipocytes [16,35]. This suggested that the Wnt/β-catenin pathway plays a key role in stem cell renewal and differentiation to the smooth muscle phenotype that is observed in UF [16].

Effects of Uterine Fibroids on the Endometrium

UFs can cause anatomical distortion and place tremendous stretch on the nearby myometrium and overlying endometrium [2]. This increase in uterine stretch can induce changes in gene expression that contribute to impaired uterine contractility [35,36]. Orisaka et al. [37] showed that women with UF have abnormal uterine contractions and peristalsis during the mid-luteal phase of the reproductive cycle, which in a follow-up study was linked to lower pregnancy rates [38].

Impaired reproduction has also been reported in women with small submucosal and intramural fibroids that do not alter or induce stretch on the endometrial cavity. So, it is likely that paracrine signaling from UF to the endometrium contributes to fibroid-related infertility. Growth factors, which are secreted by UF, are plausible mediators of endometrial effects. TGF-β3, which is produced by UF in far greater amounts than normal myometrium, has detrimental effects on signaling pathways necessary for endometrial receptivity [29,39,40]. Sinclair et al [30] showed that TGF-β3 decreases endometrial receptivity to BMP-2 by downregulating BMP receptor expression. BMP2 mediates *HOXA10* and *LIF* expression, which are key regulators of implantation [30]. Accumulating evidence is showing that *HOXA10* expression is decreased in the endometrium of women with submucosal and intramural fibroids with most prominent changes occurring in the endometrium overlying the fibroid [5,39,6]. Interestingly, the effects are observed in nearly 70% of women with UF and are reversed in patients with intramural fibroids following myomectomy [39]. So, TGF-β3 induced resistance to BMP2 likely hinders decidualization and embryo implantation. Taken together, these findings suggest that TGF-β is a paracrine mediator of UF-related infertility and pregnancy loss [40].

Heavy menstrual bleeding is one of the most common symptoms in women with UFs [3,4]. The quantity of menstrual bleeding depends on a complex interplay of vasoconstriction, angiogenesis and coagulation [5]. UF have increased production of prostaglandin $F_{2\alpha}$ and alter the expression level of endothelin-1 receptors in the myometrium, resulting in increased vasoconstriction and menstrual blood loss [41,42]. Moreover, UF increase the production of angiogenic factors such as basic fibroblast growth factor [43] and reduce the production of coagulation and thrombosis factors (i.e. thrombomodulin, antithrombin III, and plasminogen activator inhibitor 1) resulting in heavy menses [5]. Understanding the crosstalk between fibroids and the endometrium will provide key insights into implantation and menstrual biology.

Although significant strides have been made in this field in recent years, further research is needed to fully understand the pathogenesis of these common and troublesome tumors, including their growth patterns and endometrial changes. Such knowledge is needed so that gynecological and obstetric treatments can be optimized for the management of symptomatic UFs.

REFERENCES

1. Baird DD, Dunson DB, Hill MC, Cousins D, Schectman JM. High cumulative incidence of uterine leiomyoma in black and white women: Ultrasound evidence. *Am J Obstet Gynecol.* 2003;188(1):100–7.
2. Ghosh S, Naftalin J, Imrie R, Hoo W. Natural history of uterine fibroids: A radiological perspective. *Curr Obstet Gynecol Rep.* 2018;7(3):117–21.

3. Zimmermann A, Bernuit D, Gerlinger C, Schaefers M, Geppert K. Prevalence, symptoms and management of uterine fibroids: An international internet-based survey of 21,746 women. *BMC Womens Health*. 2012;12:6.
4. Okolo S. Incidence, aetiology and epidemiology of uterine fibroids. *Best Pract Res Clin Obstet Gynaecol*. 2008;22(4):571–88.
5. Ikhena DE, Bulun SE. Literature review on the role of uterine fibroids in endometrial function. *Reprod Sci*. 2018; 25(5):635–43.
6. Rackow BW, Taylor HS. Submucosal uterine leiomyomas have a global effect on molecular determinants of endometrial receptivity. *Fertil Steril*. 2010;93(6):2027–34.
7. Ishikawa H, Ishi K, Serna VA, Kakazu R, Bulun SE, Kurita T. Progesterone is essential for maintenance and growth of uterine leiomyoma. *Endocrinology*. 2010;151(6):2433–42.
8. ACOG Practice Bulletin No. 110: Noncontraceptive uses of hormonal contraceptives. *Obstet Gynecol*. 2010;115(1):206–18.
9. Zhang P, Zhang C, Hao J et al. Use of X-chromosome inactivation pattern to determine the clonal origins of uterine leiomyoma and leiomyosarcoma. *Hum Pathol*. 2006;37(10):1350–6.
10. Yin P, Ono M, Moravek MB et al. Human uterine leiomyoma stem/progenitor cells expressing CD34 and CD49b initiate tumors in vivo. *J Clin Endocrinol Metab*. 2015;100(4):E601–6.
11. Hodge JC, Park PJ, Dreyfuss JM et al. Identifying the molecular signature of the interstitial deletion 7q subgroup of uterine leiomyomata using a paired analysis. *Genes Chromosomes Cancer*. 2009;48(10):865–85.
12. Parker WH. Etiology, symptomatology, and diagnosis of uterine myomas. *Fertil Steril*. 2007;87(4):725–36.
13. Makinen N, Mehine M, Tolvanen J et al. MED12, the mediator complex subunit 12 gene, is mutated at high frequency in uterine leiomyomas. *Science*. 2011;334(6053):252–5.
14. Velagaleti GV, Tonk VS, Hakim NM et al. Fusion of HMGA2 to COG5 in uterine leiomyoma. *Cancer Genet Cytogenet*. 2010;202(1):11–6.
15. Ono M, Bulun SE, Maruyama T. Tissue-specific stem cells in the myometrium and tumor-initiating cells in leiomyoma. *Biol Reprod*. 2014;91(6):149.
16. Ono M, Yin P, Navarro A et al. Paracrine activation of WNT/beta-catenin pathway in uterine leiomyoma stem cells promotes tumor growth. *Proc Natl Acad Sci U S A*. 2013;110(42):17053–8.
17. Benassayag C, Leroy MJ, Rigourd V et al. Estrogen receptors (ERalpha/ERbeta) in normal and pathological growth of the human myometrium: Pregnancy and leiomyoma. *Am J Physiol*. 1999;276(6 Pt 1):E1112–8.
18. Moravek MB, Bulun SE. Endocrinology of uterine fibroids: Steroid hormones, stem cells, and genetic contribution. *Curr Opin Obstet Gynecol*. 2015;27(4):276–83.
19. Bulun SE, Simpson ER, Word RA. Expression of the CYP19 gene and its product aromatase cytochrome P450 in human uterine leiomyoma tissues and cells in culture. *J Clin Endocrinol Metab*. 1994;78(3):736–43.
20. Sumitani H, Shozu M, Segawa T et al. In situ estrogen synthesized by aromatase P450 in uterine leiomyoma cells promotes cell growth probably via an autocrine/intracrine mechanism. *Endocrinology*. 2000;141(10):3852–61.
21. Lamminen S, Rantala I, Helin H, Rorarius M, Tuimala R. Proliferative activity of human uterine leiomyoma cells as measured by automatic image analysis. *Gynecol Obstet Invest*. 1992;34(2):111–4.
22. Bardakhch'ian EA, Bochkov NI. Ultrastructural features of the distal portion of the nephron under conditions of thermal injury. *Tsitol Genet*. 1977;11(4):360–5.
23. Qiang W, Liu Z, Serna VA et al. Down-regulation of miR-29b is essential for pathogenesis of uterine leiomyoma. *Endocrinology*. 2014;155(3):663–9.
24. Geiger B, Bershadsky A, Pankov R, Yamada KM. Transmembrane crosstalk between the extracellular matrix--cytoskeleton crosstalk. *Nat Rev Mol Cell Biol*. 2001;2(11):793–805.
25. Cukierman E, Pankov R, Stevens DR, Yamada KM. Taking cell-matrix adhesions to the third dimension. *Science*. 2001;294(5547):1708–12.
26. Zaitseva M, Vollenhoven BJ, Rogers PA. In vitro culture significantly alters gene expression profiles and reduces differences between myometrial and fibroid smooth muscle cells. *Mol Hum Reprod*. 2006;12(3):187–207.
27. Rocha PP, Scholze M, Bleiss W, Schrewe H. Med12 is essential for early mouse development and for canonical Wnt and Wnt/PCP signaling. *Development*. 2010;137(16):2723–31.
28. Clevers H. Wnt/beta-catenin signaling in development and disease. *Cell*. 2006;127(3):469–80.
29. Tanwar PS, Lee HJ, Zhang L et al. Constitutive activation of beta-catenin in uterine stroma and smooth muscle leads to the development of mesenchymal tumors in mice. *Biol Reprod*. 2009;81(3):545–52.
30. Sinclair DC, Mastroyannis A, Taylor HS. Leiomyoma simultaneously impair endometrial BMP-2-mediated decidualization and anticoagulant expression through secretion of TGF-beta3. *J Clin Endocrinol Metab*. 2011;96(2):412–21.
31. Bulun SE. Uterine fibroids. *N Engl J Med*. 2013;369(14): 1344–55.
32. Markowski DN, Bartnitzke S, Loning T, Drieschner N, Helmke BM, Bullerdiek J. MED12 mutations in uterine fibroids – Their relationship to cytogenetic subgroups. *Int J Cancer*. 2012; 131(7):1528–36.
33. Hau X, Tan Y, Li M, Dey SK, Das SK. Canonical Wnt signaling is critical to estrogen – mediated uterine growth. *Mol Endocrinol*. 2004;18(2):3035–49.
34. Al-Hendy A, Laknaur A, Diamond MP, Ismail N, Boyer TG, Halder SK. Silencing Med12 gene reduces proliferation of human leiomyoma cells mediated via Wnt/β-catenin signaling pathway. *Endocrinology*. 2017;158(3):592–603.
35. Arango NA, Szotek PP, Manganaro TF, Oliva E, Donahoe PK, Teixeira J. Conditional deletion of beta-catenin in the mesenchyme of the developing mouse uterus results in a switch to adipogenesis in the myometrium. *Dev Biol*. 2005;288(1):276–83.
36. Payson M, Malik M, Siti-Nur Morris S, Segars JH, Chason R, Catherino WH. Activating transcription factor 3 gene expression suggests that tissue stress plays a role in leiomyoma development. *Fertil Steril*. 2009;92(2):748–55.
37. Orisaka M, Kurokawa T, Shukunami K et al. A comparison of uterine peristalsis in women with normal uteri and uterine leiomyoma by cine magnetic resonance imaging. *Eur J Obstet Gynecol Reprod Biol*. 2007;135(1):111–5.
38. Yoshino O, Hayashi T, Osuga Y et al. Decreased pregnancy rate is linked to abnormal uterine peristalsis caused by intramural fibroids. *Hum Reprod*. 2010;25(10):2475–9.
39. Matsuzaki S, Canis M, Darcha C, Pouly JL, Mage G. HOXA-10 expression in the mid-secretory endometrium of infertile patients with either endometriosis, uterine fibromas or unexplained infertility. *Hum Reprod*. 2009;24(12):3180–7.

40. Doherty LF, Taylor HS. Leiomyoma-derived transforming growth factor-beta impairs bone morphogenetic protein-2-mediated endometrial receptivity. *Fertil Steril.* 2015; 103(3):845–52.
41. Miura S, Khan KN, Kitajima M, Hiraki K, Moriyama S, Masuzaki H, Samejima T, Fujishita A, Ishimaru T. Differential infiltration of macrophages and prostaglandin production by different uterine leiomyomas. *Hum Reprod.* 2006;21(10):2545–54.
42. Fekonen F, Nyman T, Rutanen EM. Differential expression of mRNAs for endothelin-related proteins in human endometrium, myometrium and leiomyoma. *Mol Cell Endocrinol.* 1994;103(1–2):165–70.
43. Anania CA, Stewart EA, Quade BJ, Hill JA, Nowak RA. Expression of the fibroblast growth factor receptor in women with leiomyomas and abnormal uterine bleeding. *Mol Hum Reprod.* 1997;3(8):685–91.

7

Causes of Bleeding

Ophelia Yin, Carter M. Owen, Kamaria Cayton, and James H. Segars

Introduction

Abnormal uterine bleeding (AUB) is one of the most common reasons patients present to the gynecologist [1]. Fibroids are a major cause of abnormal uterine bleeding within the PALM-COEIN classification system, with "L" standing for leiomyoma [2]. Fibroids occur in multiple locations throughout the uterus (Figure 7.1), and heavy menstrual bleeding due to fibroids can result in severe anemia and decreased quality of life [3]. Despite a century of research on fibroids, there is no clear consensus on the mechanisms underlying uterine bleeding secondary to fibroids. This chapter will summarize the evolving hypotheses regarding the pathophysiology of fibroid-related bleeding.

Historical Perspectives: Structural Mechanisms

Historically, it was thought that fibroids exert mechanical forces on the uterus, causing bleeding via three main structural mechanisms: endometrial thinning/hyperplasia, venule ectasia and contractile defects. First, as early as 1918, Lockyer recognized that "as the tumor increases in size, the mucous membrane [overlying the fibroid] becomes atrophic and thinned by stretching" while endometrium at the margins of the fibroid undergo hyperplasia [4]; it was conjectured that denuding and hyperplasia of the endometrium contribute to heavy bleeding. Second, light microscopy studies revealed ectasia, or dilation, of venules in the myometrium and endometrium of fibroid uteri [5]. It was postulated that fibroids compress nearby veins to prevent drainage and lead to venous dilation, which may interfere with proper clot formation and set up an environment for hemorrhage [6]. Third, fibroids were thought to interfere with normal contractile functions involved in menstruation. Contractions in the nonpregnant uterus originate from an inner myometrium layer (junctional zone) that is adjacent to the endometrium [7]. A study using high-resolution 3 Tesla magnetic resonance imaging found that the presence and frequency of endometrial peristalsis was significantly decreased in patients with symptomatic fibroids compared to controls. Notably, the authors did not find an association between peristalsis and fibroid size [8].

Current Hypotheses: Molecular Mechanisms

Contemporary data support that neither the size nor the location of fibroids are consistently associated with symptoms of bleeding, which would be expected if mechanical forces exerted by fibroids were the entire explanation for pathogenesis of heavy menstrual bleeding [9–12]. Given this, the structural mechanisms of endometrial thinning/hyperplasia, venule ectasia and contractile defects posited earlier may not be the only explanation for causes of bleeding in the fibroid uterus. More recently, the emphasis on anatomic disturbances caused by fibroids has shifted to the study of molecular changes induced by fibroids. Of particular interest is the study of angiogenic factor dysregulation in fibroids and endometrial changes in the presence of fibroids. These molecular changes are implicated in fibroid-associated bleeding.

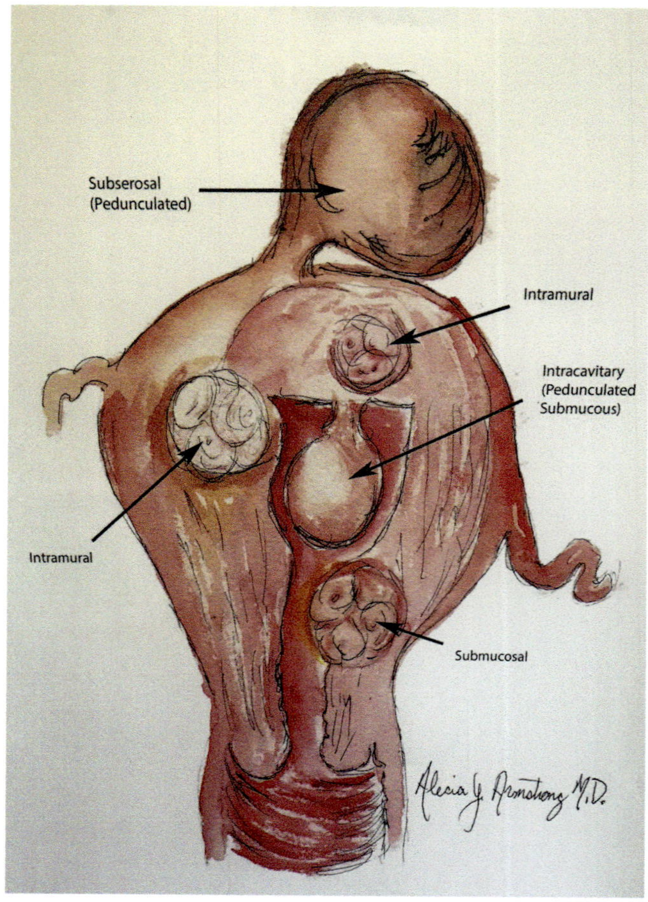

FIGURE 7.1 Illustration by Dr. Alicia Christy, a reproductive endocrinologist at the National Institutes of Health, depicting the locations that fibroids may reside in the uterus.

Angiogenic Factor Dysregulation in Fibroids

Angiogenesis, the development of new blood vessels, is normally associated with wound healing and the malignant transformation of cancer. The uterus is unique as it undergoes a cyclical angiogenesis that is associated with menstruation [13]. The primary regulators of angiogenesis in the uterus are estrogen and progesterone. Previous studies demonstrated that estrogen treatment results in upregulation of vascular endothelial growth factor (VEGF) and basic fibroblast growth factor (bFGF) mRNA and can cause doubling of microvascular density in the uterus (reviewed in [14]). Similarly, hormones that bind the progesterone receptor can also promote endometrial angiogenesis [15]. Since fibroids are known to be hyperresponsive to estrogen and have increased numbers of both estrogen and progesterone receptors, activation of fibroid hormone receptors may be key to the dysregulation of angiogenesis that has been associated with abnormal uterine bleeding [16].

There is evidence that a number of angiogenic factors are differentially expressed in fibroid tissue compared with normal myometrium, as reviewed by Tal and Segars [17]. Epidermal growth factor (EGF), EGF-receptor (EGF-R), platelet-derived growth factor (PDGF), VEGF, bFGF and finally andromedullin (ADM) were found to be more highly expressed in fibroid tissue compared with the myometrium [17]. The connection between fibroids and the majority of these angiogenic factors is likely mediated by hormones, as progesterone and estrogen are known to increase EGF, EGF-R [18], VEGF and bFGF expression [14]. Lastly, ADM expression was elevated in fibroids compared with myometrium [19], and progesterone plays a role in this process since treatment with progesterone receptor modulator ulipristal acetate (CDB-2914) decreased ADM and VEGF and their receptors in human fibroid cells [20].

The most compelling evidence supporting that differences in angiogenic factors between fibroids and normal myometrium can translate to gross changes such as blood vessel formation comes from studies by Hague et al. [19] and Di Lieto et al. [21, 22]. Hague et al. [19] assessed 52 fibroid uteri and 39 control uteri and found that ADM and VEGF were upregulated in the myometrium and endometrium of fibroid uteri. Despite the expectation that all angiogenic factors would be associated with blood vessel formation, the investigators concluded that only ADM levels correlated with higher vascular density and endothelial cell proliferation in adjacent myometrium. Di Lieto et al. [21, 22] also discovered that treatment of fibroid uteri with a gonadotropin-releasing hormone analogue (GnRH-a), a treatment often used for AUB associated with fibroids, reduced protein expression of PDGF, bFGF and VEGF, as well as vascular density and angiogenesis, demonstrating that hormone action, angiogenic factors and gross vascular changes are all interconnected. Notably, plasma iron levels and hemoglobin values improved in patients treated with GnRH-a, supporting the idea that inhibition of vascular growth can result in clinical outcomes associated with decreased bleeding.

Complicating the connections among fibroids, vascular growth and AUB, many studies have concluded that the interior of fibroids have a low vascular density but the exterior of fibroids are surrounded by a dense vascular capsule with increased blood flow (reviewed in [17]). In addition, Wei et al. showed that the concentration of VEGF displays a gradient, with a minimum in the center of the fibroid and a maximum in the outer adjacent myometrium [23]. Therefore, blood loss related to fibroids may stem from alterations in uterine angiogenesis and perivascular capsule hemorrhage rather than bleeding within the fibroid itself.

In summary, dysregulation of angiogenesis related to fibroids has been associated with gross vascular changes and clinical measures of blood loss and may be crucial to the pathogenesis of fibroid-related AUB.

Endometrial Changes in the Presence of Fibroids

While most prior studies have focused on comparing fibroids to myometrium, there are new data on how fibroids may directly affect the endometrium. Rackow and Taylor [24] compared the homeobox A10 (*HOXA10*) gene and protein expression in endometrial biopsies from 30 reproductive-age women with submucosal, intramural or no uterine fibroids in the proliferative phase of their menstrual cycle. HOXA10 is a homeobox-containing transcription factor necessary for promoting stromal decidualization and leukocyte infiltration during each menstrual cycle [25]. Endometrial samples from submucosal uteri had lower *HOXA10* expression compared with both endometrium from control patients and patients with intramural fibroids. Of utmost significance, within the same uterus, there was no difference in *HOXA10* mRNA expression in endometrial biopsies taken directly over a submucosal myoma compared to endometrium remote from the fibroid. These findings support the principle that fibroids can have both a focal and a global effect on the endometrium.

Though *HOXA10* is known to be associated with endometrial development, it is not directly associated with menstrual bleeding. More recent studies have examined changes in endometrial molecular markers of fibroid uteri more specific to AUB. It has been previously shown that women with heavy uterine bleeding have higher levels of plasminogen activator (PA), a protease that lyses fibrin blood clots, in the menstrual phase and PA inhibitor-1 (PAI-1) in the late secretory and menstrual phases. Altered timing in levels of PA and PAI-1 can tip the delicate thrombosis/anticoagulation balance of the endometrium [26]. Sinclair et al.'s [27] results corroborate that fibroids can influence levels of PAI-1 as well as two other factors essential for fibrinolysis, anti-thrombin III (ATIII) and thrombomodulin (TM). In their study, endometrial tissue was obtained from 12 patients with fibroids scheduled for hysterectomy or hysteroscopic myomectomy and 12 control patients. Protein expression of PAI-1 and TM was significantly reduced in fibroid endometrium. Furthermore, the treatment of cultured endometrial stroma cells with transforming growth factor- β3 (TGF-β3), a multifunctional cytokine secreted by fibroids that stimulates cell proliferation [28], drastically reduced PAI-1, ATIII and TM mRNA levels. Reduction in PAI-1 would lead to more thrombolysis and bleeding. Reduction in ATIII and TM, however, would allow for greater coagulation. It appears that fibroids, possibly through secretion of TGF-β3, may shift the balance of hemostatic factors found within the endometrium and thus contribute to AUB.

Conclusion

There is an urgent need for improved understanding of the causes of fibroid-associated uterine bleeding in order to accelerate the discovery of effective, safe and long-lasting nonsurgical therapies. There is a paucity of data connecting alterations associated with fibroids on a molecular level with clinical parameters of AUB. Interdisciplinary research spanning multiple scales of study will be critical for developing targeted treatments for fibroid-associated AUB and improving patient care.

REFERENCES

1. Munro MG. *Abnormal Uterine Bleeding*. Cambridge: Cambridge University Press; 2010.
2. Munro MG, Critchley HOD, and Fraser IS. The FIGO systems for nomenclature and classification of causes of abnormal uterine bleeding in the reproductive years: Who needs them? *Am J Obstet Gynecol*. 2012;207(4):259–65.
3. Stovall DW. Clinical symptomatology of uterine leiomyomas. *Clin Obstet Gynecol*. 2001;44(2):364–71.
4. Myoma LC. In: Cuthbert Lockyer, ed. *Fibroids and Allied Tumours*. London: MacMillan and Co., Limited; 1918:14–5.
5. Farrer-Brown G, Beilby JO, and Tarbit MH. Venous changes in the endometrium of myomatous uteri. *Obstet Gynecol*. 1971;38(5):743–51.
6. Stewart EA and Nowak RA. Leiomyoma-related bleeding: A classic hypothesis updated for the molecular era. *Hum Reprod Update*. 1996;2(4):295–306.
7. Aguilar HN and Mitchell BF. Physiological pathways and molecular mechanisms regulating uterine contractility. *Hum Reprod Update*. 2010;16(6):725–44.
8. Kido A, Ascher SM, Hahn W et al. 3T MRI uterine peristalsis: Comparison of symptomatic fibroid patients versus controls. *Clin Radiol*. 2014;69(5):468–72.
9. Peddada SD, Laughlin SK, Miner K et al. Growth of uterine leiomyomata among premenopausal black and white women. *Proc Natl Acad Sci USA*. 2008;105(50):19887–92.
10. Tsiligiannis SE, Zaitseva M, Coombs PR et al. Fibroid-associated heavy menstrual bleeding: Correlation between clinical features, Doppler ultrasound assessment of vasculature, and tissue gene expression profiles. *Reprod Sci*. 2013;20(4):361–70.
11. Parker WH. Etiology, symptomatology, and diagnosis of uterine myomas. *Fertil Steril*. 2007;87(4):725–36.
12. Hickey M and Fraser I. Human uterine vascular structures in normal and diseased states. *Microsc Res Tech*. 2003;60(4):377–89.
13. Fraser HM and Lunn SF. Angiogenesis and its control in the female reproductive system. *Br Med Bull*. 2000;56(3):787–97.
14. Reynolds LP, Grazul-Bilska AT, and Redmer DA. Angiogenesis in the female reproductive organs: Pathological implications. *Int J Exp Pathol*. 2002;83(4):151–63.
15. Hague S, MacKenzie IZ, Bicknell R, and Rees MCP. *In-vivo* angiogenesis and progestogens. *Hum Reprod*. 2002;17(3):786–93.
16. Hickey M and Fraser I. The Clinical Relevance of Disturbances of Uterine Vascular Growth, Remodeling, and Repair. In: Augustin HGI-A, Smith SKML, and Rogers PAW, eds. *Vascular Morphogenesis in the Female Reproductive System*. US: Birkhauser Boston; 2001, pp. 223–44.
17. Tal R and Segars JH. The role of angiogenic factors in fibroid pathogenesis: Potential implications for future therapy. *Hum Reprod Update*. 2014;20(2):194–216.
18. Shimomura Y, Matsuo H, Samoto T, and Maruo T. Up-regulation by progesterone of proliferating cell nuclear antigen and epidermal growth factor expression in human uterine leiomyoma. *J Clin Endocrinol Metab*. 1998;83(6):2192–8.
19. Hague S, Zhang L, Oehler MK et al. Expression of the hypoxically regulated angiogenic factor adrenomedullin correlates with uterine leiomyoma vascular density. *Clin Cancer Res*. 2000;6(7):2808–14.
20. Xu Q, Ohara N, Chen W et al. Progesterone receptor modulator CDB-2914 down-regulates vascular endothelial growth factor, adrenomedullin and their receptors and modulates progesterone receptor content in cultured human uterine leiomyoma cells. *Hum Reprod*. 2006;21(9):2408–16.
21. Di Lieto A, Falco M, Pollio F et al. Clinical response, vascular change, and angiogenesis in gonadotropin-releasing hormone analogue-treated women with uterine myomas. *J Soc Gynecol Investig*. 2005;12(2):123–8.
22. Di Lieto A, De Falco M, Mansueto G, De Rosa G, Pollio F, and Staibano S. Preoperative administration of GnRH-a plus tibolone to premenopausal women with uterine fibroids: Evaluation of the clinical response, the immunohistochemical expression of PDGF, bFGF and VEGF and the vascular pattern. *Steroids*. 2005;70(2):95–102.
23. Wei J-J, Zhang X-M, Chiriboga L, Yee H, Perle MA, and Mittal K. Spatial differences in biologic activity of large uterine leiomyomata. *Fertil Steril*. 2006;85(1):179–87.
24. Rackow BW and Taylor HS. Submucosal uterine leiomyomas have a global effect on molecular determinants of endometrial receptivity. *Fertil Steril*. 2010;93(6):2027–34.
25. Daftary GS and Taylor HS. Pleiotropic effects of *Hoxa10* on the functional development of peri-implantation endometrium. *Mol Reprod Dev*. 2004;67(1):8–14.
26. Gleeson NC. Cyclic changes in endometrial tissue plasminogen activator and plasminogen activator inhibitor type 1 in women with normal menstruation and essential menorrhagia. *Am J Obstet Gynecol*. 1994;171(1):178–83.
27. Sinclair DC, Mastroyannis A, and Taylor HS. Leiomyoma simultaneously impair endometrial BMP-2-mediated decidualization and anticoagulant expression through secretion of TGF-β3. *J Clin Endocrinol Metab*. 2011;96(2):412–21.
28. Arici A and Sozen I. Transforming growth factor-beta3 is expressed at high levels in leiomyoma where it stimulates fibronectin expression and cell proliferation. *Fertil Steril*. 2000;73(5):1006–11.

8

Ultrasound

Caitlin R. Sacha and Bryann Bromley

Ultrasound Modalities

The use of ultrasound in gynecology was first described in the 1950s, at which time the technology was capable of outlining the borders of a fibroid and estimating its thickness [1]. Since then, numerous advances have made ultrasound the first-line method of evaluation for women with suspected fibroids. Compared to other imaging modalities, ultrasound is less expensive, readily available, allows real-time interaction between the patient and sonologist and does not expose the patient to radiation [2].

Transabdominal and transvaginal ultrasound are the most common modalities for the investigation of uterine fibroids. Initial evaluation with a transabdominal approach provides a global view of the pelvis with better tissue penetration and is compulsory for uteri that extend beyond the pelvis, especially when evaluating subserosal, pedunculated or parasitic fibroids [3]. Endocavitary imaging, usually performed transvaginally, provides enhanced resolution when compared with transabdominal imaging and is critical in evaluating uteri within the pelvis and mapping fibroid location with respect to the myometrium and endometrial cavity [2]. Real-time imaging should include a physical exam at the same time as the organs are being viewed in gray scale, which provides the sonologist the opportunity to examine the movement of lesions relative to adjacent organs and focus on areas of pain or tenderness. In a retrospective study by Hanafi et al., transvaginal ultrasound was found to have a positive predictive value of 99% and a sensitivity of 96% for leiomyoma, based on correlation with pathology [4]. In cases where transvaginal ultrasound is not possible, the transrectal approach has been useful to visualize the uterus [5].

In addition to standard two-dimensional (2D) ultrasound, modern evaluation of fibroids includes three-dimensional (3D) ultrasound, sonohysterography and color or power Doppler. Three-dimensional ultrasound captures a volume of information in three orthogonal planes and can be manipulated to display images in any plane and in multiple formats. This type of imaging is particularly useful in mapping intramural and submucosal fibroids [6]. Three-dimensional imaging for fibroid location with respect to the endometrium is optimally performed in the later luteal phase when the endometrium provides a contrasting appearance to fibroids. An adjunctive technique to transvaginal sonography for the assessment of the endometrial cavity is sonohysterography, which is performed early in the menstrual cycle. The endometrial cavity is distended with saline, offering a contrasting imaging parameter that optimizes characterization of fibroid location with respect to the endometrial cavity, as well as discrimination between other intracavitary lesions such as polyps [7].

Color or power Doppler allows for characterization of the vascular flow within a lesion using parameters of blood-flow impedance. In general, power Doppler is preferred as it optimally demonstrates small vessels with low blood flow velocities. Leiomyomas have been shown in several studies to have higher blood-flow velocity around the periphery than in the center, due to rich peripheral vascularization, which distinguishes them from other pathologies such as adenomyosis, which has diffusely distributed vasculature and low-velocity flow in the central part of the lesion [3,6].

Characteristics of Leiomyomas on Ultrasound

Uterine fibroids are composed of smooth muscle and fibrous stroma. Sonographically, they appear as rounded, well-circumscribed, solid masses within, or contiguous with, the myometrium that are hypoechoic, echogenic or heterogeneous in echotexture, depending on their cellular composition [8] (Figure 8.1). The variable penetration and transmission of ultrasound waves due to tissue characteristics result in radial shadowing in what has been coined a "venetian blind effect" (Figure 8.2). Fibroids may cause the outer contour of the uterus to be irregular and lobulated and obscure the inner endometrial shape (Figure 8.3). In addition, constriction of blood supply, as occurs with degeneration, can lead to cystic spaces within the fibroid [8] (Figure 8.4a, b and c). Finally, fatty infiltration and calcification of a fibroid, caused by deposition of calcium salts, which occurs more commonly in postmenopausal women, are characterized by hyperechoic components [8] (Figure 8.5a, b and c).

Individual fibroids (typically up to three of the largest clinically relevant fibroids) are described in terms of size by measuring the fibroid diameter in three orthogonal planes [9] (Figure 8.6). These are generally well-defined by a pseudocapsule that forms around the fibroid due to the compression of the surrounding myometrium [3,8]. The position of the fibroid(s) within the uterus (corpus, lower segment, cervix, anterior or posterior to the endometrial cavity), as well as the location with respect to the myometrium and endometrial cavity, can then be assessed. Fibroid location can be further described as intramural, submucosal or subserosal, and may be pedunculated or parasitic. In

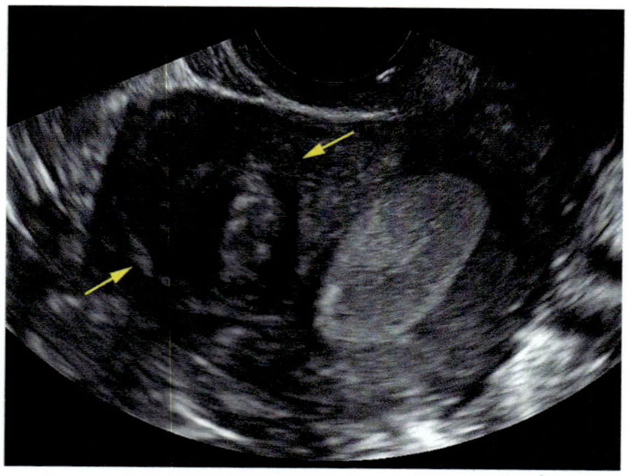

FIGURE 8.1 Transvaginal sagittal image of a uterus demonstrating a well-circumscribed mass characteristic of a fibroid (arrow). The mass is in the anterior myometrium extending to the serosa. Note the uniform endometrium characteristic of the late luteal phase in the menstrual cycle.

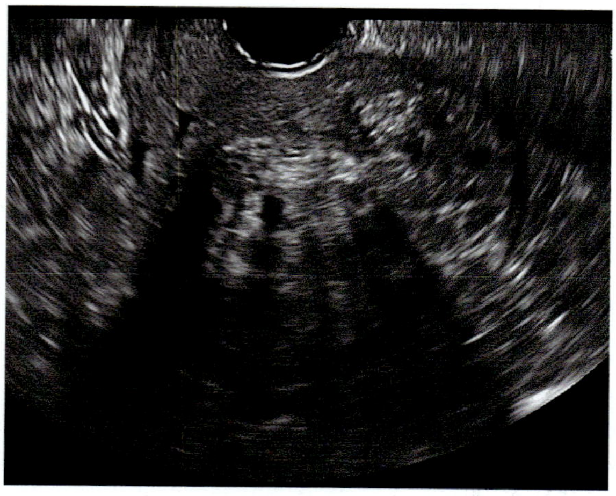

FIGURE 8.2 Transvaginal scan demonstrating a heterogeneous fibroid with radial acoustic shadowing (venetian blind effect) due to variable acoustic properties associated with fibroid composition.

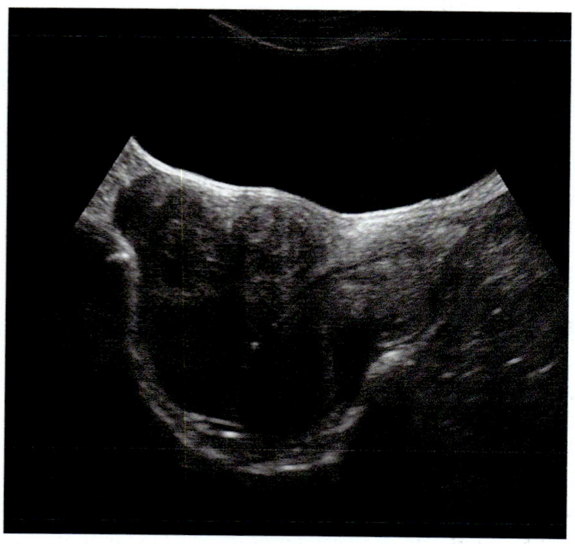

FIGURE 8.3 Transabdominal sagittal view of a retroverted uterus containing multiple fibroids that distort the contour of the uterus.

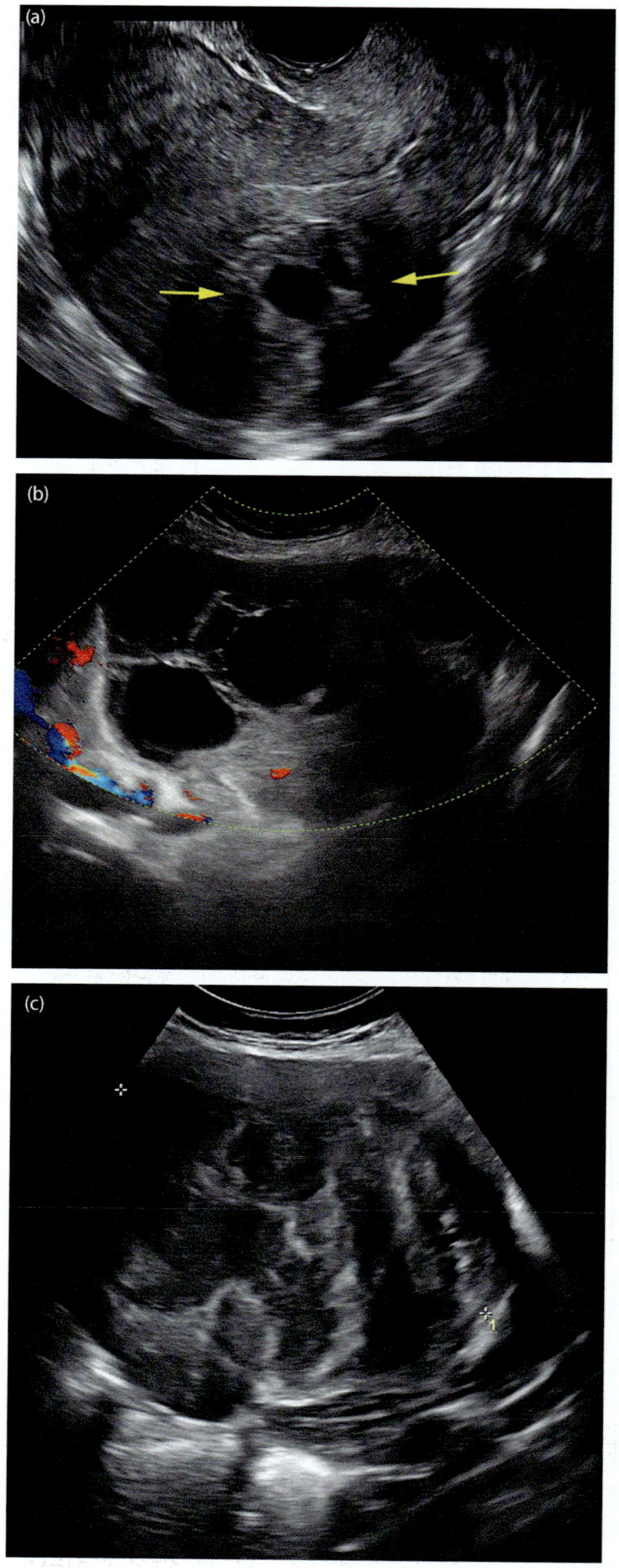

FIGURE 8.4 (a) Transvaginal sagittal image of the uterus demonstrating a posterior intramural fibroid (arrows) that contains internal cystic spaces consistent with degeneration. (b) Transabdominal scan showing a pedunculated fibroid with solid and cystic areas and no significant color flow, characteristic of degeneration. A normal left ovary was documented (not shown), eliminating the possibility of an ovarian mass. (c) Transabdominal scan showing mixed echogenicity in a degenerating fibroid.

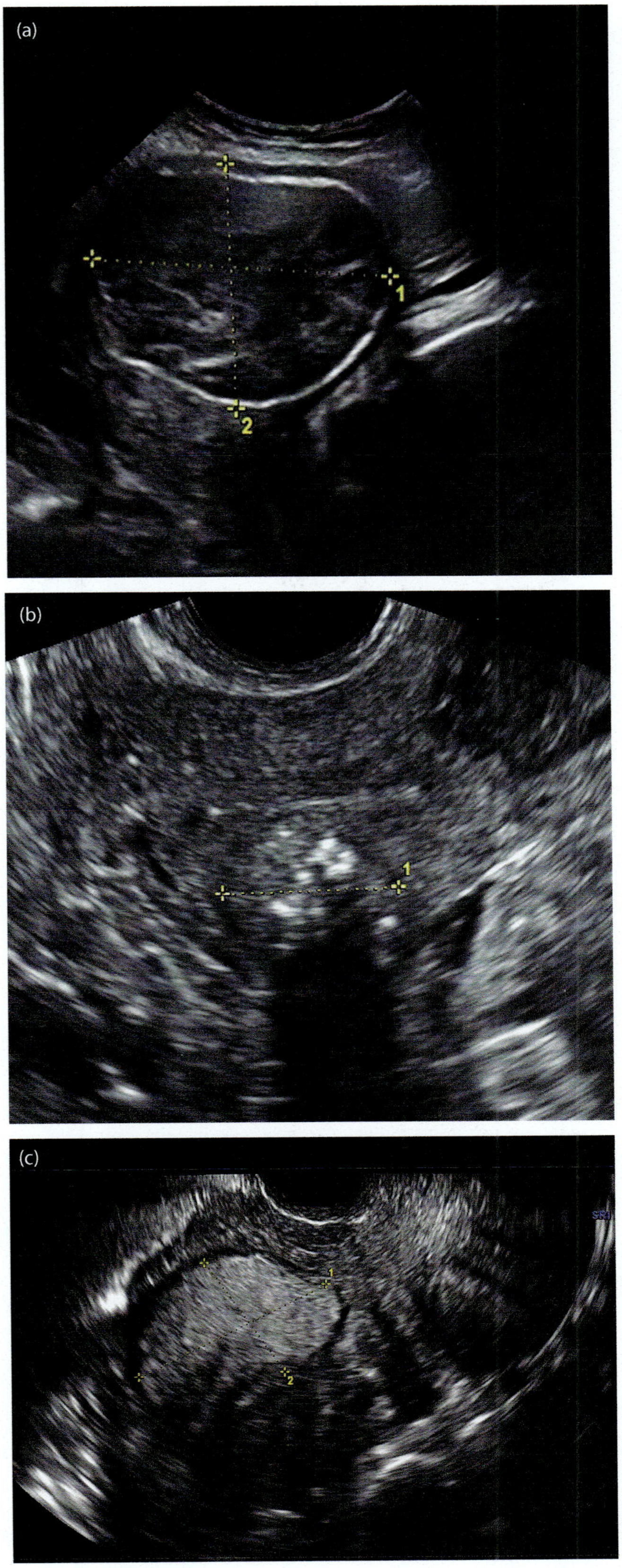

FIGURE 8.5 (a) Transabdominal scan in a pregnant patient showing a fibroid with a calcified rim. (b) Transvaginal image of the uterus showing a fibroid (calipers) with punctate calcifications. (c) Transvaginal scan demonstrating a sagittal view of the uterus and an echogenic fibroid (calipers) in the anterior myometrium.

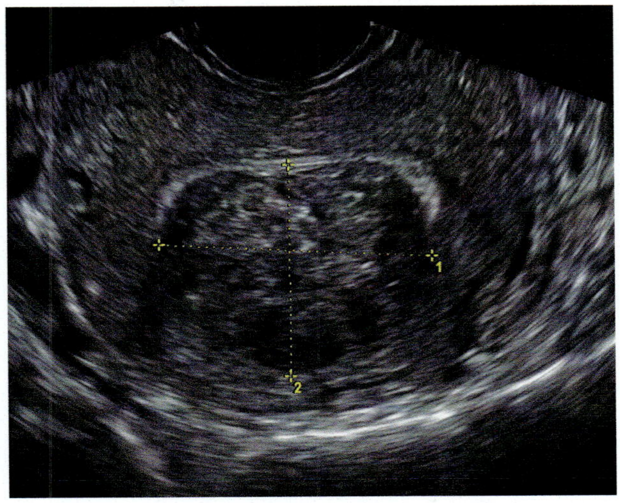

FIGURE 8.6 Transvaginal transverse view of the uterus demonstrating the measurements of a submucosal fibroid in two of the three orthogonal planes. Note the echogenic endometrium draped around the fibroid.

patients with numerous fibroids that distort the uterine architecture, the overall size of the uterus and appearance of the myometrium should be reported [9,10]. Of note, myometrial lesions that are asymmetric and diffuse with cysts or hyperechogenic islands are consistent with adenomyosis rather than fibroids [9]. A staging system has been developed for women with irregular bleeding by the International Federation of Gynecology and Obstetrics (FIGO), indicating the location of the fibroids relative to the serosal and mucosal surface [9,11]. Furthermore, a consensus opinion on standard nomenclature for describing myometrial findings has been suggested and is relevant both for daily practice and research [9].

Submucosal fibroids are in close proximity to the endometrial cavity and protrude into the cavity to variable degrees [11]. Submucosal fibroids are a cause of abnormal uterine bleeding, and distortion of the endometrial cavity is associated with infertility [3,8] (Figure 8.6, Figure 8.7a and b). Although transvaginal ultrasound is highly sensitive for submucosal fibroids, diagnostic accuracy for intracavitary lesions is improved with the addition of sonohysterography, which allows enhanced visualization of fibroid location, base of attachment and degree of protrusion into the endometrial cavity [7,8] (Figure 8.8). The use of color or power Doppler is helpful in distinguishing a submucosal fibroid with peripheral flow from a polyp which may have a single feeder vessel (Figure 8.7a) [3]. On occasion, submucosal fibroids may prolapse through the cervix (Figure 8.9).

Subserosal fibroids are located between the serosa and the myometrium (Figure 8.10). Some subserosal fibroids become pedunculated, and the stalk attachment typically has a feeder vessel (Figure 8.11a and b). The stalk may not be visible with ultrasound if the pedicle is thin. Broad ligament fibroids may extend from the uterus into the peritoneum and can be confused with adnexal masses. In these cases, the identification of the normal ovary separate from the mass is critical. Additionally, ultrasound can potentially delineate lesion attachment to the uterus (or ovary) using gentle prodding with the probe as an extension of a bimanual exam to evaluate whether or not the lesion moves independently from the uterus or ovary [2]. If delineation

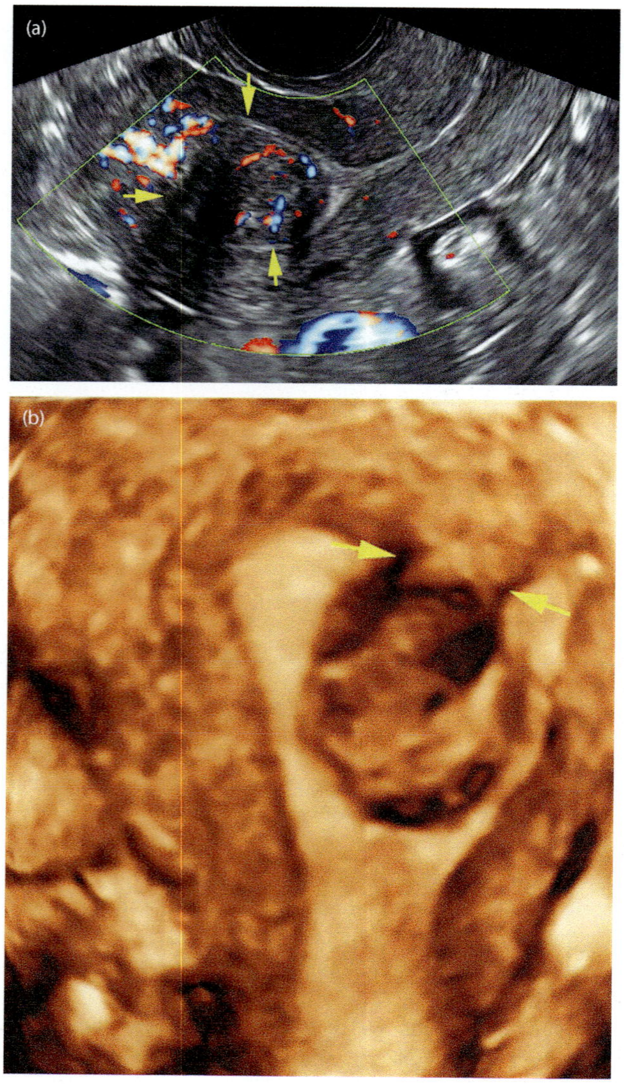

FIGURE 8.7 (a) Transvaginal sagittal view of an anteverted uterus containing a submucosal fibroid (arrows). Note the splaying of the echogenic endometrial echo around the hypoechoic solid fibroid. Vascular flow is shown by Doppler. (b) 3D rendering of the endometrial cavity showing the fibroid protrudes into the cavity and is attached by a stalk (arrows).

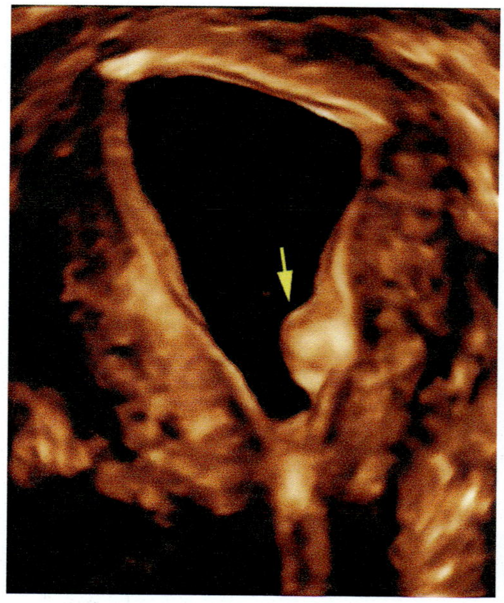

FIGURE 8.8 3D coronal image of the endometrial cavity obtained with adjunctive sonohysterography demonstrating the position and location of a submucosal fibroid (arrow).

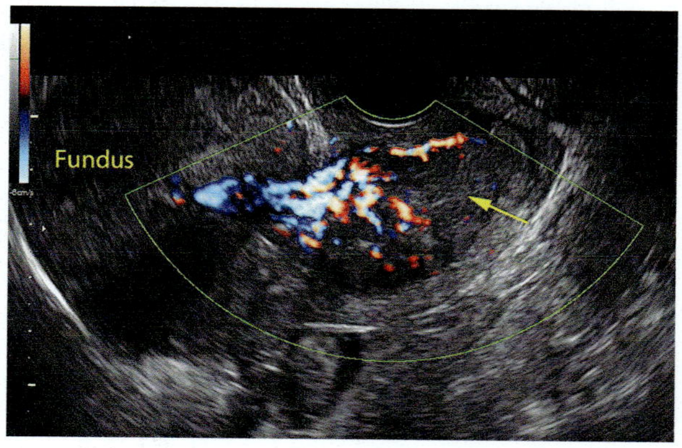

FIGURE 8.9 Transvaginal sagittal view of the uterus demonstrating a fibroid (arrow) prolapsing through the endocervix into the vagina. Note the vascular stalk.

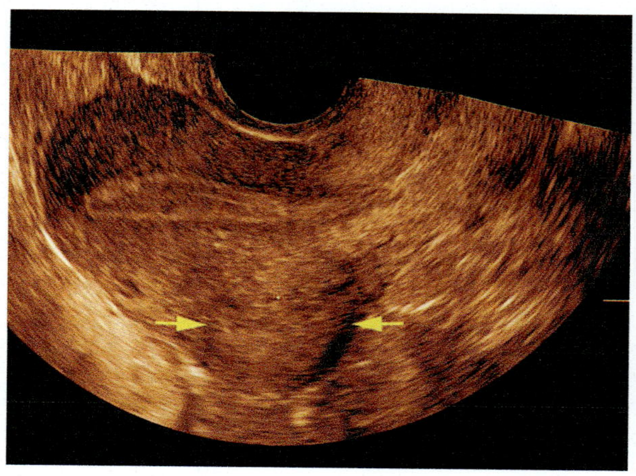

FIGURE 8.10 Transvaginal image of an anteverted uterus demonstrating a subserosal fibroid in the posterior wall (arrows) distorting the outer contour of the uterus.

between a solid ovarian mass and a pedunculated or parasitic fibroid remains uncertain, MRI may potentially be helpful [3] (see Chapter 29).

Retrospective case series have examined whether or not ultrasound parameters such as size, heterogeneity and vascularization can be used to differentiate benign leiomyomas from malignant tumors such as leiomyosarcomas and carcinosarcomas. Some data suggest that larger lesions with increased heterogeneity and irregular centralized vascularization are more concerning for malignancy [3,12]. However, there are currently no definitive guidelines, and more studies are needed to better differentiate these lesions preoperatively, especially when considering morcellation procedures [13] (Figure 8.12a and b). Ultrasound features of unusual types of leiomyoma, such as intravascular leiomyomatosis and disseminated peritoneal leiomyomatosis, are similar to those of benign fibroids [9] (Figure 8.13a and b).

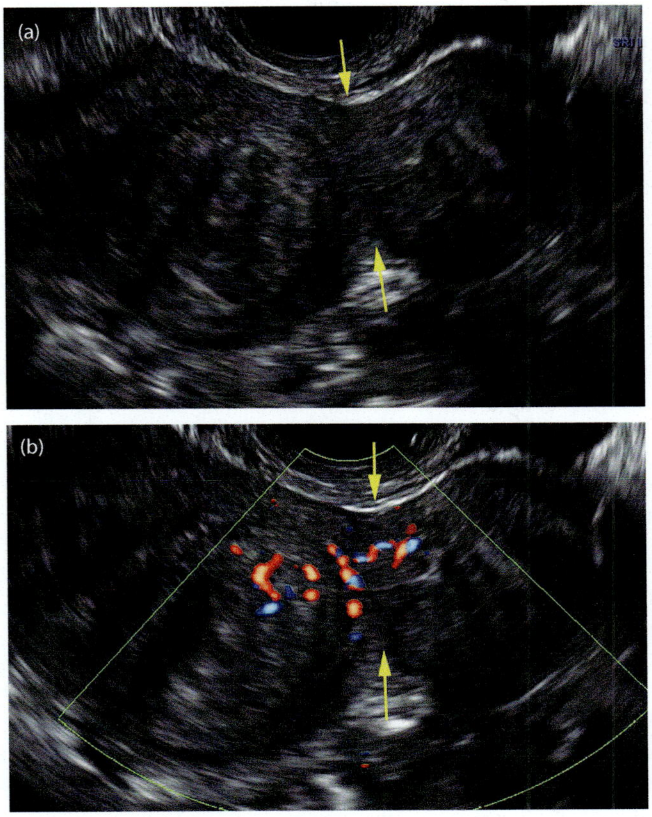

FIGURE 8.11 (a) Transvaginal scan demonstrating a pedunculated fibroid attached to the uterus with a stalk (arrows). (b) Corresponding image demonstrating color flow to the fibroid.

Sonography of Leiomyoma in the Gravid Uterus

Fibroids are diagnosed by ultrasound in pregnancy in up to 4% of patients, a significantly lower fraction than in nongravid patients, potentially due to the effects of increased uterine size and myometrial changes during pregnancy [14]. Braxton-Hicks contractions may have a similar appearance to fibroids on ultrasound, but several features can tell them apart: fibroids possess a pseudocapsule and may distort the uterus itself, while contractions move unidirectionally and typically resolve over a short period of time; contractions do not create the shadowing effect that fibroids do; and fibroids possess peripheral blood flow while contractions have flow throughout on color Doppler [14]. Given the potential effects of fibroids on pregnancy outcome depending on location, an attempt should be made to characterize uterine fibroids on routine prenatal ultrasound to inform patient counseling (see Chapter 9).

Operative Planning

Ultrasound is the first step in operative planning for women with symptomatic fibroids. A prospective study by Baird et al. demonstrated that randomly selected premenopausal women with fibroids identified on a screening ultrasound were at increased risk of requiring a surgical procedure within the following 8 years, and this risk increased with fibroid size [15]. The number, size and location of leiomyomas are all important characteristics to know prior to surgery in order to plan the safest approach for excision. In patients with infertility, the identification of fibroids on ultrasound and mapping their position relative to the endometrial cavity by 3D imaging is imperative as distortion of the endometrial cavity or alteration of the intracavity milieu may impact fertility. Additionally, 3D imaging is reliable in depicting the shape of the endometrial cavity, which may be relevant to infertility evaluation (Figure 8.14). In some patients with numerous fibroids, there may be no normal-appearing myometrium, and this should be communicated, as surgery may not be an appropriate choice.

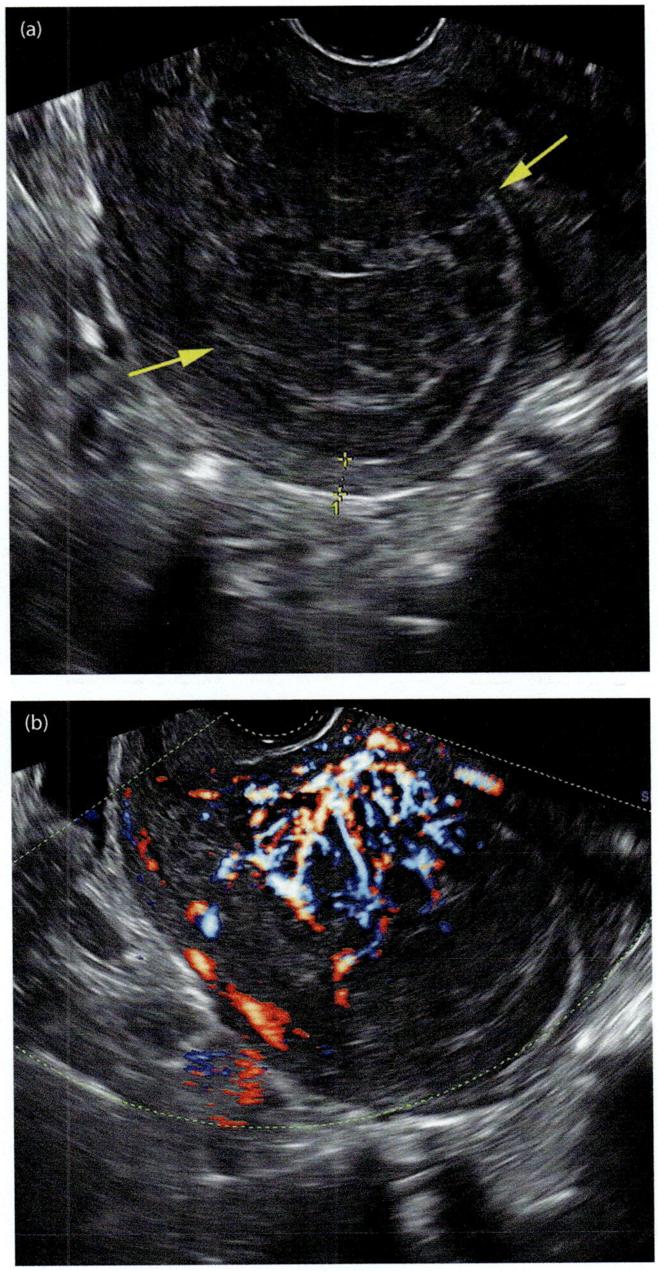

FIGURE 8.12 (a) Transvaginal image demonstrating a solid mass in the uterus characteristic of a fibroid (arrows). Calipers demonstrate the distance between the mass and the serosa. (b) Doppler revealed extensive vascularity. Pathology confirmed leiomyosarcoma in this patient.

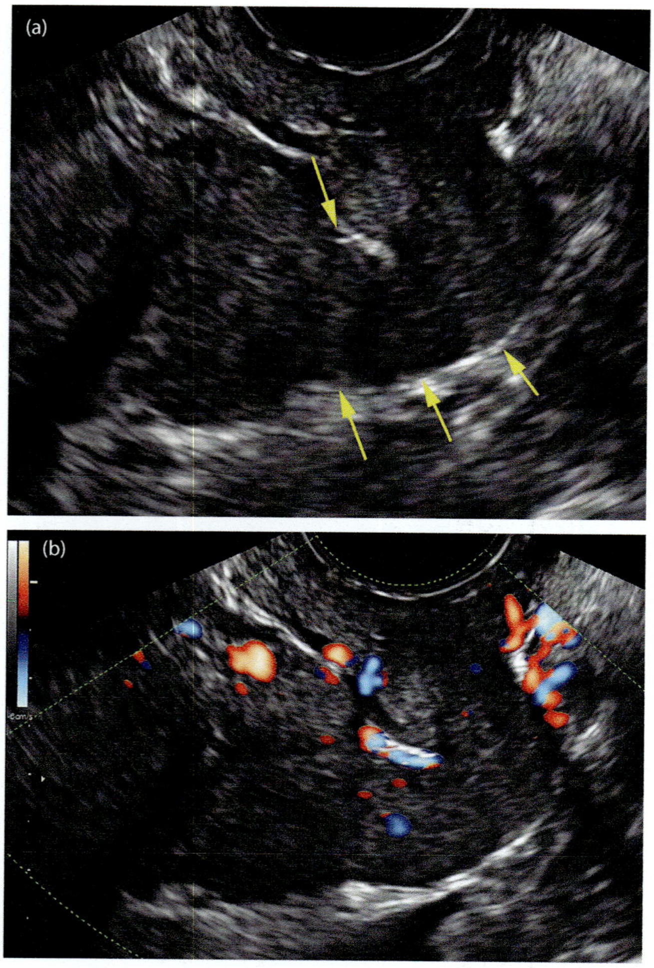

FIGURE 8.13 (a) Transvaginal image demonstrating a solid tubular mass (arrows) in a patient with fibroids, suggesting intravascular leiomyomatosis. (b) Corresponding image demonstrating vascular flow.

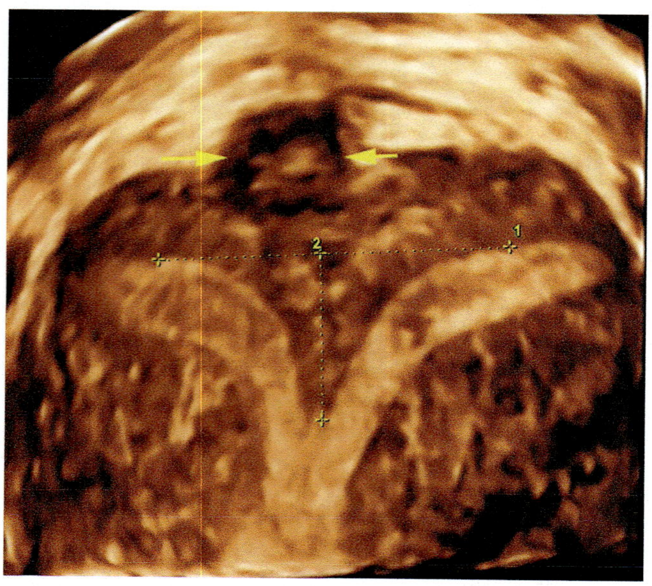

FIGURE 8.14 3D coronal view of a subseptate uterus demonstrating a small subserosal fibroid (arrows).

Limitations

Despite its relatively easy accessibility and low cost, a limitation of ultrasound in the diagnosis and characterization of fibroids is operator experience. Individuals performing ultrasounds must take advantage of educational and practical advances in 2D and 3D sonographic imaging techniques. Importantly, 3D volume imaging allows review off-line with the opportunity for specialized consultation. Finally, while transvaginal ultrasound is as sensitive as MRI in diagnosing the presence of uterine fibroids, its ability to fully characterize fibroids decreases when the uterus is extremely large, when there are numerous fibroids or when fibroids are smaller in size [16]. In these cases, MRI may help to map the fibroids.

Conclusions

Transabdominal and transvaginal ultrasound are the first steps in the initial imaging evaluation of a patient with gynecologic complaints [2]. The majority of fibroids have a characteristic appearance on ultrasound, and their position and location can be elucidated with real-time 2D imaging. The addition of 3D imaging and power Doppler improves visualization of fibroid location relative to the uterine tissues and endometrial cavity and is part of the modern sonographic armamentarium to evaluate fibroids. Enhanced visualization using adjunctive sonohysterography can improve diagnostic performance for preoperative planning. Standard nomenclature should be used to communicate the sonographic findings [9]. Ultrasound is the primary and often only imaging modality necessary for most gynecologic patients, playing a critical role in fibroid mapping for both medical and surgical therapies.

REFERENCES

1. Donald I, MacVicar J, and Brown TG. Investigation of abdominal masses by pulsed ultrasound. *The Lancet*. 1958; 271(7032):1188–95.
2. Benacerraf BR, Abuhamad AZ, Bromley B et al. Consider ultrasound first for imaging the female pelvis. *J Obstet Gynaecol*. 2015;212(4):450–5.
3. Testa AC, LDi Legge A, Bonatti M, Manfredi R, and Scambia G. Imaging techniques for evaluation of uterine myomas. *Best Pract Res Clin Obstet Gynaecol*. 2016;34:1–17.
4. Hanafi M. Ultrasound diagnosis of adenomyosis, leiomyoma, or combined with histopathological correlation. *J Hum Reprod Sci*. 2013;6(3):189–93.
5. Timor-Tritsch IE, Monteagudo A, Rebarber A, Goldstein SR, and Tsymbal T. Transrectal scanning: An alternative when transvaginal scanning is not feasible. *Ultrasound Obstet Gynecol*. 2003;21:473–9.
6. Sharma K, Bora MK, Venkatesh BP et al. Role of 3D ultrasound and doppler in differentiating clinically suspected cases of leiomyoma and adenomyosis of uterus. *J Clin Diagn Res*. 2015;9(4):8–12.
7. Grimbizis GF, Tsolakidis D, Mikos T et al. A prospective comparison of transvaginal ultrasound, saline infusion sonohysterography, and diagnostic hysteroscopy in the evaluation of endometrial pathology. *Fert Steril*. 2010;94(7):2720–5.

8. Shwayder J and Sakhel K. Imaging for uterine myomas and adenomyosis. *J Minim Invasive Gynecol.* 2013;21(3):362–74.
9. Van Den Bosch A, Dueholm M, Leone FPG et al. Terms, definitions and measurements to describe sonographic features of myometrium and uterine masses: A consensus opinion from the Morphological Uterus Sonographic Assessment (MUSA) group. *Ultrasound Obstet Gynecol.* 2015;46:284–98.
10. American Institute of Ultrasound in Medicine. AIUM practice parameter for the performance of an ultrasound examination of the female pelvis. *J Ultrasound Med.* 2020; 9999:1–7.
11. Munro MG, Critchley HOD, Fraser IS, for the FIGO Menstrual Disorders Committee. The two FIGO systems for normal and abnormal uterine bleeding symptoms and classification of causes of abnormal uterine bleeding in the reproductive years: 2018 revisions. *Int J Gynecol Obstet.* 2018;143:393–408.
12. Exacoustos C, Romanini ME, Amadio A et al. Can gray-scale and color Doppler sonography differentiate between uterine leiomyosarcoma and leiomyoma? *J Clin Ultrasound.* 2007;35(8):449–57.
13. Rodriguez AM, Asoglu MR, Sak ME, Tan A, Borahay MA, and Kilic GS. Incidence of occult leiomyosarcoma in presumed morcellation cases: A database study. *Eur J Obstet Gynecol Reprod Biol.* 2016;197:31–5.
14. Coldwell B, Steinkeler J, and Warner M. Ultrasound of the gravid uterus. *Ultrasound Q.* 2012;28(2):87–95.
15. Baird DD, Saldana TM, Shore DL, Hill MC, and Schectman JM. A single baseline ultrasound assessment of fibroid presence and size is strongly predictive of future uterine procedure: 8-year follow-up of randomly sampled premenopausal women aged 35–49 years. *Hum Reprod.* 2015;30(12):2936–44.
16. Wise LA and Laughlin-Tommaso SK. Epidemiology of uterine fibroids: From menarche to menopause. *Clin Obstet Gynecol.* 2016;59(1):2–24.

9

Leiomyomata and Reproduction

Amy L. Harris and Aaron K. Styer

Prevalence

Fibroids (leiomyomata) are the most common gynecologic tumor, with a prevalence of 20%–80% in reproductive-aged women and 5%–10% in women with infertility [1]. Although 26%–30% of patients are asymptomatic [2,3], it has been estimated that in approximately 1%–2.4% of women, fibroids are the primary infertility diagnosis (uterine factor infertility) [4,5].

Physiology

Despite the significant prevalence of leiomyomata, the association of this reproductive disorder and infertility has been incompletely studied. There has been significant controversy regarding the impact of uterine myomas on fertility and pregnancy outcomes. Several putative mechanisms for their possible negative impact on fertility have been proposed. However, mechanism-based causative relationships between fibroids and infertility and pregnancy loss, respectively, have not been established. Table 9.1 lists the proposed mechanisms for fibroid-related infertility. Fibroids cause distortion of uterine anatomy and alter the uterine environment and implantation potential of the endometrium. Cervical fibroids can cause obstruction or displacement of the cervix. Similarly, submucosal and intramural leiomyomata may cause cavity deformity that can potentially hinder sperm and embryo transport and fallopian tube function. Magnetic resonance imaging (MRI) studies suggest that intramural leiomyomata alter uterine peristalsis in the midluteal phase when embryos transport and implant [6]. Fibroids located near the uterine cornua can obstruct fallopian tube transport and oocyte capture. Submucosal fibroids may distort the endometrium, impair endometrial blood flow and potentially reduce implantation [7]. Pathologic specimens of endometrium overlying submucosal fibroids demonstrate abnormal pathological changes including atrophy and endometritis [8]. Notably, Horcajadas et al. found that the implantation window was delayed by 1.8 days on endometrial biopsy in those with large intramural fibroids (≥5 cm) [9].

Leiomyomata are responsive to sex steroids and secrete and respond to inflammatory and vasoactive factors. Aberrant excessive production of transforming growth factor-beta (TGF-β), a multifunctional cytokine, from fibroids has been reported by several investigators [10,11] and has been implicated in altered implantation of the embryo [12]. Homeobox A10 (*HOXA-10*) is one of the most recognized gene sequences in mammalian implantation.

TABLE 9.1

Proposed Mechanisms of the Impacts of Fibroids on Infertility

Pathophysiology of Fibroids & Infertility:

Anatomic:
- Displaced cervix (reduced sperm exposure)
- Cavity deformity/enlargement
- Tubal obstruction
- Compression/distortion of endometrium

Impede migration:
- Dysfunctional uterine peristalsis/contractility
- Interference with sperm migration
- Disturbance of junctional myometrial zone

Secretory factors:
- Abnormal vascularity/Impaired blood flow/disruption of angiogenesis
- Inflammation
  - TGF-B
  - HOXA-10
  - IL-10
  - EGF
- Impaired endometrial receptivity

Lower levels of expression have been identified in endometrial specimens in patients with fibroids [13,14]. Altered growth-factor secretion may lead to abnormal vasculature, characterized by dilated venous plexuses and disordered angiogenesis [15,16].

Evaluation

Assessment for the presence of uterine fibroids or an enlarged uterus due to fibroids should be performed during routine physical examination and bimanual examination during the initial fertility consultation [17]. Diagnosis is confirmed by transvaginal ultrasonography. Fibroids traditionally appear as hypoechoic, well-circumscribed spheres on transvaginal ultrasound. The location and degree of endometrial involvement may be determined by hysterosalpingogram, saline-infusion sonogram, hysteroscopy and/or MRI, respectively. Hysteroscopy is the gold standard for direct assessment of the endometrial cavity. This procedure can be performed both in office and the operating room and uses an endoscope with a camera that instills saline or gas in the uterus as a distending medium. Direct visualization facilitates diagnosis and may guide treatment of FIGO type 0 (pedunculated intracavitary) and 1 (≥50% intracavitary) submucosal fibroids.

Hysterosalpingogram (HSG) is a common screening test for uterine cavity and tubal abnormalities. During this procedure, radiopaque contrast is injected into the uterus, and the cavity and fallopian tubes are evaluated by X-ray. However, its relatively low sensitivity (50%) to differentiate different uterine-cavity lesions limits its function as the sole screening test for those at risk for fibroids [17]. Saline-infusion sonohysterogram (SIS) is an ultrasound performed after the instillation of saline in the uterus. The positive predictive value for SIS in diagnosing uterine abnormalities is 100%, with reportedly 77% sensitivity [18]. Advances in technology allowing for three-dimensional renderings of the uterus done during SIS have improved diagnosis of submucosal fibroids, allowing for better characterization than by traditional two-dimensional SIS [19]. The hystero-contrast sonography (HyCoSy), which utilizes contrast medium or agitated saline has enhanced the positive and negative predictive values of fallopian tube evaluation [20], making the HyCoSy a promising "single comprehensive" screening tool for both uterine and tubal factor infertility[21]. Leiomyomata have a low-intensity signal compared with surrounding myometrium on both T1- and T2-weighted MRI images. Although MRIs are more sensitive than sonograms for diagnosis of fibroids, they are significantly more costly than the other modalities. MRI imaging can be useful in describing the size and location of fibroids and may be best utilized for preoperative planning and to determine the best surgical approach for the surgical removal (myomectomy) of fibroids [22].

Treatment Indications

The classic indication for myomectomy includes symptomatic women who experience heavy menstrual bleeding or bulk symptoms. Patients with leiomyomata that are rapidly growing may benefit from further evaluation and treatment to exclude an occult malignancy such as leiomyosarcoma [7]. There has been significant controversy regarding the impact of uterine myomas on fertility and pregnancy outcome. As a result, the benefit (likelihood of conception, pregnancy loss, live birth and obstetrical complications) of myomectomy in women with asymptomatic myomas has also been uncertain. Data regarding the association of fecundity and fibroid size, location and conception (spontaneous vs. undergo ART—assisted reproductive technology) after myomectomy are inconsistent. In addition, most individual studies were retrospective or insufficiently powered, and meta-analyses evaluate very heterogeneous studies. As a result, the interpretation of conflicting results has been challenging.

Fibroid Characteristics

A 2009 meta-analysis of 18 studies demonstrated that patients with fibroids had a decreased clinical pregnancy rate (CPR) and ongoing pregnancy/live birth rate (LBR). However, most authors had not included size or location of fibroids [23]. Stratified by location, a comprehensive meta-analysis reported that the presence of submucosal fibroids are associated with a reduced likelihood of CPR (RR = 0.36, CI: 0.18–0.73, $p = 0.005$) and ongoing pregnancy/LBR (RR = 0.32, CI: 0.12–0.85, $p < 0.001$), respectively. In a comparison of 249 patients with intramural (without endometrial cavity distortion) or subserosal fibroids, there was no difference in CPR for LBR compared to controls [24]. A recent secondary analysis of a prospective randomized trial of 900 women undergoing ovarian stimulation with intrauterine insemination for unexplained infertility showed no difference in conception or live birth rates in women with fibroids that did not distort the cavity [25].

Myomectomy and Spontaneous Conception

The effect of myomectomy on patients with infertility who are not planning on undergoing ART is uncertain. Removal of submucosal fibroids has been shown to improve pregnancy rates [26]. In 1999, Bulletti et al. demonstrated that laparoscopic myomectomy resulted in an almost fourfold higher delivery rate than those who underwent expectant management ($p < 0.001$). However, this study included fibroids of varying sizes and locations. In a randomized controlled trial, Casini et al. randomized 181 patients with 1 year of infertility with a solitary fibroid <4 cm to surgical versus expectant management. Higher clinical pregnancy rates in the year following the randomization were appreciated in those who underwent surgical intervention for submucosal (43.3% vs. 27.2%, $p < 0.05$) and submucosal-intramural (36.4% vs. 15%, $p < 0.05$) fibroids. Although pregnancy rates were also higher in those with intramural-subserosal (35.3% vs. 21.4%, NS) and intramural alone (56.6 vs 40.9, NS) fibroids, they did not reach statistical significance [27]. A retrospective cohort study suggests a potential benefit of myomectomies in younger white women with larger fibroids (<7CM) suggesting a role for individualized medicine [28].

Myomectomy and Assisted Reproductive Technologies

Much of the early data that evaluated the role of fibroids prior to ART included small studies with significant heterogeneity with respect to patient demographics, size and location of fibroids and observational duration. In 1995, the first retrospective analysis of 46 women who underwent in-vitro fertilization (IVF) found that there were decreased implantation rates in those with hysteroscopic evidence of fibroids distorting uterine cavities [29]. Since that time, there have been many conflicting studies with regard to infertility and ART [30].

Several studies suggests that submucosal fibroids negatively impact fertility and report a benefit for the removal of submucosal fibroids prior to IVF [23,31]. Submucosal fibroids are primarily resected by minimally invasive hysteroscopic resection of fibroids (see Chapter 20).

In contrast, there are conflicting data for pregnancy outcomes in women with intramural fibroids with normal cavities (no cavity distortion) prior to IVF. Specifically, some studies show reduced pregnancy success, while other studies do not demonstrate a difference in conception or live birth rates in those with fibroids that do not encroach on the cavity [32–34]. Pooled data from 19 studies show a reduction in CPR and LBR of 15% and 21%, respectfully ($p = 0.002$) [35]. Recent case-cohort and retrospective cohort studies showed decreased live birth rates after IVF in patients with FIGO Class 3 fibroids [36,37]. However, there are little data evaluating whether or not myomectomy improves their outcomes. Procedures for intramural or subserosal fibroids are more invasive than the hysteroscopic approaches used for subserosal fibroids (see Chapter 20). A recent Cochrane review concluded that there was no benefit of myomectomy on pregnancy rates irrespective of type of fibroid [38].

Nonsurgical Intervention

Surgery has long been the mainstay treatment of uterine fibroids in those desiring pregnancy. Recently, less-invasive procedures have been introduced. Uterine artery ablation (UAE) utilizes fluoroscopy to place embolic particles in the uterine vasculature, occluding blood flow to fibroids. UAE has been shown to reduce heavy uterine bleeding and dysmenorrhea, especially in multiple-fibroid uteri [39,40]. Although pregnancy has been reported after UAE, complications such as malplacentation, fetal growth restriction and diminished ovarian blood flow have been reported [41]. Ultrasound-guided radiofrequency ablation (RFA) employs laparoscopic or transcervical placement of radiofrequency electrodes that destroy the fibroid. Few pregnancies have been reported after this procedure [42].

Ulipristal acetate (UPA) is an oral selective progesterone receptor modulator that been successful in treating heavy bleeding and bulk symptoms due to fibroids in phase 3 trials [43,44]. In the first review of 21 women attempting pregnancy, stopping UPA treatment resulted in high pregnancy and live birth rates [45]. Based on available data, there are insufficient data to access conception rates and pregnancy safety after UAE, RFA or UPA.

Miscarriage

The association between fibroids and miscarriage is also controversial. Retrospective studies, including Buttram and Reiter, described an increased prevalence of spontaneous abortions in those with fibroids [5]. However, a large epidemiologic study showed no increased risk of pregnancy loss with one or more fibroids [46]. Bulletti et al. showed that patients who underwent a laparoscopic myomectomy had a lower rate of miscarriage compared with those who had expectant management [47]. No definitive data exist to demonstrate that a preemptive myomectomy reduces the risk of primary miscarriage. However, in patients with recurrent miscarriage, one study showed resection of fibroids that invade the cavity may increase the likelihood of live birth [48]. In a randomized controlled trial that investigated the role of surgical intervention on removal of a solitary <4cm fibroid versus expectant management demonstrated a reduced rate in miscarriages in those with myomectomies of submucosal fibroids (38% vs. 50%, $p<0.05$). They did not find any significant differences in those with myomectomies after intramural or subserosal myomectomies [27]. However, owing to a lack of high-quality studies, it is unknown if hysteroscopic myomectomy reduces the rate of early pregnancy loss or increases the rate of live birth pregnancy in women with infertility.

Conclusion

The management of asymptomatic patients with uterine leiomyomata is complex. The mechanisms by which fibroids may contribute to infertility have not been completely elicited. Although patients with cavity-altering submucosal or intramural fibroids would likely benefit from intervention, the impact of other fibroids on fertility or miscarriages is unclear. These findings lead to the guidelines from the American Society of Reproductive Medicine published in 2017 recommending against routine myomectomy for asymptomatic women with non-cavity deforming myomas [49]. Studies investigating myomectomy outcomes are heterogeneous, making them difficult to interpret. There is no evidence that subserosal fibroids impact fertility outcomes. Prospective studies should be designed to address the surgical and nonsurgical interventions in women with reproductive desires.

REFERENCES

1. Makker A and Goel MM. Uterine leiomyomas effects on architectural, cellular, and molecular determinants of endometrial receptivity. *Reprod Sci.* 2013;20(6):631–8.
2. Selo-Ojeme D, Lawal O, Shah J et al. The incidence of uterine leiomyoma and other pelvic ultrasonographic findings in 2,034 consecutive women in a north London hospital. *J Obstet Gynaecol.* 2008;28(4):421–3.
3. Harmon Q and Baird D. Use of depot medroxyprogesterone acetate and prevalent leiomyoma in young African American women. *Hum Reprod.* 30(6):1499–504.
4. Buttram VC Jr, Reiter RC. Uterine leiomyomata: Etiology, symptomatology, and management. *Fertil Steril.* 1981; 36:433–5.
5. Buttram Jr VC and Reiter RC. Uterine leiomyomata: Etiology, symptomatology, and management. *Fertil Steril.* 1981;36(4):433.
6. Yoshino O, Hayashi T, Osuga Y et al. Decreased pregnancy rate is linked to abnormal uterine peristalsis caused by intramural fibroids. *Hum Reprod.* 25(10):2475–479.
7. Medicine PCotASfR. Myomas and reproductive function. *Fertil Steril.* 2008;90(5):S125–S30.
8. Deligdish L and Loewenthal M. Endometrial changes associated with myomata of the uterus. *J Clin Pathol.* 1970;23(8):676–80.
9. Horcajadas JA, Goyri E, Higón MaA, Martínez-Conejero JA et al. Endometrial receptivity and implantation are not affected by the presence of uterine intramural leiomyomas: A clinical and functional genomics analysis. *J Clin Endocrinol Metab.* 2008;93(9):3490–8.
10. Maybin JA, Critchley HO, and Jabbour HN. Inflammatory pathways in endometrial disorders. *Mol Cell Endocrinol.* 2011;335(1):42–51.
11. Leppert PC, Catherino WH, and Segars JH. A new hypothesis about the origin of uterine fibroids based on gene expression profiling with microarrays. *Am J Obstet Gynecol.* 2006;195(2):415–20.
12. Dimitriadis E, White C, Jones R, and Salamonsen L. Cytokines, chemokines and growth factors in endometrium related to implantation. *Hum Reprod Update.* 2005;11(6):613–30.
13. Matsuzaki S, Canis M, Darcha C, Pouly J-L, and Mage G. HOXA-10 expression in the mid-secretory endometrium of infertile patients with either endometriosis, uterine fibromas or unexplained infertility. *Hum Reprod.* 2009: 24(12); 3180–3187.
14. Rackow BW and Taylor HS. Submucosal uterine leiomyomas have a global effect on molecular determinants of endometrial receptivity. *Fertil Steril.* 2010;93(6):2027–34.
15. Stewart EA and Nowak RA. Leiomyoma-related bleeding: A classic hypothesis updated for the molecular era. *Hum Reprod Update.* 1996;2(4):295–306.

16. Ben-Nagi J, Miell J, Mavrelos D, Naftalin J, Lee C, and Jurkovic D. Endometrial implantation factors in women with submucous uterine fibroids. *Reprod Biomed Online.* 2010;21(5):610–5.
17. Medicine PCotASfR. Diagnostic evaluation of the infertile female: A committee opinion. *Fertil Steril.* 2015;103(6):e44–e50.
18. Soares SR, dos Reis MMBB, and Camargos AF. Diagnostic accuracy of sonohysterography, transvaginal sonography, and hysterosalpingography in patients with uterine cavity diseases. *Fertil Steril.* 2000;73(2):406–11.
19. Salim R, Lee C, Davies A, Jolaoso B, Ofuasia E, and Jurkovic D. A comparative study of three-dimensional saline infusion sonohysterography and diagnostic hysteroscopy for the classification of submucous fibroids. *Hum Reprod.* 2005;20(1):253–7.
20. Maheux-Lacroix S, Boutin A, Moore L, Bergeron ME, Bujold E, Laberge P, Lemyre M, Dodin S. Hysterosalpingosonography for diagnosing tubal occlusion in subfertile women: A systematic review with meta-analysis. *Hum Reprod.* 2014;29(5):953–63.
21. Groszmann YS, Benacerraf BR. Complete evaluation of anatomy and morphology of the infertile patient in a single visit; the modern infertility pelvic ultrasound examination. *Fertil Steril.* 2016;105(6):1381–93.
22. Dudiak C, Turner D, Patel S, Archie J, Silver B, and Norusis M. Uterine leiomyomas in the infertile patient: Preoperative localization with MR imaging versus US and hysterosalpingography. *Radiology.* 1988;167(3):627–30.
23. Pritts EA, Parker WH, and Olive DL. Fibroids and infertility: An updated systematic review of the evidence. *Fertil Steril.* 2009;91(4):1215–23.
24. Yan L, Ding L, Li C, Wang Y, Tang R, and Chen Z-J. Effect of fibroids not distorting the endometrial cavity on the outcome of in vitro fertilization treatment: A retrospective cohort study. *Fertil Steril.* 2014;101(3):716–21. e6.
25. Styer AK, Jin S, Liu D, Wang B, Polotsky AJ, Christianson MS et al. Association of uterine fibroids and pregnancy outcomes after ovarian stimulation-intrauterine insemination for unexplained infertility. *Fertil Steril.* 107(3):756–62.
26. Goldenberg M, Sivan E, Sharabi Z, Bider D, Rabinovici J, and Seidman DS. Outcome of hysteroscopic resection of submucous myomas for infertility. *Fertil Steril.* 1995;64(4):714–6.
27. Casini ML, Rossi F, Agostini R, and Unfer V. Effects of the position of fibroids on fertility. *Gynecol Endocrinol.* 2006;22(2):106–9.
28. Lebovitz O, Orvieto R, James KE, Styer AK, Brown DN. Predictors of reproductive outcomes following myomectomy for intramural fibroids. *Reproductive biomedicine online.* 2019 Sep 1;39(3):484-91.
29. Farhi J, Ashkenazi J, Feldberg D, Dicker D, Orvieto R, and Ben Rafael Z. Effect of uterine leiomyomata on the results of in-vitro fertilization treatment. *Hum Reprod.* 1995;10(10):2576–8.
30. Bulletti C, De Ziegler D, Levi Setti P, Cicinelli E, Polli V, and Stefanetti M. Myomas, pregnancy outcome, and in vitro fertilization. *Ann N Y Acad Sci.* 2004;1034(1):84–92.
31. Narayan R and Goswamy RK. Treatment of submucous fibroids, and outcome of assisted conception. *J Am Assoc Gynecol Laparosc.* 1994;1(4):307–11.
32. Surrey ES, Lietz AK, and Schoolcraft WB. Impact of intramural leiomyomata in patients with a normal endometrial cavity on in vitro fertilization–embryo transfer cycle outcome. *Fertil Steril.* 2001;75(2):405–10.
33. Somigliana E, De Benedictis S, Vercellini P et al. Fibroids not encroaching the endometrial cavity and IVF success rate: A prospective study. *Hum Reprod.* 2011: 26(4), 834-839.
34. Jun SH, Ginsburg ES, Racowsky C, Wise LA, and Hornstein MD. Uterine leiomyomas and their effect on in vitro fertilization outcome: A retrospective study. *J Assist Reprod Genet.* 2001;18(3):139–43.
35. Sunkara SK, Khairy M, El-Toukhy T, Khalaf Y, and Coomarasamy A. The effect of intramural fibroids without uterine cavity involvement on the outcome of IVF treatment: A systematic review and meta-analysis. *Hum Reprod.* 2009: 25(2), 418-429.
36. Yan L, Yu Q, Zhang YN, Guo Z, Li Z, Niu J, and Ma J. Effect of type 3 intramural fibroids on in vitro fertilization–intracytoplasmic sperm injection outcomes: a retrospective cohort study. *Fertil Steril.* 2018;109(5):817–22.
37. Bai X, Lin Y, Chen Y, and Ma C. The impact of FIGO type 3 fibroids on in-vitro fertilization outcomes: A nested retrospective case-control study. *Eur J Obstet Gynecol Reprod Biol.* 2020;247:176–80.
38. Metwally M, Raybould G, Cheong YC, and Horne AW. Surgical treatment of fibroids for subfertility. *Cochrane Database Syst Rev.* 2020;1(1):CD003857.doi:10 1002/14651858.CD003857.pub4
39. Pron G, Bennett J, Common A et al. The Ontario Uterine Fibroid Embolization Trial. Part 2. Uterine fibroid reduction and symptom relief after uterine artery embolization for fibroids. *Fertility and sterility.* 2003;79(1):120–7.
40. Torre A, Paillusson B, Fain V, Labauge P, Pelage J, and Fauconnier A. Uterine artery embolization for severe symptomatic fibroids: Effects on fertility and symptoms. *Hum Reprod.* 2014;29(3):490–501.
41. Pron G, Mocarski E, Bennett J, Vilos G, Common A, and Vanderburgh L. Pregnancy after uterine artery embolization for leiomyomata: The Ontario Multicenter Trial. *Obstet Gynecol.* 2005;105(1):67–76.
42. Jones S, O'Donovan P, and Toub D. Radiofrequency ablation for treatment of symptomatic uterine fibroids. *Obstetrics and gynecology international.* 2011;2012.
43. Donnez J, Tatarchuk TF, Bouchard P et al. Ulipristal acetate versus placebo for fibroid treatment before surgery. *N Engl J Med.* 2012;366(5):409–20.
44. Donnez J, Tomaszewski J, Vázquez F et al. Ulipristal acetate versus leuprolide acetate for uterine fibroids. *N Engl J Med.* 2012;366(5):421–32.
45. Luyckx M, Squifflet J-L, Jadoul P, Votino R, Dolmans M-M, and Donnez J. First series of 18 pregnancies after ulipristal acetate treatment for uterine fibroids. *Fertil Steril.* 2014;102(5):1404–9.
46. Hartmann KE, Velez Edwards DR, Savitz DA, Jonsson-Funk ML, Wu P, Sundermann AC, Baird DD. Prospective cohort study of uterine fibroids and miscarriage risk. *Am J Epidemiol.* 2017;186(10):1140–8.
47. Bulletti C, De Ziegler D, Polli V, and Flamigni C. The role of leiomyomas in infertility. *J Am Assoc Gynecol Laparosc.* 1999;6(4):441–5.
48. Saravelos SH, Yan J, Rehmani H, and Li T-C. The prevalence and impact of fibroids and their treatment on the outcome of pregnancy in women with recurrent miscarriage. *Hum Reprod.* 2011;26(12):3274–9.
49. Practice Committee of the American Society for Reproductive Medicine. Removal of myomas in asymptomatic patients to improve fertility and/or reduce miscarriage rate: A guideline. *Fertil Steril.* 2017;108(3):416–25.

10

Hormonal Regulation in the Treatment of Fibroids

Victoria Fitz and Steven L. Young

Introduction

Leiomyomata (fibroids) are common, monoclonal, proliferative and fibrotic lesions of the uterine smooth muscle. Although fibroid pathogenesis remains unclear, genetics and micronutrients appear to play a role. Additionally, fibroids are highly dependent on sex steroids for growth and maintenance. The aim of this chapter is to review current knowledge regarding the pathophysiological mechanisms of sex steroid action and the current and future role of sex steroid-receptor modulating agents (SSMAs) for therapeutic benefit.

Hormone Dependence of Fibroids

Uterine fibroids grow after puberty and regress with menopause and earlier menarche is a further risk factor for fibroid development, strongly implicating sex steroids in their growth [1]. Fibroids often regress postpartum, a period of uterine remodeling and a time when sex-steroid levels fall to postmenopausal levels. Interestingly, during pregnancy, a state of elevated sex-steroid levels, only about one-third of fibroids increase in size after the first trimester [2].

Estrogens signal primarily through two specific nuclear receptors, ER-alpha and ER-beta, though additional membrane-bound ER-alpha and the G-protein-coupled estrogen receptor (GPER) on the cell surface can also mediate estrogen responses. Estrogen is able to induce human fibroid cell proliferation *in vitro* [3] as well as fibroid growth in a rat model *in vivo* and in rat leiomyoma cells *in vitro* [4,5]. The production of estradiol by some leiomyomas [6] also suggests autocrine or intracrine pathways for estrogen to promote growth. Estrogen receptors alpha and beta are found in higher concentration in leiomyoma cells compared with surrounding normal myometrium. Estrogen activates fibroblasts within leiomyomas leading to proliferation and ECM deposition [7]. These and many other studies strongly implicate a role for estradiol in leiomyoma growth.

Additionally, progesterone appears to be of at least equal importance to estradiol in leimyoma pathophysiology as supported by clinical and laboratory observations. Human mitotic activity in fibroids is maximal during the secretory phase of the menstrual cycle, when serum progesterone is highest [8]. Progesterone receptor expression is increased in leiomyomas, likely because of estrogen action, and progesterone receptor agonists can increase leiomyoma cell proliferation *in vitro* [9].

Human leiomyoma tissue xenograft studies further support the role of progesterone. When immunodeficient mice are xenografted with human leiomyoma tissue and treated with estradiol, leiomyoma ER-alpha and PR expression is increased, but growth is not stimulated. Similarly, progesterone treatment, alone, does not result in growth. However, treatment with both progesterone and estrogen results in both cellular proliferation and leiomyoma volume growth [11].

Virtually all physiological and pathophysiological effects of progesterone are exerted through two nuclear receptors, progesterone receptor alpha (PR-A) and beta (PR-B). The two proteins are transcribed from the same gene and are identical, except PR-B has an extra 165 N-terminal amino acids, significantly complicating separate analysis in human tissues. Thus, most of the published information in leiomyomata includes undifferentiated analysis of PR, without regard to subtype, though both subtypes appear to be upregulated in leiomyomata [10].

Leiomyoma growth and pathophysiological impact is determined not only by cellular proliferation, but also by extensive fibrosis [12]. The fibrotic component is due to extensive production of extracellular matrix (ECM) proteins, such as collagens, fibronectin, laminins and proteoglycans. The biology of ECM is complex and beyond the scope of this chapter, but it is clear that ECM can act as a reservoir of specific growth factors as well as alter cellular signaling directly through mechano-transduction receptors, such as integrins, to promote proliferation and further ECM changes. Estrogen may play an important role in leiomyoma fibrosis, by stimulating ECM biosynthesis as well as altering growth factors, such as platelet-derived growth factor (PDGF), that modulate ECM. Progesterone again contributes, altering ECM and stimulating expression of TGF-beta, a potent pro-fibrotic factor that has a near-ubiquitous role in fibrotic disease, and inducing microRNA species that may drive further fibrosis. Taken together, *in vivo*, *ex vivo*, *in vitro* and xenograft data demonstrate that estrogens and progesterone work in concert to stimulate leiomyoma cell proliferation and alter production of ECM to support leiomyoma growth.

Hormonal Management of Fibroids

As summarized earlier, sex steroids play a necessary and critical role in fibroid biology, which allows an opportunity to clinically target sex steroids and their receptors to provide a medical alternative to surgical therapy for fibroids. However, currently available medical therapies have limited effectiveness and/or significant adverse effects, leaving surgical therapy as the most definitive and effective option for many patients. The relative balance between medical and surgical therapies may change with the advent of newer SSMAs under development, which may provide similar or improved benefit over conservative surgical therapy, but with greatly reduced complications. This section will review currently available and potential future medications that act via modulation of sex-steroid signaling pathways (see Table 10.1).

Progesterone Receptor and Estrogen Receptor Agonists

An important consideration when approaching the treatment of fibroids is whether the treatment is addressing the fibroids directly by reducing their size or volume, or if the treatment is addressing the symptoms that result from fibroids such as heavy menstrual bleeding or bulk symptoms. Estrogen and progesterone agonist therapy fall into the category of symptomatic treatment. A well-established practice is the use of high-dose estrogen, such as intravenous conjugated equine estrogens or various protocols using multiple doses of combined oral contraceptives to temporize acute uterine hemorrhage caused by a submucous myoma [50]. These treatments carry significant risk of thrombosis and are only used as temporizing measures to stabilize bleeding. Combined oral contraceptive pills (COCs), containing highly potent estrogen and progesterone receptor agonists at standard doses, are commonly used to treat the symptoms of leiomyoma-associated abnormal uterine bleeding (AUB-L). COCs achieve this goal by suppressing pituitary gonadotropins and providing high-dose estrogens and progestins to achieve a stable, compact endometrium, which is less likely to shed. AUB-L can often be controlled using COCs, but these medications do not lead to a decrease in the size of uterine fibroids. Despite COC treatment, abnormal uterine bleeding often returns over time and fibroids may continue to grow, resulting in increased bleeding despite COC treatment. Counterintuitively, fibroid growth is not consistently demonstrated in clinical studies of COC use, and in fact, some observational studies suggest that COC use may be protective against development of uterine fibroids, while others have demonstrated increased risk for development of fibroids with COC use in early adolescence [13,14,51].

Treatment with progestins, such as norethindrone, levonorgestrel and medroxyprogesterone, alone is another method used to control abnormal uterine bleeding that results from fibroids. Oral progestins or those delivered via intrauterine device (IUD) can reduce bleeding associated with uterine fibroids by inducing decidualization of the endometrium [52]. Oral progestins have not been observed to decrease the size of leiomyoma or alleviate symptoms, while the levonorgestrel IUD was shown to significantly reduce menstrual blood loss associated with uterine fibroids. There have been varying reports of the impact of the levonorgestrel IUD on leiomyoma size. Kriplani et al. found that levonorgestrel IUD use has different effects on normal myometrium and leiomyoma tissue, reducing uterine volume, but not leiomyoma volume [15], while Maruo et al. reported that some myomas increased in size after levonorgestrel IUD placement though menorrhagia was controlled [16]. Depot medroxyprogesterone acetate (DMPA) has long been used as a therapy for heavy menstrual bleeding. Interestingly, epidemiologic studies have found that use of DMPA is inversely associated with the development of symptomatic fibroids [17,18].

A 2013 Cochrane review of oral and IUD delivery of progestins concluded that there is insufficient evidence to support the use of either for the treatment of uterine fibroids [19]; however, our clinical experience suggests that the use of progestins either alone or in combination with an estrogen is warranted for temporizing bleeding prior to surgical management. In general, we do not favor long-acting progestin therapy (e.g., DMPA) for this purpose, because progestins can sometimes worsen bleeding. Given that the progestin effects of DMPA cannot be practically reversed and the lowered response of progestin-treated endometrium to estrogen action, further medical therapy is unlikely to be successful in patients with increased bleeding after DMPA. Thus, we favor use of COCs, oral progestins or an easily removable IUD, if progestin agonists are used.

Estrogen Reduction

Given the previously described role of estrogen in promoting leiomyoma growth, investigators have targeted suppression of the hypothalamic-pituitary-ovarian axis as a potential therapy to reduce leiomyoma size and associated bulk symptoms as well as AUB-L. The first agents used to reduce estrogen production were gonadotropin releasing hormone agonists (GnRHa). These agents induce a hypoestrogenic state by downregulating GnRH receptor function in pituitary gonadotroph cells, resulting in little to no FSH stimulation of ovarian estrogen production. GnRHa treatment is effective: Leuprolide acetate treatment for 3–6 months has been found to stop AUB-L in up to 80% of women and reduce both uterine and fibroid volume by about 36%–50% compared with placebo [20,21]. Side effects of therapy with GnRHa include hot flushes and other menopausal symptoms and are observed in 60%–95% of patients treated with this medication. Long-term side effects include a marked reduction in bone density. Thus, therapy with GnRHa is primarily a short-term bridge to surgical management or menopause. It is also important to note that GnRHa can lead to fibroid degeneration, and subsequent acute hemorrhage, though incidence is likely low.

There have been investigations of long-term GnRH treatment with low-dose add-back of estrogen and/or progesterone in an effort to mitigate the menopausal symptoms and bone loss. The goal of such a regimen is long-term use with fewer side effects while still decreasing vaginal bleeding and leiomyoma size. A 2015 Cochrane review of 12 small studies included treatment with leuprolide acetate and add-back with medroxyprogesterone, raloxifene, tibolone or conjugated estrogens. Loss of bone mass was reduced and vasomotor symptoms were improved with add-back, but uterine size was not reduced to the same extent as with GnRHa alone, suggesting an overlap between estrogen levels therapeutic for leiomyomata and those needed to alleviate symptoms [22].

Recently, elagolix, an orally administered GnRH antagonist currently in development, was found to be safe and effective at reducing circulating estrogen levels [23]. Given its oral administration, incomplete antagonism and ability to titrate

TABLE 10.1
Comparison of Hormonal Medications

Class	Mechanism of Action	Names	Route	FDA Approved Treatment of Fibroids?	Clinical Impact	Side Effects	Length of Therapy
Hormonal contraceptives (estrogen+progestin or progestin only)	Suppresses pituitary gonadotropin production; also agonist effect at level of ER and PR receptors	CHCs (many varieties), norethindrone, medroxyprogesterone	PO, transdermal, vaginal ring, and IM	Yes, for contraception. Use for AUB is off-label	Varied, may reduce volume of menstrual blood loss; unlikely to impact fibroid size	Risk of VTE	Variable
Levonorgestrel intrauterine system	Proposed mechanism for reduction of AUB is decidualization of the endometrium	Mirena, Liletta	Intrauterine	Yes, for contraception and AUB	Reduction in menstrual blood loss, uterine volume, possibly fibroid volume	Risks of device placement, expulsion, irregular bleeding	Variable up to 5 years
GnRH agonist	Induces hypoestrogenic state by downregulating the pituitary GnRH receptor	Leuprolide, Goserelin	IM	Yes, leuprolide for preoperative anemia only	Decrease leiomyoma size and induce amenorrhea[a]	Menopausal symptoms • Bone loss • Vasomotor	3–6 months (or longer with add back)
GnRH antagonist	Induces hypoestrogenic state by competitive inhibition of GnRH	Ganerelix, Elagolix	IM or PO	No	Reduce leiomyoma volume and improve anemia[b]	Same as above	3 months (or longer with add-back)
SPRM	Agonist, antagonist, or mixed effects on PR depending on the target tissue	Mifespristone, asoprisnil, ulipristal, telapristone, vilaprisan	PO	No	Reduce leiomyoma size and induce amenorrhea [c]	Endometrial thickening, PAEC, liver toxicity (telapristone only)	3 months Intermittent and longer duration therapy under investigation

Abbreviations: PR, progesterone receptor; PAEC, progesterone receptor modulator-associated endometrial changes.
[a] Reduction in volume of leiomyoma by 36%–50% and amenorrhea in 80% of patients.
[b] Reduction in volume of leiomyoma by 30%; improvement in hemoglobin by $\geq$1 g/dL in 50%–70% of patients.
[c] 30% reduction of leiomyoma volume; amenorrhea in 70% of patients.

hypoestrogenism somewhat by dose, elagolix may allow refinement of GnRHa therapy, but only a phase 2 trial for fibroids has been reported [24]. Other orally active GnRH antagonists, including relugolix, OBE2109 and ASP-1707 are also being actively developed, suggesting that a number of related medications in this class will be available in the near future.

Investigators have also attempted to target estrogen action using an aromatase inhibitor (letrozole) to partially block estrogen synthesis. Since fibroids may, themselves, produce estrogen via aromatase expression [25], such an approach could reduce autocrine/intracrine estrogen action as well as the endocrine action of ovarian estrogens inhibited by GnRHa medications. Furthermore, these agents may be helpful for treating postmenopausal fibroids that may be maintained mainly by endogenous estrogen production. Encouragingly, small trials have suggested a similar effect of aromatase inhibitors to that of a GnRHa, triptorelin, but with a greatly reduced incidence of vasomotor symptoms [26].

Though effective at decreasing uterine and leiomyoma volume and reducing vaginal bleeding, GnRH agonists have had significant adverse effects that limit their long-term use as therapy of uterine fibroids. Early results of aromatase inhibitors and the partial inhibition of the oral GnRH antagonists are encouraging, but long-term and larger studies will be needed to better evaluate efficacy and limitations of these approaches.

Selective Progesterone Receptor Modulators (SPRMs)

Given the limitations (vide supra) of progestin receptor agonists and GnRH agonists, investigators have recently turned their attention to selective progesterone receptor modulators (SPRMs), including ligands such as mifepristone, ulipristal and asoprisnil, which have agonist, antagonist or mixed effects on progesterone receptors, depending on the target tissue and its physiological state. The SPRM ligand binds to PR-A or PR-B (both found in higher concentrations in leiomyoma tissue compared with surrounding myometrium), and initiates interactions with co-repressors or co-activators that dictate whether the SPRM is an agonist or antagonist in that cellular environment.

Several different SPRMs have been clinically investigated for efficacy in fibroid treatment: mifepristone and ulipristal, strong PR antagonists with very little or no agonist activity; asoprisnil and telapristone, more complex, tissue-specific antagonist/agonists. Each acts at the level of the fibroid, the endometrium and the pituitary to influence fibroid symptomatology [27]. At the level of the fibroid, they decrease size through induction of apoptosis and inhibition of cellular proliferation. Action on the endometrium reduces bleeding and results in cellular changes discussed later. These agents also act to suppress pituitary gonadotropin production, but not nearly to the level seen with GnRHa, keeping serum estradiol concentrations at a mid-follicular level [28] and inducing anovulation in up to 80% of patients at therapeutic doses for fibroid management [29]. Currently, none of these SPRMs are FDA approved for use in the US for the purpose of uterine fibroid treatment.

Mifepristone was originally developed as an abortifacient, but has recently been investigated as a possible treatment for uterine fibroids. When administered orally at doses ranging from 2.5 to 25 mg daily for 3–6 months, it reduces menstrual blood loss, pelvic pain, pressure and dysmenorrhea. Individual studies also report reduction of uterine and leiomyoma volume when compared with placebo [30,31]; however, this was not supported by a 2012 Cochrane Review [32]. Vaginal administration of mifepristone also resulted in decreased leiomyoma volume of approximately 20% over 2–3 months, and 44% of patients achieved amenorrhea [33].

At least three factors limit mifepristone's appeal for long-term treatment of fibroids. First, endometrial hyperplasia has been reported with mifepristone use, though the incidence varies widely by study. Additionally, much of the reported "hyperplasia" was actually an unusual endometrial morphology (also seen with ulipristal and asoprisnil) that mimics hyperplasia on ultrasound, but is associated with very low mitotic activity [34]. Another concern with mifepristone is its anti-glucocorticoid effect that could potentially lead to clinically significant adrenal insufficiency [35]. In the United States, mifepristone's abortifacient effects are another potential barrier to wide introduction for fibroid therapy.

Ulipristal is a SPRM that is currently approved for use in the United States as an emergency contraceptive but not yet for fibroid treatment. It has been studied as a therapy for uterine fibroids in a series of large clinical trials [36]. When taken daily for 3 months at 5 or 10 mg doses, ulipristal treatment led to amenorrhea in 70%–80% of patients and 30%–42% decrease in fibroid volume. Ulipristal was non-inferior to leuprolide acetate in reducing bleeding associated with fibroids prior to surgery. Patients taking ulipristal maintained normal serum estradiol levels in the midfollicular phase range and did not experience hot flashes with the same frequency as patients treated with GnRH agonist (11% of ulipristal group compared with 40% of patients treated with leuprolide). Notably, the reduction of leiomyoma volume after taking ulipristal was sustained for 6 months post-treatment compared to 1 month in patients treated with leuprolide acetate. Although not approved for treatment of fibroids in the United States, approval for short-term use for this purpose has been given in Canada and Europe. Furthermore, longer-term intermittent therapy seems to increase efficacy and maintain safety with the longest study including eight 3-month-long courses, with each course separated by one menses [37].

Asoprisnil was found to have similar effects [38]. There was a dose-dependent decrease in uterine bleeding with suppression of bleeding in 85% of participants for the duration of treatment at the highest dose of 25 mg daily and a 17% reduction in uterine volume [39]. Since asoprisnil has no significant abortifacient properties, it has potential to be a more widely accepted therapy in the United States, but lower efficacy at currently tested routes and doses remains a concern and its clinical development was discontinued in 2009 [37].

Telapristone was shown in *in vitro* studies to induce apoptosis and inhibit proliferation in uterine leiomyoma cells [40]. Clinical trials in women with fibroids were initiated but discontinued owing to concerns for liver toxicity in 2009. Development has since restarted with lower doses of the medication [37]. Vilaprisan is another SPRM which is currently being investigated with Phase III trials.

Mechanism of Action

The mechanisms of SPRM therapeutic properties are a topic of ongoing investigation [41]. Multiple growth factors have been identified as possible targets of SPRM activity, including EGF, IGF-I, TGF-beta-3. Expression of these growth factors was downregulated in leiomyoma cells treated with asoprisnil, but not in cells from the surrounding normal myometrium [42]. Bcl-2, an anti-apoptotic protein, is expressed at much higher levels in uterine leiomyoma compared with normal myometrium and is upregulated by progesterone [43]. Both mifepristone and asoprisnil suppress Bcl-2, suggesting apoptosis as another possible mechanism for SPRM reduction of leiomyoma size [44,45]; however, doubts regarding the relevance of this mechanism *in vivo* have been raised [46].

Endometrial Changes with SPRMs

One of the main concerns with SPRMs is that anti-progestin activity at the level of the endometrium will lead to hyperplasia, atypia and other sequela of unopposed estrogen stimulation. The endometrial changes associated with SPRM therapy have been termed PRM-associated endometrial changes (PAEC) [47]. These changes include cystic glandular dilation, asymmetry of stromal and epithelial growth, with admixed estrogen (mitotic) and progestin (secretory) epithelial effects. There was low mitotic activity and <1% incidence of hyperplasia [48]. Reassuringly, most studies of mifepristone, ulipristal and asoprisnil treatment of women have involved post-treatment follow-up with endometrial biopsy and have found that the PAEC regress and normal endometrium is found within 6 months of discontinuing treatment [36].

Clinical Use of SPRMs

While there is mounting evidence in support SPRMs for the treatment of uterine fibroids, in the United States, SPRMs have not yet become a widely used therapy. The initial clinical trials with ulipristal established the use of SPRMs as an effective option for short-term therapy prior to definitive surgery. In this role, it can serve to improve anemia, improve bleeding profile and decrease uterine size while awaiting definitive therapy and possibly allowing for a minimally invasive approach to surgery.

The follow-up long-term trials of ulipristal have demonstrated efficacy of repeating 3-month courses for up to 1 year. This resulted in sustained amenorrhea in >70% of patients, with decreased uterine size, while maintaining safety. These findings have led to expansion of ulipristal use to include management of fibroids regardless of plan for surgery. Several algorithms have been proposed incorporating ulipristal into management options, with varied endpoints including preoperative management, as a substitution for surgery, to decrease fibroid size prior to conception, or as a bridge to menopause for different patients [40,27].

ACOG has not yet weighed in on the role of SPRMs in medical management of uterine fibroids. The last practice bulletin from 2008 advises consideration of mifepristone for short-term preoperative management but calls for additional research and does not mention other SPRMs [49]. It will be interesting to see the application of SPRM therapy to fibroid management evolve over the coming years as additional research is performed and novel medications continue to be developed.

Summary and Conclusions

Sex-steroid action is a critical determinant of leiomyoma cell survival, proliferation and ECM production. Modulation of sex-steroid production and action can significantly reduce leiomyoma size. Currently used SSMAs all have significant limitations for long-term use, but emerging agents such as the aromatase inhibitors, oral GnRH antagonists and SPRMs show significant potential for controlling leiomyoma symptoms on a long-term basis and thus reducing the number of needed surgeries.

REFERENCES

1. Wise LA and Laughlin-Tommaso SK. Epidemiology of uterine fibroids: From menarche to menopause. *Clin Obstet Gynecol.* 2016 Mar;59:2–24.
2. Rosati P, Exacoustòs C, and Mancuso S. Longitudinal evaluation of uterine myoma growth during pregnancy. A sonographic study. *J Ultrasound Med.* 1992 Oct;11:511–5.
3. Barbarisi A, Petillo O, Di Lieto A et al. 17-beta estradiol elicits an autocrine leiomyoma cell proliferation: Evidence for a stimulation of protein kinase-dependent pathway. *J Cell Physiol.* 2001 Mar;186:414–24.
4. Burroughs KD, Fuchs-Young R, Davis B, and Walker CL. Altered hormonal responsiveness of proliferation and apoptosis during myometrial maturation and the development of uterine leiomyomas in the rat. *Biol Reprod.* 2000 Nov;63:1322–30.
5. Howe SR, Gottardis MM, Everitt JI, and Walker C. Estrogen stimulation and tamoxifen inhibition of leiomyoma cell growth *in vitro* and *in vivo*. *Endocrinology.* 1995 Nov; 136:4996–5003.
6. Bulun SE, Simpson ER, and Word RA. Expression of the CYP19 gene and its product aromatase cytochrome P450 in human uterine leiomyoma tissues and cells in culture. *J Clin Endocrinol Metab.* 1994 Mar;78:736–43.
7. Luo N, Guan Q, Zheng L, Qu X, Dai H, and Cheng Z. Estrogen-mediated activation of fibroblasts and its effects on the fibroid cell proliferation. *Transl Res.* 2014 Mar;163:232–41.
8. Kawaguchi K, Fujii S, Konishi I, Nanbu Y, Nonogaki H, and Mori T. Mitotic activity in uterine leiomyomas during the menstrual cycle. *Am J Obstet Gynecol.* 1989 Mar;160:637–41.
9. Hoekstra AV, Sefton EC, Berry E et al. Progestins activate the AKT pathway in leiomyoma cells and promote survival. *J Clin Endocrinol Metab.* 2009 May;94:1768–74.
10. Viville B, Charnock-Jones DS, Sharkey AM, Wetzka B, and Smith SK. Distribution of the A and B forms of the progesterone receptor messenger ribonucleic acid and protein in uterine leiomyomata and adjacent myometrium. *Hum Reprod.* 1997 Apr;12:815–22.
11. Ishikawa H, Ishi K, Serna VA, Kakazu R, Bulun SE, and Kurita T. Progesterone is essential for maintenance and growth of uterine leiomyoma. *Endocrinology.* 2010 Jun;151:2433–42.
12. Islam MS, Ciavattini A, Petraglia F, Castellucci M, and Ciarmela P. Extracellular matrix in uterine leiomyoma pathogenesis: A potential target for future therapeutics. *Hum Reprod Update.* 2018 Jan 1;24:59–85.

13. Qin J, Yang T, Kong F, and Zhou Q. Oral contraceptive use and uterine leiomyoma risk: A meta-analysis based on cohort and case-control studies. *Arch Gynecol Obstet.* 2013 Jul;288:139–48.
14. Moroni RM, Martins WP, Dias SV et al. Combined oral contraceptive for treatment of women with uterine fibroids and abnormal uterine bleeding: A systematic review. *Gynecol Obstet Invest.* 2015;79(3):145–52.
15. Kriplani A, Awasthi D, Kulshrestha V, and Agarwal N. Efficacy of the levonorgestrel-releasing intrauterine system in uterine leiomyoma. *Int J Gynaecol Obstet.* 2012 Jan;116:35–8.
16. Maruo T, Ohara N, Matsuo H et al. Effects of levonorgestrel-releasing IUS and progesterone receptor modulator PRM CDB-2914 on uterine leiomyomas. *Contraception.* 2007 Jun;75:S99–103.
17. Lumbiganon P, Rugpao S, Phandhu-fung S, Laopaiboon M, Vudhikamraksa N, and Werawatakul Y. Protective effect of depot-medroxyprogesterone acetate on surgically treated uterine leiomyomas: A multicentre case--control study. *Br J Obstet Gynaecol.* 1996 Sep;103:909–14.
18. Harmon QE and Baird DD. Use of depot medroxyprogesterone acetate and prevalent leiomyoma in young African American women. *Hum Reprod.* 2015 Jun;30:1499–504.
19. Lethaby A, Hussain M, Rishworth JR, and Rees MC. Progesterone or progestogen-releasing intrauterine systems for heavy menstrual bleeding. *Cochrane Database Syst Rev.* 2015;(4);CD002126.
20. Friedman AJ, Daly M, Juneau-Norcross M, Gleason R, Rein MS, and LeBoff M. Long-term medical therapy for leiomyomata uteri: A prospective, randomized study of leuprolide acetate depot plus either oestrogen-progestin or progestin "add-back" for 2 years. *Hum Reprod.* 1994 Sep;9:1618–25.
21. Stovall TG, Muneyyirci-Delale O, Summitt RL, and Scialli AR. GnRH agonist and iron versus placebo and iron in the anemic patient before surgery for leiomyomas: A randomized controlled trial. Leuprolide Acetate Study Group. *Obstet Gynecol.* 1995 Jul;86:65–71.
22. Moroni RM, Martins WP, Ferriani RA et al. Add-back therapy with GnRH analogues for uterine fibroids. *Cochrane Database Syst Rev.* 2015;(3);CD010854.
23. Struthers RS, Nicholls AJ, Grundy J et al. Suppression of gonadotropins and estradiol in premenopausal women by oral administration of the nonpeptide gonadotropin-releasing hormone antagonist elagolix. *J Clin Endocrinol Metab.* 2009 Feb;94:545–51.
24. Archer DF, Stewart EA, Jain RI et al. Elagolix for the management of heavy menstrual bleeding associated with uterine fibroids: Results from a phase 2a proof-of-concept study. *Fertil Steril.* 2017 Jul;108:152–60.e4.
25. Sumitani H, Shozu M, Segawa T et al. *In situ* estrogen synthesized by aromatase P450 in uterine leiomyoma cells promotes cell growth probably via an autocrine/intracrine mechanism. *Endocrinology.* 2000 Oct;141:3852–61.
26. Hilário SG, Bozzini N, Borsari R and Baracat EC. Action of aromatase inhibitor for treatment of uterine leiomyoma in perimenopausal patients. *Fertil Steril.* 2009 Jan;91:240–3.
27. Donnez J and Dolmans M-M. Uterine fibroid management: From the present to the future. *Hum Reprod Update.* 2016;22(6):665–86.
28. Donnez J, Tomaszewski J, Vázquez F et al. Ulipristal acetate versus leuprolide acetate for uterine fibroids. *N Engl J Med.* 2012 Feb 2;366:421–32.
29. Chabbert-Buffet N, Pintiaux-Kairis A, and Bouchard P. Effects of the progesterone receptor modulator VA2914 in a continuous low dose on the hypothalamic-pituitary-ovarian axis and endometrium in normal women: A prospective, randomized, placebo-controlled trial *J Clin Endocrinol Metab.* 2007 Sep 1;92(9):3582–9.
30. Shen Q, Hua Y, Jiang W, Zhang W, Chen M, and Zhu X. Effects of mifepristone on uterine leiomyoma in premenopausal women: A meta-analysis. *Fertil Steril.* 2013 Dec;100(6):1722–6.e1–10.
31. Chabbert-Buffet N, Esber N, Bouchard P. Fibroid growth and medical options for treatment. *Fertil Steril.* 2014 Sep;102:630–9.
32. Tristan M, Orozco LJ, Steed A, Ramírez-Morera A, and Stone P. Mifepristone for uterine fibroids. *Cochrane Database Syst Rev.* 2012;(8):CD007687.
33. Yerushalmi GM, Gilboa Y, Jakobson-Setton A et al. Vaginal mifepristone for the treatment of symptomatic uterine leiomyomata: An open-label study. *Fertil Steril.* 2014 Feb;101:496–500.
34. Wilkens J, Male V, Ghazal P et al. Uterine NK cells regulate endometrial bleeding in women and are suppressed by the progesterone receptor modulator asoprisnil. *J Immunol.* 2013 Sep 9;191:2226–35.
35. Agarwai MK. The antiglucocorticoid action of mifepristone. *Pharmacol Ther.* 1996;70:183–213.
36. Donnez J, Donnez O, Dolmans M-M. The current place of medical therapy in uterine fibroid management. *Best Pr Res Clin Obstet Gynaecol.* 2018 Jan;46:57–65.
37. Singh SS, Belland L, Leyland N, von Riedemann S, and Murji A. The past, present, and future of selective progesterone receptor modulators in the management of uterine fibroids. *Am J Obstet Gynecol.* 2018 Dec;218(6):563–72.
38. Bartels CB, Cayton KC, Chuong FS et al. An evidence-based approach to the medical management of fibroids: A systematic review. *Clin Obstet Gynecol.* 2016;59:30–52.
39. Chwalisz K, Larsen L, Mattia-Goldberg C, Edmonds A, Elger W, and Winkel CA. A randomized, controlled trial of asoprisnil, a novel selective progesterone receptor modulator, in women with uterine leiomyomata. *Fertil Steril.* 2007 Jun;87(6):1399–412.
40. Luo X, Yin P, Coon V JS, Cheng Y-H, Wiehle RD, and Bulun SE. The selective progesterone receptor modulator CDB4124 inhibits proliferation and induces apoptosis in uterine leiomyoma cells. *Fertil Steril.* 2010 May 15;93(8):2668–73.
41. Wagenfeld A, Saunders PTK, Whitaker L, and Critchley HOD. Selective progesterone receptor modulators (SPRMs): Progesterone receptor action, mode of action on the endometrium and treatment options in gynecological therapies. *Expert Opin Ther Targets.* 2016 Sep;20:1045–54.
42. Wang J, Ohara N, Wang Z et al. A novel selective progesterone receptor modulator asoprisnil (J867) down-regulates the expression of EGF, IGF-I, TGFbeta3 and their receptors in cultured uterine leiomyoma cells. *Hum Reprod.* 2006 Jul;21:1869–77.
43. Matsuo H, Maruo T, and Samoto T. Increased expression of Bcl-2 protein in human uterine leiomyoma and its up-regulation by progesterone. *J Clin Endocrinol Metab.* 1997 Jan;82:293–9.
44. Chen W, Ohara N, Wang J et al. A novel selective progesterone receptor modulator asoprisnil (J867) inhibits proliferation and induces apoptosis in cultured human uterine leiomyoma cells in the absence of comparable effects on myometrial cells. *J Clin Endocrinol Metab.* 2006 Apr;91:1296–304.

45. Chung Y-J, Chae B, Kwak S-H et al. Comparison of the inhibitory effect of gonadotropin releasing hormone (GnRH) agonist, selective estrogen receptor modulator (SERM), anti-progesterone on myoma cell proliferation *in vitro*. *Int J Med Sci*. 2014;11:276–81.
46. Courtoy GE, Donnez J, Marbaix E, Barreira M, Luyckx M, Dolmans M-M. Progesterone receptor isoforms, nuclear corepressor-1 and steroid receptor coactivator-1 and B-cell lymphoma 2 and Akt and Akt phosphorylation status in uterine myomas after ulipristal acetate treatment: A systematic immunohistochemical evaluation. *Gynecol Obstet Invest*. 2018;83(5):443–54.
47. Mutter GL, Bergeron C, Deligdisch L et al. The spectrum of endometrial pathology induced by progesterone receptor modulators. *Mod Pathol*. 2008 May;21:591–8.
48. Horne FM, Blithe DL. Progesterone receptor modulators and the endometrium: Changes and consequences. *Hum Reprod Update*. 2007;13(6):567–80.
49. American College of Obstetrics and Gynecology. Alternatives to hysterectomy for the management of leiomyomas. Practice Bullectin No 96 [Internet]. 2008. Available from: https://www.acog.org/Clinical%20Guidance%20and%20Publications/Practice%20Bulletins/Committee%20on%20Practice%20Bulletins%20Gynecology/Alternatives%20to%20Hysterectomy%20in%20the%20Management%20of%20Leiomyomas.aspx
50. DeVore GR, Owens O, Kase N. Use of intravenous Premarin in the treatment of dysfunctional uterine bleeding—A double-blind randomized control study. *Obstet Gynecol*. 1982;59(3):285–291.
51. Marshall LM, Spiegelman D, Goldman MB et al. A prospective study of reproductive factors and oral contraceptive use in relation to the risk of uterine leiomyomata. *Fertil Steril*. 1998;70(3):432–39.
52. Silverberg SG, Haukkamaa M, Arko H, Nilsson CG, Luukkainen T. Endometrial morphology during long-term use of levonorgestrel-releasing intrauterine devices. *Int J Gynecol Pathol*. 1986;5(3):235–41.

11

The Role of Gonadotropin-Releasing Hormone (GnRH) Agonists in the Treatment of Uterine Fibroids

Whitney A. Leonard and Alexander M. Quaas

Introduction

Mechanism of Action of GnRH-Agonist Medications

Gonadotropin-releasing hormone (GnRH) is the primary hormonal stimulus of the hypothalamic-pituitary-gonadal axis. GnRH is produced in the arcuate nucleus of the hypothalamus and released to the hypophysial portal system, which connects the hypothalamus to the pituitary. GnRH then binds to the GnRH receptor on gonadotrophs in the anterior pituitary, stimulating the release of luteinizing hormone (LH), as well as follicle stimulating hormone (FSH), from the pituitary. These hormones then act on the ovaries to help control the menstrual cycle. Hormonal control of the reproductive organs has been utilized by the medical field to treat human disease and dysregulation of endocrine functions [1].

Landmark experiments from the last century have helped to understand the physiology of the hypothalamic–pituitary–ovarian (HPO) axis [2]. In 1969, Ernst Knobil's laboratory studied ovariectomized rhesus monkeys and discovered that LH was secreted in a pulsatile manner and proposed that there was a releasing factor from the brain that stimulated the pituitary to release LH [3]. Andrew Schally and Roger Guillemin, who shared the 1977 Nobel Prize, actually independently discovered the decapeptide structure and described the chemical makeup of GnRH after Knobil's groundwork [4,5].

Figures 11.1 and 11.2 demonstrate and compare the amino acid sequence and structure of gonadotropin-releasing hormones [6,7].

GnRH is relatively dormant during childhood and attains its normal pulsatile nature in puberty. This pulsatile release continues throughout the reproductive years and menopause. Its short duration of action and pulsatile release allows continuous GnRH-agonist therapy to desensitize pituitary receptors and downregulate the HPO axis. Amino acid substitution at position six of the decapeptide has allowed for biologically active analogues of GnRH [1,8]. Further substitutions and additions have led to the creation of over 2000 GnRH analogues since its isolation in 1971. New research has revealed that kisspeptin, a polypeptide that binds to a G-protein-coupled receptor in the hypothalamus, plays a central role in the control of GnRH secretion [9]. Mutations in kisspeptin may be involved in the pathogenesis of disease, and research is ongoing to understand the kisspeptin–GnRH relationship and its impact on human endocrinology and disease [10].

Pharmacology of GnRH Agonists

Major types of GnRH analogues include those with substitutions at the sixth amino acid position. More commonly utilized agonists include leuprolide acetate (Lupron, Abbvie), nafarelin acetate (Synarel, Pfizer); and goserelin acetate (Zoladex, AstraZeneca). Leuprolide acetate was first approved in the United States in 1985 for the treatment of prostate cancer, using the same principle of downregulation of gonadal hormones used for treatment of fibroids [11].

GnRH agonists induce a pseudomenopausal state with continued usage. Hot flashes are a common complaint from patients and concerns of bone demineralization are warranted with long-term use. Because of these adverse effects, many providers prescribe "add-back" therapy with hormonal medications to prevent these outcomes. Currently, consensus does suggest prescribing some sort of add-back therapy when treating patients for long durations, that is, greater than 6 months. A recent Cochrane review on the various types of add-back therapies (raloxifene, medroxyprogesterate acetate, tibolone, estriol, ipriflavone and conjugated estrogen) was limited by low-quality evidence but did suggest that use of tibolone with leuprolide resulted in higher quality-of-life scores [12].

GnRH-Agonist Treatment of Leiomyomas as Primary Therapy

Leiomyomata form during the reproductive years, due to the presence of higher levels of estrogen and progesterone compared with prepubescent and menopausal years. These benign tumors are highly dependent on estrogen and progesterone; thus, their growth is correlated with the reproductive years only [13,14]. While there are many medical treatment options for symptomatic leiomyomas causing abnormal uterine bleeding, anemia, pelvic pain and infertility, GnRH agonists are likely the most-effective nonsurgical treatment available to clinicians. Within the first month of use, hemoglobin and hematocrit levels rise and bleeding decreases. Patients report better quality-of-life scores due to decreased uterine bleeding [15].

GnRH-Agonist Treatment of Leiomyomas as Adjunct Therapy Prior to Surgery

The rationale behind GnRH-agonist use prior to surgery is to downregulate the hypothalamic–pituitary–gonadal axis by

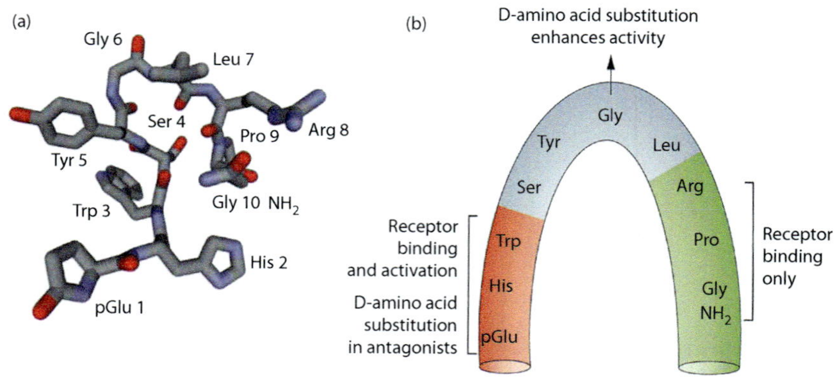

FIGURE 11.1 Amino acid sequence and structure of gonadotropin-releasing hormone. (From Kafarski P and Lipok M, Structural Analogy — Direct Similarity Versus Topographical Complementarity, in Vallisuta O and Olimat S, eds., *Drug Discovery and Development* , In Tech 2015, reproduced under Open License. Available from http://www.intechopen.com/books/drug-discovery-and-development-from-molecules-to-medicine/structural-analogy-direct-similarity-versus-topographical-complementarity.)

non-pulsatile release of GnRH and binding to the pituitary receptors. Use of these for 2–3 months before leiomyomectomy decreases estrogen and progesterone levels, causing decreased size of the benign fibroid growths. This leads to decreased operative risk and morbidity associated with the procedure. One recent Cochrane systematic review states there is no definitive recommendation for using "add-back therapy" along with GnRH agonists in this setting [12].

The mechanism of size reduction is postulated to be from ischemic necrosis due to the hypoestrogenic state induced by GnRH agonists. The decreased estrogen levels cause decreased blood flow and decreased abnormal uterine bleeding prior to surgery [16].

Studies have demonstrated a 35%–65% reduction in leiomyoma size after 3 months of GnRH-agonist therapy [9]. Leiomyoma location plays an important role in the resulting symptoms and determines the treatment approach. Increased fibroid protrusion into the uterine cavity results in increased blood loss [15]. The resulting anemia can be more quickly reversed with GnRH-agonist therapy followed by an interval myomectomy after a state of amenorrhea is induced and fibroid size is reduced [17].

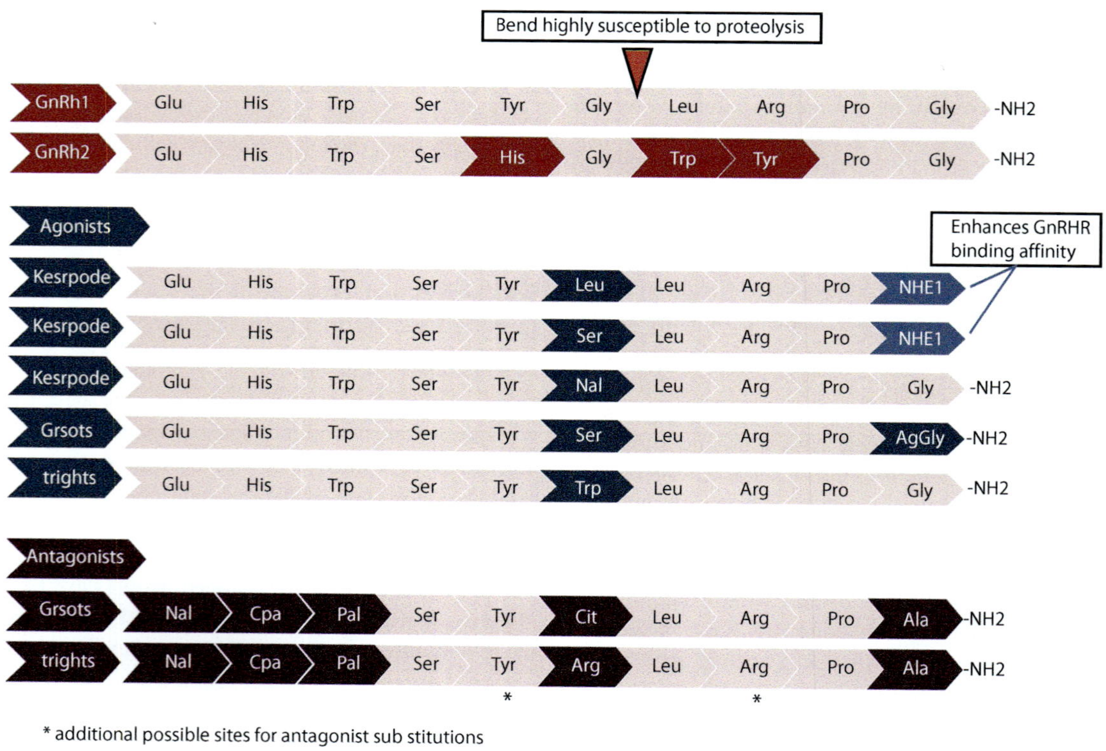

FIGURE 11.2 Comparison of the amino acid compositions of GnRH1 and GnRH2 with commonly used agonists and antagonists. Amino acid variations as compared with GnRH1 are color coded. Nal, napthyl-alanine; Aza-Gly, Aza-glycine (alpha carbon replaced with a nitrogen); CpA, cyanopropionic amino acid; Pal, pyridyl-alanine. (From Ehlers K, Halvorson L, Gonadotropin-releasing Hormone (GnRH) and the GnRH Receptor (GnRHR), in Arulkumaran S, ed., *Global Library of Women's Medicine* 2013, reproduced with permission. Available from http://resources.ama.uk.com/glowm_www/uploads/1359275965_Ch_5.8_fig_1.JPG.)

However, there is some evidence to suggest an increased recurrence of fibroids after myomectomy when patients are pretreated with GnRH agonists. In one clinical trial, 17 patients (14.4%) had symptomatic recurrence as early as 5 months to as late as 30 months postoperatively [18]. The symptomatic recurrence group had significantly higher preoperative GnRH use (35% vs. 9% nonrecurrence; $p = 0.009$). A total of 7.6% of all patients underwent reoperation. GnRH-agonist use was significantly higher in the reoperation group (56% vs. 9% no reoperation; $p = 0.002$).

In a prospective randomized multicenter clinical study, GnRH treatment before hysteroscopic resection of fibroids resulted in decreased operative time and reduction in absorbed fluid compared with no preoperative medical treatment in hysteroscopic resection [19]. Pretreatment also resulted in decreased difficulty of the procedure from the surgeon's perspective.

A systematic review and meta-analysis of pretreatment with GnRH agonists prior to laparoscopic myomectomy showed statistically significant decreases in intraoperative blood loss and postoperative hemoglobin drop, but no significant difference in operative time in those pretreated with GnRH agonists [20].

In another meta-analysis, GnRH-agonist pretreatment was shown to reduce preoperative pelvic symptoms and the need for a vertical skin incision [21]. Patients were also more likely to receive a vaginal procedure, without significant difference in postoperative complications when comparing with other preoperative treatments [21].

REFERENCES

1. Conn PM and Crowle WF, Jr. Gonadotropin-releasing hormone and its analogues. *N Engl J Med*. 1991;324(2):93–103.
2. Plant TM. 60 years of neuroendocrinology: The hypothalamo-pituitary-gonadal axis. *J Endocrinol*. 2015;226(2):T41–54.
3. Atkinson LE, Bhattacharya AN, Monroe SE et al. Effects of gonadectomy on plasma LH concentration in the rhesus monkey. *Endocrinology*. 1970;87(5):847–9.
4. Schally AV, Arimura A, Kastin AJ et al. Gonadotropin-releasing hormone: One polypeptide regulates secretion of luteinizing and follicle-stimulating hormones. *Science*. 1971;173(4001):1036–8.
5. Matsuo HY, Baba Y, Nair RG et al. Structure of the porcine LH- and FSH-releasing hormone. I. The proposed amino acid sequence. *Biochem Biophys Res Commun*. 1971;43(6):1334–9.
6. Kafarski P and Lipok M. Structural analogy — Direct similarity versus topographical complementarity, in Vallisuta O and Olimat S, eds., *Drug Discovery and Development* , In Tech 2015. Available from: http://www.intechopen.com/books/drug-discovery-and-development-from-molecules-to-medicine/structural-analogy-direct-similarity-versus-topographical-complementarity
7. Ehlers K and Halvorson L. *Gonadotropin-releasing hormone (GnRH) and the GnRH receptor (GnRHR)*, in Arulkumaran S, ed., *Global Library of Women's Medicine* 2013. Available from: http://resources.ama.uk.com/glowm_www/uploads/1359275965_Ch_5.8_fig_1.JPG
8. Karten MJ and Rivier JE. Gonadotropin-releasing hormone analog design. Structure-function studies toward the development of agonists and antagonists: Rationale and perspective. *Endocr Rev*. 1986;7(1):44–66.
9. Skorupskaite K, George JT, and Anderson RA. The kisspeptin-GnRH pathway in human reproductive health and disease. *Hum Reprod Update*. 2014;20(4):485–500.
10. Millar RP and Newton CL. Current and future applications of GnRH, kisspeptin and neurokinin B analogues. *Nat Rev Endocrinol*. 2013;9(8):451–66.
11. American College of Obstetricians and Gynecologists. Alternatives to hysterectomy in the management of leiomyomas. ACOG Practice Bulletin No. 96. *Obstet Gynecol*. 2008;112(2 Part 1):387–99.
12. Moroni RM, Martins WP, Ferriani RA et al. Add-back therapy with GnRH analogues for uterine fibroids. *Cochrane Database Syst Rev*. 2015;(3):CD010854.
13. Ishikawa H, Ishi K, Serna VA et al. Progesterone is essential for maintenance and growth of uterine leiomyoma. *Endocrinology*. 2010;151(6):2433–42.
14. Kim JJ and Sefton EC. The role of progesterone signaling in the pathogenesis of uterine leiomyoma. *Mol Cell Endocrinol*. 2012;358(2):223–31.
15. Cetin NN, Karabacak O, Korucuoglu U et al. Gonadotropin-releasing hormone analog combined with a low-dose oral contraceptive to treat heavy menstrual bleeding. *Int J Gynaecol Obstet*. 2009;104(3):236–9.
16. Grigoriadis C, Papaconstantinou E, Mellou A et al. Clinicopathological changes of uterine leiomyomas after GnRH agonist therapy. *Clin Exp Obstet Gynecol*. 2012;39(2):191–4.
17. Yang JH, Chen MJ, Chen CD et al. Impact of submucous myoma on the severity of anemia. *Fertil Steril*. 2011;95(5):1769–72 e1.
18. Sangha R, Katukuri V, Palmer M et al. Recurrence after robotic myomectomy: Is it associated with use of GnRH agonist? *J Robot Surg*. 2016;10(3):245–9.
19. Muzii L, Boni T, Bellati F et al. GnRH analogue treatment before hysteroscopic resection of submucous myomas: A prospective, randomized, multicenter study. *Fertil Steril*. 2010;94(4):1496–9.
20. Chen I, Motan T, and Kiddoo D. Gonadotropin-releasing hormone agonist in laparoscopic myomectomy: Systematic review and meta-analysis of randomized controlled trials. *J Minim Invasive Gynecol*. 2011;18(3):303–9.
21. Zhang Y, Sun L, Guo Y et al. The impact of preoperative gonadotropin-releasing hormone agonist treatment on women with uterine fibroids: A meta-analysis. *Obstet Gynecol Surv*. 2014;69(2):100–8.

12

GnRH Antagonists in the Treatment of Uterine Fibroids

Tejumola Adegoke and Shruthi Mahalingaiah

Introduction

Fibroids are the most common solid tumor of the female genital tract, occurring in up to 70% of reproductive-age women [1]. These benign monoclonal tumors are composed of smooth muscle and large amounts of extracellular matrix, arising via chromosomal abnormalities in a single smooth muscle cell followed by clonal expansion. Sex steroids and receptor expression likely play a significant role [2], as fibroids appear to respond to hormonal changes [3]. Common genetic disruptions in fibroids and the resulting changes in the uterine microenvironment are summarized in Figure 12.1.

Clinically significant fibroid disease occurs in up to 35% of Caucasian and 50% of African American women [11] and is the leading indication for hysterectomy. Gonadotropin-releasing hormone (GnRH) antagonists are currently under investigation as a nonsurgical option for the treatment of uterine fibroids, but have not become part of common practice.

Mechanism of Action

GnRH antagonists primarily function by competitive blockade, reversibly binding to GnRH receptors in the pituitary gland and causing an immediate (within 4–24 hours), dose-dependent, and rapidly reversible (24–72 hours) decrease in serum gonadotropins, with a greater suppression of luteinizing hormone (LH) compared with follicle stimulating hormone (FSH) [12–19]. The effects of GnRH antagonists on fibroids are illustrated in Figure 12.2.

Pharmacodynamics and Pharmacokinetics

GnRH antagonists have linear pharmacokinetics: their serum concentration increases proportionally with dose rate. Clearance is via hepatic metabolism; and excretion occurs through feces or urine. The plasma half-life of non-depot formulations ranges from 5 to 30 hours after administration of a single dose [14–16,24–26]. Table 12.1 depicts the structures of various GnRH antagonists.

Adverse Reactions and Contraindications

Adverse reactions to newer GnRH antagonists are rare and mild. They include injection site reactions (bruising, erythema, pruritus and swelling), nausea, headache, ovarian hyperstimulation syndrome, mood changes and decreased libido. Ganirelix (Antagon, Organon International) is associated with pelvic pain and vaginal bleeding [27]. Elevations of hepatobiliary enzymes were observed with use of cetrorelix acetate (Cetrotide; Serono) [28]. Use is contraindicated in anyone with known hypersensitivity to GnRH or GnRH analogues.

Pregnancy and Lactation

No effect on embryonic development has been detected in animal models, but use should be avoided in pregnant and breastfeeding women [29,30].

Literature Review

A literature search was performed of the PubMed, MedLine and Cochrane databases for English language articles related to fibroids and GnRH antagonists. Search terms used included "GnRH antagonist," "fibroid" and "leiomyoma." Studies included in this review are summarized in Table 12.2.

Prospective Cohort Studies

In the first study of its kind, Kettel et al. [31] administered daily subcutaneous Nal-Glu (50 μg/kg) to seven women with symptomatic fibroids for 3 months. Monthly ultrasound detected a 52.8% mean decrease in leiomyoma size that mostly occurred within the first month of therapy. The authors also noted rapid and persistent decreases in serum estradiol (E2), estrone and progesterone. Conversely, serum levels of FSH, LH, androstenedione, testosterone and dehydroepiandrosterone (DHEA) remained stable. Five patients subsequently underwent surgical removal of their fibroids. In the remaining two patients, leiomyomata returned to their original size within 1 month.

In 1997, Gonzalez-Barcena et al. [32] treated 18 premenopausal candidates for hysterectomy with cetrorelix for 3–10 months. Patients received 5 mg of subcutaneous cetrorelix twice daily for 2 days, followed by 0.8 mg twice daily. Serum LH, FSH and E2 were assessed on days 1, 3 and 5 of treatment and then monthly. Ultrasound examination illustrated a 39% reduction in mean uterine volume ($p < 0.001$) after 3 months of therapy and a 44% reduction ($p < 0.001$) by the end of the study. Thirteen women exhibited a clear decrease in uterine volume after just

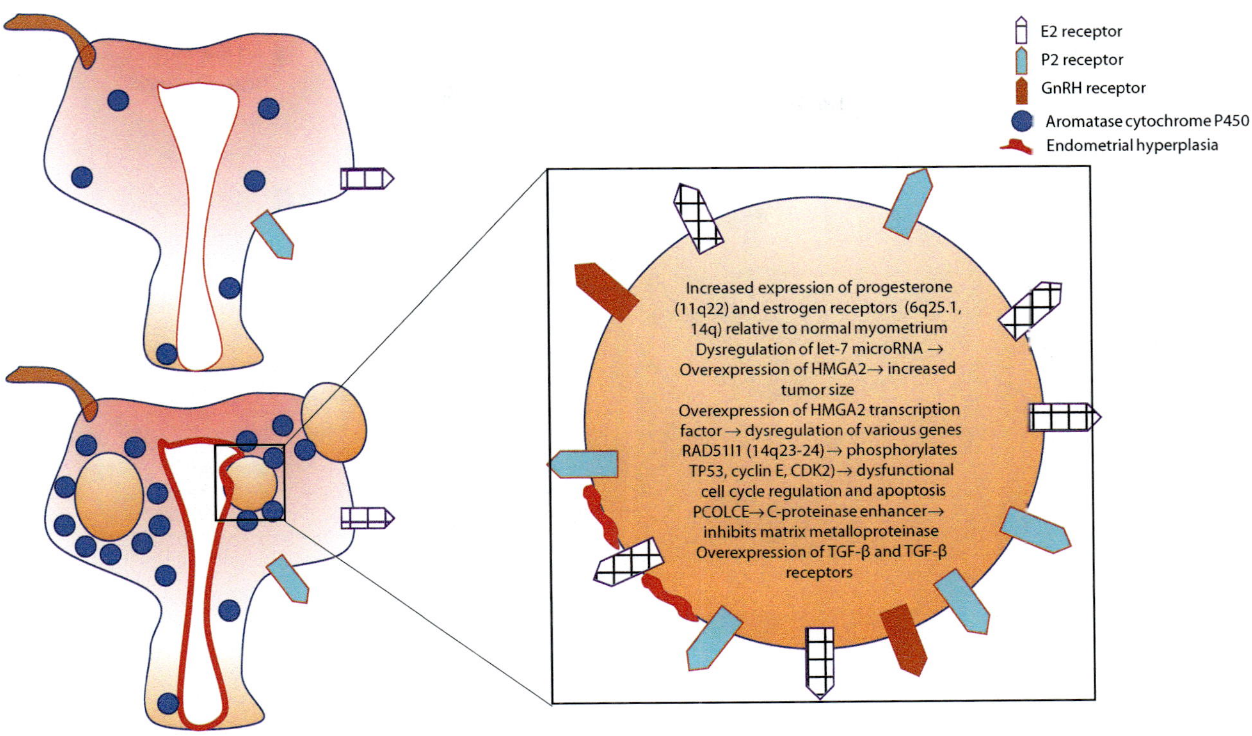

FIGURE 12.1 Top left: Normal uterus. Bottom left: Fibroid uterus. Myometrial cells contain binding sites for gonadotropin-releasing hormone [4]; and estrogen and progesterone receptors are expressed at higher levels in fibroids compared to normal myometrial tissue [5,6]. Elevated aromatase cytochrome p450 levels [7,8] and endometrial glandular hyperplasia in tissue adjacent to fibroids also suggest a surrounding hyperestrogenic environment [9]. Right: Uterine fibroid depicting expression of GnRH receptors, increased expression of estrogen and progesterone receptors and common genetic abnormalities associated with various fibroid characteristics [10].

1 month of treatment. One patient did not show any response to treatment for the first 3 months but achieved a 24% decrease in uterine volume after 8 months of continuous therapy. Another patient did not respond even after 10 months of treatment.

Timing of the initial cetrorelix dose (follicular phase vs. luteal phase) did not appear to affect the degree of uterine shrinkage. Most patients showed a progressive decrease in serum gonadotropins and estradiol to subnormal levels after the first dose of cetrorelix. However, four patients experienced decreases in uterine volume (mean 225 mL) after 3–4.5 months of treatment despite little or no depression in gonadotropin or estradiol levels. Twelve of fourteen patients who were anemic at the start of the study were observed to have normal hemoglobin levels after 3 months of treatment. Fifteen patients became amenorrheic. Among women who did not undergo hysterectomy, menstrual function returned 1 month after completion of treatment. Reported side effects included hot flashes, increased appetite and decreased libido. These resolved within 2 weeks of discontinuing therapy. Following treatment, three women underwent hysterectomy and 12 were treated with myomectomy. Repeat ultrasound illustrated a recurrence in one myomectomy patient and an increase in uterine volume (77 mL) in one patient who was expectantly managed.

Felberbaum et al. [33] used cetrorelix as an intermediate depot preparation prior to myomectomy. Ten premenopausal women received 3 mg of subcutaneous cetrorelix at 4-day intervals (days 1, 5, 9 and 13). Magnetic resonance imaging (MRI) was used to monitor fibroid size. Six patients had observable decreases in fibroid size, with a mean reduction of 31%, while three patients did not respond to treatment. Fibroid size could not be effectively assessed in one subject. All patients demonstrated sufficient pituitary downregulation. Myomectomy was performed after final MRI for all participants.

Flierman et al. [34] observed similar results with the use of ganirelix. Nineteen premenopausal women were treated using 2 mg daily, subcutaneous injections for a maximum of 12 weeks (median 19 days). Leiomyoma size and uterine volume were monitored using weekly ultrasound and pre- and post-treatment MRI. Serum LH, FSH, E2 and progesterone were assessed weekly. Treatment was discontinued when a 10% decrease in fibroid or uterine size was detected over four consecutive ultrasound measurements. For 11 subjects over 6 weeks, ultrasound revealed a median 42.7% (14%–77%) decrease in leiomyoma volume and a 46.6% (6.1%–78.6%) decrease in uterine volume. MRI revealed a median 29.2% (35.6%–62.2%) decrease in leiomyoma volume and a 25.2% (28.9%–63.6%) decrease in uterine volume. Six of these subjects noted a reduction in fibroid volume by one-third within 16 days of treatment. Serum LH and E2 levels dropped below limits of detection within 1 week in nearly all subjects. FSH and progesterone levels also remained low throughout treatment. Furthermore, the authors noted that tumor echogenicity changed with treatment. Of note, one patient had an increase in leiomyoma and uterine volume, in spite of decreasing estrogen levels. The most common reported side effects were hot flashes (75%) and headache (45%), though none were reported prior to week 3 of treatment. All participants underwent surgery within 2 weeks of their final dose of ganirelix.

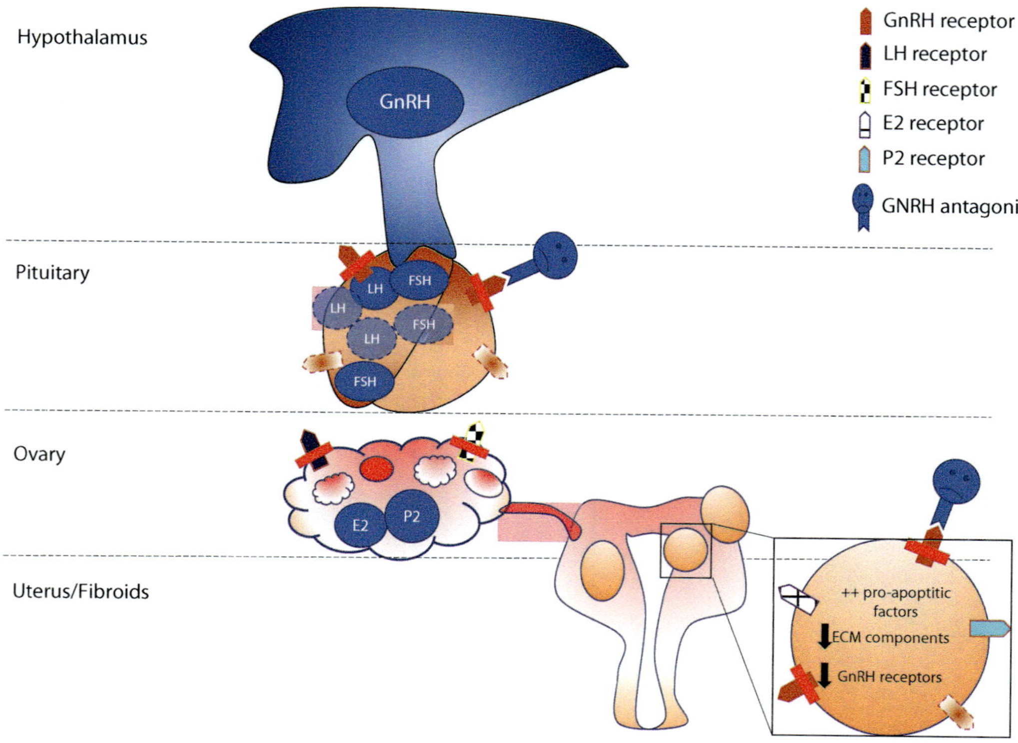

FIGURE 12.2 Gonadotropins secretion in the anterior pituitary is stimulated by GnRH. Gonadotropins LH (luteinizing hormone) and FSH (follicle-stimulating hormone) in turn stimulate production of estrogen and progesterone. GnRH antagonists reversibly bind to GnRH receptors and cause an immediate-dose-dependent decreases in LH and FSH, as well as a decrease in GnRH receptor expression. There is a resulting decrease in circulating estrogen and progesterone. They may also decrease the concentration of pituitary GnRH receptors [20]. *In vitro* studies suggest that GnRH antagonists also increase expression of pro-apoptotic factors in leiomyoma cells [21,22]; and downregulate gene expression of extracellular matrix components that modulate cell proliferation and leiomyoma bulk such as fibronectin and vesicant [23]. - - - - - Dashed lines signify receptor and hormone downregulation in the presence of GnRH antagonists. (red) indicates receptors with decreased activity following binding of GnRH antagonist.

Randomized Clinical Trials

Felberbaum et al. [12] performed a prospective randomized phase II trial of cetrorelix for preoperative treatment in twenty premenopausal patients. Each subject received 60 mg of intramuscular cetrorelix pamoate salt on day 2 of their menstrual cycle. Patients were then randomized to a second dose of either 30 or 60 mg of cetrorelix administered on day 21 in subjects with day 21 estradiol >50 pg/mL (n = 4), or on day 28. Outcome measures included weekly serum levels of gonadotropins, estradiol, progesterone, and cetrorelix. The authors also assessed volume of the 4 largest fibroids and the uterus using weekly transvaginal ultrasound and pre- and post-treatment MRI. Sixteen patients completed the study.

By the end of treatment, MRI fibroid volume decreased by an average of 25% and ultrasound volume decreased by 33.46%. Of note, by 2 weeks on treatment, the mean shrinkage was 31.3% by transvaginal ultrasound (TVUS). Mean reduction in fibroid size correlated positively with total cetrorelix dose: 20.5% ± 20% in subjects who received 90 mg versus 30.4% ± 15.2% in subjects given 120 mg. All 16 patients exhibited maximum LH suppression to <2 mIU/mL and estradiol suppression on day 7. Serum cetrorelix fell below levels required for pituitary suppression within 1 week of administration. There were no differences in uterine artery Doppler studies or leiomyoma estrogen-receptor expression between patients who demonstrated <20% decrease in fibroid or uterine volume compared with patients with a more dramatic response. Eight subjects reported hot flashes within the first 4 weeks. All subjects underwent surgical removal of their fibroids within 3 weeks of their final MRI.

In a double-blind randomized trial, Engel et al. [35] compared reduction in fibroid size in 109 premenopausal women treated with placebo (group 1), four weekly doses of 5 mg (group 2) or 10 mg of cetrorelix (group 3) and two doses of 10 mg every 14 days (group 4). MRI was performed at the beginning of the study and on day 29 of the treatment cycle. Pre- and post-treatment hemoglobin and hematocrit levels were also obtained. Among 107 patients who completed the study, the authors observed a mean decrease in uterine volume of 5.1% ± 32.1% in group 1, 15.6% ± 20.2% in group 2, 15.4% ± 34.6% in group 3 and 0.6% ± 30.6% in group 4. Fibroid volume decreased by 2%, 9.2%, 14.3% and 21.9%, respectively. "Significant response," defined as a decrease in uterine volume of at least 30%, occurred more often in group 4 compared with group 1 (42.3% vs. 11.1%, $p < 0.05$). Side effects included injection site reaction (two cases in treatment groups, one in the placebo group), hot flashes (two cases) and a single case of sleep disturbance. Hemoglobin levels did not significantly differ by treatment group, but showed a more favorable trend and were lower at the end of the study in group 4 compared with groups 2 and 3. The treatment groups also reported greater improvements

TABLE 12.1

Amino Acid Sequences of GnRH Antagonists

Name	Amino Acid Sequence
GnRH	pGlu-His-Trp-Ser-Tyr-Gly-Leu-Arg-Pro-Gly-NH_2
First Generation	
Substitution of His at position 2 and Trp at position 3 of the GnRH protein sequence.	
Hydrophilic, low potency, anaphylaxis	
4F Ant	NAc⊗1, 1Pro-D4FPhe-DTrp-Ser-Tyr-DTrp-Leu-Arg-Pro-GlyNH_2
Second Generation	
Substitution of D-arginine or other basic proteins at position 6.	
Higher potency, anaphylaxis	
Detirelix	NACD2Nal-D4ClPhe-pTrp-Ser-Tyr-DHarg(Et2)-Leu-Arg-Pro-DAlaNH_2
NalArg	NACD2Nal-D4lFPhe-pTrp-Ser-Tyr-DArg-Leu-Arg-Pro-GlyNH_2
Third Generation	
Substitution of neutral D-ureidoalkyl amino acids for D-Arg at position 6.	
Decreased allergenic effect	
Abarelix	NACD2Ala-D4ClPhe-DAla-Ser-Tyr-DAsp-Leu-Lys(iPr)-Pro-DAlaNH_2
Antarelix	NACD2Nal-D4ClPhe-D3Pal-Ser-Tyr-DHcit-Leu-Lys(Isp)-Pro-DAlaNH_2
Antide (Iturelix)	NACD2Nal-D4ClPhe-D3Pal-Ser-Lys(Nic)-DDLys(Nic)-Leu-Lys(Isp) Pro-DAlaNH_2
Azaline B	NACD2Nal-D4ClPhe-D3Pal-Ser-Aph(atz)-DAph(atz)-Leu-Lys(Isp)-Pro-DAlaNH_2
Cetrorelix	NACD2Nal-D4ClPhe-D3Pal-Ser-Tyr-DCit-Leu-Arg-Pro-DAlaNH_2
Ganirelix	NACD2Nal-D4ClPhe-D3Pal-Ser-Tyr-DHarg(Et2)-Leu-Hart(Et2)-Pro-DAlaNH_2
Org30850	NACD4ClPhe-D4ClPhe-DBal-Ser-Tyr-DLys-Leu-Arg-Pro-DAlaNH_2
Ramorelix	NACD2Nal-D4ClPhe-DTrp-Ser-Tyr-DSet(Rha)-Leu-Arg-Pro-AzaglyNH_2
NalGlu	NACD2Nal-D4C7Phe-D3Pal-Ser-Arg-DGlut(AA)-Leu-Arg-Pro-DAlaNH_2
Fourth Generation	
A-75998	NACD2-Nal-D4ClPhe-D3Pal-Ser-NMeTyr-DLys(Nic)-Leu-Lys(Isp)-Pro- DAlaNH_2
Ozarelix	AcD2Nal-D4Cpa-D3Pal-Ser-NMe-Tyr-DHciNleArg-Pro-DAlaNH_2

in symptoms of menorrhagia, dysmenorrhea, uterine pressure or pain and spotting compared with the placebo group.

Comparison to GnRH Agonists

GnRH agonists, such as leuprolide acetate (Lupron), activate the pituitary gland before they cause pituitary desensitization, leading to a gradual decline in estrogen levels after an initial stimulatory phase in which gonadotropin levels become supraphysiologic [36]. As a result, it may take 4–8 weeks to achieve the desired suppression with GnRH agonists [37]. Furthermore, fibroids tend to grow back to their original size within 3–6 months of discontinuing treatment.

Conversely, the literature indicates that GnRH antagonists induce near-immediate pituitary inhibition without initial stimulation. They thus avoid the associated vasomotor symptoms and exacerbation of hormone-sensitive disease. Furthermore, it appears that fibroid shrinkage can occur in the absence of gonadotropin suppression, suggesting that GnRH antagonists function through alternative mechanisms. The change in fibroid echogenicity observed by Flierman et al. [34] implies that these agents affect fibroid tissue composition as well as size. Their dose-dependent effect can be exploited to obtain the desired degree of suppression while avoiding the adverse effects of hypoestrogenism [34]. Lastly, significant decrease in uterine and fibroid size can be achieved with short courses of treatment and may be a superior alternative for short-term preoperative fibroid suppression.

Directions for Future Research

Fibroid and hormonal response to GnRH antagonists can vary widely between individual women [31]. It also appears that fibroid size may diminish in the absence of pituitary suppression, or continue to grow in a hypoestrogenic environment [32,34]. Further study may elucidate what factors, if any, predict treatment response. Additional investigation is needed to understand alterative pathways through which these agents affect fibroid size and/or tissue composition.

Currently available formulations of GnRH antagonists are injectable. Two orally administered GnRH antagonists, elagolix sodium (elagolix) and TAK-385 (Relugolix) have not yet been tested for treatment of fibroids but seem well-tolerated for other conditions [38,39]. Innovations in GnRH antagonists include trials of oral nonpeptide formulations.

Lastly, fibroids create significant surgical burden, with over 200,000 hysterectomies performed for this indication in 2010 [40]. The results of at least one study [32] suggest that treatment with GnRH antagonists may eliminate or delay the need for surgery. Further research is required to determine the duration and frequency of long-term suppressive effects and the side effects of

TABLE 12.2

GnRH Antagonist Literature

Authors/Agonist	N[a]	Dose/Duration	Results
Prospective Cohort Studies			
Kettle et al. [31] Nal-Glu	7	50 μg/kg daily 3 months	52.8% ± 7.3% reduction in mean fibroid size after 1 month Decrease in serum estradiol, estrone, progesterone No change in serum FSH, LH, androstenedione, testosterone, DHEA Return to original size within one month in patients who did not undergo surgical removal
Gonzales-Barcena [32] Cetrorelix acetate	18	5 mg twice daily 2 days, 0.8 mg twice daily 3–10 months	39% reduction in mean uterine volume after 3 months ($p < 0.001$) 44% reduction in mean uterine volume after treatment ($p < 0.001$) Normalization of hemoglobin in 12 of 14 participants with anemia after 3 month Persistent decrease in uterine size in 11 of 12 patients who underwent myomectomy after therapy
Felberbaum et al. [33] Cetrorelix acetate	9	3 mg on days 1, 5, 9, 13 28 days	31% ± 19.53% mean reduction in fibroid size in 6 patients 3 patients with no response to therapy (stable or increased uterine volume) 1 patient excluded for unreliable measurements Sustained reduction in FSH, LH, estradiol, progesterone
Flierman et al. [34] Ganirelix acetate	19	2 mg daily ≤12 weeks[b]	42.7% median decrease in fibroid volume, 46.6% decrease in uterine volume by ultrasound 29.2% decrease in fibroid volume, 25.2% decrease in uterine volume by MRI
Randomized Controlled Studies			
Felberbaum et al. [12] Cetrorelix Acetate	16	All groups	33.46% ± 7% mean reduction in fibroid volume, mostly in the initial 14 days of study duration. LH suppression for 14 days, FSH suppression for 21 days. Estradiol and progesterone suppression (nadir on day 7)
	8	60 mg/30 mg day 2 & day 21/28	20.5% ± 20% mean reduction in fibroid volume
	8	60 mg/60 mg day 2 & day 21/28	30.4% ± 15.2% mean reduction in fibroid volume
Engel et al. [35] Cetrorelix acetate	27	Placebo[c] weekly 4 weeks	5.1% ± 32.1% mean decrease in uterine volume 2% decrease in fibroid volume
	25	5 mg weekly 4 weeks	15.6% ± 20.2% mean decrease in uterine volume 9.2% decrease in fibroid volume
	29	10 mg weekly 4 weeks	15.4% ± 34.6% mean decrease in uterine volume 14.3% decrease in fibroid volume 42.3% significant response[d] compared to placebo (11.1%), $p = 0.014$
	26	10 mg days 1 & 15	0.6% ± 30.6% mean decrease in uterine volume 21.9% decrease in uterine volume

[a]Number of participants included in analysis.
[b]Treatment continued until 4 consecutive measurements showed a <10% decrease or treatment discontinued at 12 weeks.
[c]Mannitol lyophilisate.
[d]Significant response defined by authors as >30% reduction in uterine size by MRI from day 2 to day 29.

long-term use. More randomized and sufficiently powered studies comparing different antagonists and dosing regimens, with representation from multiple ethnicities, are needed to ascertain the most effective treatment protocols.

REFERENCES

1. Baird DD, Dunson DB, Hill MC, Cousins D, and Schectman JM. High cumulative incidence of uterine leiomyoma in black and white women: Ultrasound evidence. *Am J Obstet Gynecol.* 2003 January;188(1):100–7.
2. Pollow K, Geilfuss J, Boquoi E, and Pollow B. Estrogen and progesterone binding proteins in normal human myometrium and leiomyoma tissue. *J Clin Chem Clin Biochem.* 1978 September;16(9):503–11.
3. Frankel T and Benjamin F. (1975) Rapid enlargement of a uterine fibroid after clomiphene therapy. *J Obstet Gynaecol Br Commonw.* 1973 August;80(8):764–5.
4. Wiznitzer A, Marbach M, Hazum E, Insler V, Sharoni Y, and Levy J. Gonadotropin-releasing hormone specific binding sites in uterine leiomyomata. *Biochem Biophys Res Commun.* 1998 May;152(3):1326–31.
5. Rein MS, Friedman AJ, Stuart JM, MacLaughlin DT. Fibroid and myometrial steroid receptors in women treated with gonadotropin-releasing hormone agonist leuprolide acetate. *Fertil Steril*;1990 June;53(6):1018–23.
6. Nisolle M, Gillerot S, Casanas-Roux F, Squifflet J, Berliere M, and Donnez J. Immunohistochemical study of the proliferation index, oestrogen receptors and progesterone receptors A and B in leiomyomata and normal myometrium during the menstrual cycle and under gonadotrophin-releasing hormone agonist therapy. *Hum Reprod.* 1999 November;14(11):2844–50.
7. Folkerd EJ, Newton CJ, Davidson K, Anderson MC, and James VH. Aromatase activity in uterine leiomyomata. *J Steroid Biochem.* 1984 May;20(5):1195–200.
8. Bulun SE, Simpson ER, and Word RA. Expression of the CYP19 gene and its product aromatase cytochrome P450 in human uterine leiomyoma tissues and cells in culture. *J Clin Endocrinol Metab.* 1999 March;78(3):736–43.
9. Deligdish L and Loewenthal M. Endometrial changes associated with myomata of the uterus. *J Clin Pathol.* 1970 November;23(8):676–80.
10. Medikare V. Kandukuri LR, Anathapur V, Deendayal M, and Nallari P. The genetic bases of uterine fibroids; A review. *J Reprod Inferil.* 2011 July–September;12(3):181–91.
11. Cramer SF and Patel A. The frequency of uterine leiomyomas. *Am J Clin Pathol.* 1990 October;94(4):435–8.
12. Felberbaum, RE, Germer U, Ludwig M et al. Treatment of uterine fibroids with a slow-release formulation of the gonadotrophin releasing hormone antagonist Cetrorelix. *Human Reprod.* 1998 June;13(6):1660–8.
13. Reismman T, Felberbaum R, Diedrich K, Engel J, Comary-Schally AM, and Schally AV. Development and applications of luteinizing hormone-releasing hormone antagonists in the treatment of infertility. *Hum Reprod.* 1995 Aug ust;10(8):1974–81.
14. Erb K, Klipping C, Dujkers I, Pechstein B, Schueler A, and Hermann R. Pharmacodynamic effects and plasma pharmacokinetics of single doses of cetrorelix acetate in healthy premenopausal women. *Fertil Steril.* 2001 February;75(2):316–23.
15. Oberyé JJ, Mannaerts BM, Kleijn HJ, and Timmer CJ. Pharmacokinetic and pharmacodynamics characteristics of ganirelix (Antagon/Orgalutran). Part I. Absolute bioavailability of 0.25 mg of ganirelix after a single subcutaneous injection in healthy female volunteers. *Fertil Steril.* 1999 December;72(6):1001–5.
16. Oberyé JJ, Mannaerts BM, Huisman JA, and Timmer CJ. Pharmacokinetic and pharmacodynamics characteristics of ganirelix (Antagon/Orgalutran). Part II. Dose-proportionality and gonadotropin suppression after multiple doses of ganirelix in healthy female volunteers. *Fertil Steril.* 1999 December;72(6):1006–12.
17. Tomera K, Gleason D, Gittleman M et al. The gonadotropin-releasing hormone antagonist abarelix depot versus luteinizing hormone releasing hormone agonists leuprolide or goserelin: Initial results of endocrinological and biochemical efficacies in patients with prostate cancer. *J Urol.* 2001 May;165(5):1585–9.
18. Sommer L, Zanger K, Dyong T et al. Seven-day administration of the gonadotropin-releasing hormone antagonist Cetrorelix in normal cycling women. *Eur J Endocrinol.* 1994 September; 131(3):280–5.
19. Couzinet B, Lahlou N, Thomas G et al. Effects of gonadotrophin releasing hormone antagonist and agonist on the pulsatile release of gonadotrophins and alpha-subunit in postmenopausal women. *Clin Endocrinol (Oxf).* 1991 June;34(6):477–83.
20. Halmos G, Schally AV, Pinski J, Vadilo-Buenfil M, and Groot K. Down-regulation of pituitary receptors for luteinizing hormone-releasing hormone (LH-RH) in rats by LH-RH antagonist Cetrorelix. *Proc Natl Acad Sci USA.* 1996 March;93(6):2398–402.
21. Kwon JY, Park KH, Park YN, and Cho NH. Effect of cetrorelix acetate on apoptosis and apoptosis regulatory factors in cultured uterine leiomyoma cells. *Fertil Steril.* 2005 November;84(5):1526–8.
22. Chen W, Yoshida S, Ohara N, Matsuo H, Morizane M, and Maruo T. Gonadotropin-releasing hormone antagonist cetrorelix down-regulates proliferating cell nuclear antigen and epidermal growth factor expression and up-regulates apoptosis in association with enhanced poly(adenosine 5'-diphosphate-ribose) polymerase expression in cultured human leiomyoma cells. *J Clin Endocrinol Metab.* 2005 February;90(2):884–92.
23. Britten JL, Malik M, Levy G, Mendoza, M, and Catherino WH. Gonadotropin-releasing hormone (GnRH) agonist leuprolide acetate and GnRH antagonist cetrorelix acetate directly inhibit leiomyoma extracellular matrix production. *Fertil Steril.* 2012 November;98(5):1299–307.
24. Huirne JA and Lambalk CB. Gonadotropin-releasing-hormone antagonists. *Lancet.* 2001 November;358(9295):1793–803.
25. Duijkers IJM, Klipping C, Willemsen WNP, Krone D, Schneider E, Niebch G, and Hermann R. Single and multiple dose pharmacokinetics and pharmacodynamics of the gonadotrophin-releasing hormone antagonist Cetrorelix in healthy female volunteers. *Human Reproduction.* 1998;13(9):2392–8.
26. Wong, SL, Lau DTW, Baughman SA, Fotheringham N, Menchaca D, and Garnick M. Pharmacokineticsa and Pharmacodynamics of a novel depot formulation of abarelix, a gonadotropin-releasing hormone (GnRH) antagonists, in healthy men ages 50 to 75. *J Clin Pharmacol.* 2004;44:495–502.
27. *Ganirelix Acetate Injection [Prescribing Information]. Whitehouse Station.* NJ: Merck & Co, August 2015.

28. Cetrotide® 0.25 mg [Internet]. Place unknown. Available from: http://tinyurl.com/zgwhzbd
29. Anon. Ganirelix acetate GnRH antagonist treatment of female infertility. *Drugs Future.* 2000;24:3939–403.
30. Anon. Cetrorelix, LHRH antagonist. *Drugs Future.* 1994;19:228–37.
31. Kettel LM, Murphy AA, Morales AJ, River J, Vale W, and Yen SS. Rapid regression of uterine leiomyomas in response to daily administration of gonadotropin-releasing hormone antagonist. *Fertil Steril.* 1993 October;60(4):642–6.
32. Gonzalez-Barcena D, Alvarea RB, Ochoa EP et al. Treatment of uterine leiomyomas with luteinizing-hormone releasing hormone antagonist Cetrorelix. *Hum Reprod.* 1997 September;12(9):2028–35.
33. Felberbaum RE, Kupker W, Krapp M, Gehl B, Ludwig M, and Diedrich K. Preoperative reduction of uterine fibroids in only 16 days by administration of a gonadotrophin-releasing hormone antagonist (Cetrotide). *Reprod Biomed Online.* 2001;3(1):14–8.
34. Flierman PA, Oberyé JJ, van der Hulst VP, and de Blok S. Rapid reduction of leiomyoma volume during treatment with the GnRH antagonist ganirelix. *BJOG.* 2005 May;112(5):638–42.
35. Engel JB, Audebert A, Frydman R, Zivny J, and Diedrich K. Presurgical short term treatment of uterine fibroids with different doses of cetrorelix acetate: A double-blind, placebo-controlled multicenter study. *Eur J Obstet Gynecolo Reprod Biol.* 2007 October;134(2):225–32.
36. Lemay A, Maheux R, Faure N, Jean C, and Fazekas AT. Reversible hypogonadism induced by a luteinizing hormone-releasing hormone (LH-RH) agonist (Buserelin) as a new therapeutic approach for endometriosis. *Fertil Steril.* 1984 June;41(6):863–71.
37. Letterie, GS, Coddington, CC, Winkel CA, Shawker, TH, Loriaux DP, and Collins RL. Efficacy of a gonadotropin-releasing hormone antagonist in the treatment of uterine leiomyomata: Long-term follow-up. *Fertil Steril.* 1998 June;51(6):951–6.
38. Struthers RS, Nicholls AJ, Grundy J, Chen T, Jimenez R, Yen SS, and Bozigian HP. Suppression of gonadotropins and estradiol in premenopausal women by oral administration of the nonpeptide gonadotropin-releasing hormone antagonist elagolix. *J Clin Endocrinol Metab.* 2009 February;94(2):545–51.
39. MacLean D, Shi H, Faessel H, and Saad F. Medical castration using the investigational oral GnRH antagonist TAK-385 (Relugolix): Phase 1 study in healthy males. *J Clin Endocrinol Metab.* 2015 December;100(12):4579–87.
40. Wright JD, Herzog TJ, Tsui J et al. Nationwide trends in the performance of inpatient hysterectomy in the United States. *Obstet Gynecol.* 2013 August;122(2 Pt 1):233–41.

13

Role of Aromatase Inhibitors (AIs) and Selective Estrogen Receptor Modulators (SERMs) in the Treatment of Uterine Leiomyoma

Luis S. Noble and Diego Ramirez

Aromatase Inhibitors (AIs)

Background

Estrogen dependence is unquestionably the common denominator among uterine leiomyoma, endometriosis, adenomyosis and endometrial polyps. 17-β estradiol (E2) stimulates the growth and maintenance of these uterine and endometrial disorders. Uterine leiomyoma's estrogen dependence is well understood; however, the intricate molecular mechanisms involving cell division under estrogen representation is complicated, to say the least. Decreased apoptosis and increased rate of mitosis-stimulated cell division have been documented under estrogen influence; moreover, progesterone's stimulation of the Kruppel-like transcription factor 11 (KLF11) has been implicated as another of the molecular-mediated effects of E2 as well as progesterone [1–3].

E2 is primarily supplemented to uterine leiomyoma from the circulation of ovarian origin, stimulating the growth and simultaneously increasing the secretion of vascular endothelial growth factor (VEGF) by the myoma cells, which in turn enhances the delivery of estrogen in a refined synchronized fashion, promoting leiomyoma growth and maintenance.

Bulun and Word et al. in 1994 described the expression of the CYP19 gene and its product aromatase cytochrome P450 (P450arom) in uterine leiomyoma. The presence of P450arom transcripts were also identified in myometria adjacent to the leiomyoma, whereas the expression of P450arom was absent in disease-free myometrium, describing for the first time the inherent ability of uterine leiomyoma to locally synthesize estrone (E1) from circulating androstenedione. P450arom catalyzes the conversion of circulating C19 steroids to estrogens and is expressed physiologically in many human cells such as ovarian granulosa cells, syncytiothrophoblast of the placenta, testicular Leydig cells and adipose tissue [4]. The aberrant expression of aromatase in uterine leiomyoma and adjacent myometrium, as well as endometriosis and endometrial cancer, is stimulated by cAMP-dependent signaling pathway using primarily promoter II of the CYP19 gene, which is exactly the same ovarian promoter for P450arom expression [4–7].

The role of *in situ* E1 and possibly E2 production could promote tumor growth in a paracrine, autocrine or potentially intracrine fashion. In addition, E2 representation via increased estrogen and progesterone receptors has been well documented in uterine leiomyoma [8–10]. In simplistic terms, these neoplasms have immense resources to sustain accelerated growth under E2 influence.

Aromatase Inhibitor (AI) Types and Generation

There are only a few medical treatments for uterine leiomyoma that are proved to be effective. The data supporting the use of aromatase inhibitors (AIs) are scant; however, some of the results are promising. Aromatase inhibition can be accomplished by two subclasses of compounds: the ones that form an irreversible bound to aromatase (exemestane) and the ones that have reversible competition such as letrozole and anastrazole [11]. There are three generations of aromatase inhibitors (Table 13.1). Anastrazole and letrozole are the most commonly used in clinical practice, resulting in 98%–99% suppression of aromatase activity [11].

Clinical Evidence of the use of AIs in Uterine Fibroids

Hilário et al. treated 20 premenopausal patients using anastrazole 1 mg/day for 12 weeks, resulting in a decrease of 9.2% of uterine volume and 32% reduction in symptoms (menstrual duration and dysmenorrhea). They also reported no alterations in gonadotropin measurements, and group concluded that the use of anastrazole was effective; however, it was inferior to GnRH analogues [12]. In another study, Parsanezhad et al. randomized 70 premenopausal women who had a single fibroid 5 cm or greater to treatment with either letrozole 2.5 mg a day or the gonadotropin release-hormone analogue (GnRHa) triptorelin (3.75 mg/month) for 12 weeks. They observed a statistically significant reduction in leiomyoma size in the letrozole group compared with the triptorelin (46% vs. 33%). In addition, serum E2 levels were significantly reduced in the triptorelin arm compared with letrozole; they concluded that there was rapid onset of action of the aromatase inhibitor with the avoidance of the initial flare associated with GnRH analogues [13]. In another study, Gurates et al. treated 16 premenopausal women with uterine leiomyoma measuring 2 cm or greater using a higher dose of letrozole (5 mg daily) for 3 months, resulting in a 47% reduction in uterine leiomyoma size compared with baseline and a mean volume reduction of uterine size of 22%

TABLE 13.1 Aromatase Inhibitors Type

Type 1: Irreversible bound (steroidal)		**Type 2**: Competitive inhibition (nonsteroidal)
Generation:		
1st		Aminoglutethemide
2nd		Fadrazole, Formestane
3rd	Exemestane	Anastrazole, Letrozole, Vorozole

[14]. In this particular study, the mean FSH and LH levels were noted to be statistically higher as the treatment advanced with a significant decrease in serum E2 levels [14]. In addition, there was a significant reduction in blood loss after 3 months of treatment, with no apparent effect on lumbar bone density measurements compared to baseline [14]. Shozu et al. presented a case report in a perimenopausal woman with large uterine fibroids and urinary retention where they used fadrozole 2 mg daily for 8 weeks followed by 1 mg for 4 weeks, resulting in a significant improvement of symptoms and a volume reduction of 71% at 12 weeks [15].

GnRHa use has been the gold standard in treating uterine leiomyoma; these agents have been shown to provide a significant reduction in uterine size of 35%–65% [16]. GnRHa use has significant side effects derived from hypoestrogenism, including hot flashes, amenorrhea and significant bone loss with prolonged use. In contrast, based on the previously presented evidence, AIs have been shown to have a similar reduction in uterine volumes and leiomyoma size compared with GnRHa without the initial flare associated with GnRHa and secondary bone loss. The rapid onset of action (decreased E2 levels) of AIs may be advantageous over GnRHa. There are many questions that remain to be answered by further studies using AIs in the arena of pre-surgical treatment or as adjuvants to GnRHa; for example, using AIs for the first 4 weeks in order to minimize the flare of GnRHa, continuation of AIs to shorten the treatment of GnRHa or combining AIs with progestational agents for long-term use.

In conclusion, the results of the studies using AIs appear to be promising; however, further randomized studies are necessary to establish its indications in the treatment of uterine leiomyoma.

Selective Estrogen Receptor Modulators (SERMs)

Currently selective estrogen receptor modulators (SERMs) are more frequently used for the treatment of osteoporosis and breast cancer, with documented proven benefits [17]. Early generation SERMs such as clomiphene citrate have been used for ovulation induction in polycystic ovarian syndrome (PCOS) related infertility. Newer SERM therapies have been developed for the treatment of postmenopausal vasomotor symptoms in patients with an intact uterus and are also indicated in the treatment of vaginal atrophy and dyspareunia associated with hypoestrogenism. Most of the estrogen representation is mediated by either estrogen receptor (ER)-α or ERβ receptors [17–19]. SERMs are chemically diverse nonsteroidal compounds that belong to one of two different chemical families: the triphenylethylenes and the benzothiophenes, with the exception of fulvestran (downregulator) that acts on the ligand binding domain (LBD) located in the ER carboxyl-terminal site, causing conformational changes which facilitate interactions as a co-activator or co-repressor proteins, and subsequently initiate or suppress the transcription of target genes [17–19]. Different types of SERMs can have both agonist and antagonist action in different target tissues; for example, tamoxifen has agonist action on bone and is an antagonist on the breast ERs and, in addition, it can also have an agonist effect on endometrial tissue.

The available components of SERMs being used today are summarized in Table 13.2.

TABLE 13.2 Summay of Available Components of SERMs Being Used Today

SERM	Clinical Data	Bone	Breast	Endometrium
Tamoxifen	Invasive breast cancer risk reduction 49% vs. placebo. Endometrial CA risk vs. placebo (RR 2.53 95% CI 1.35–4.97) [20]	Agonist	+antagonist	Agonist
Clomiphene	Antiestrogenic effect mostly in the hypothalamus, clinical indication is infertility [19].	Agonist	N/A	+antagonist
Raloxifene	Increases bone density, lowers LDL, no significant effect on the endometrium vs. controls [21], no increased risks of endometrial CA (RR 0.8 95% CI 0.2–2.7), reduced invasive breast cancer risk (RR 0.35 95% CI 0.21–0.58 vs. placebo) [20].	Agonist	++antagonist	+antagonist
Basedoxifene	No increase in endometrial thickness or endometrial CA risk. Blocked stimulatory effects of estradiol or conjugated estrogen (CE) in MCF7 cells [20].	Agonist	+++antagonist	++antagonist
Ospemifene	Increased uterine weight in rats, despite *in vitro* antagonist effects in the endometrium [20]. Agonist effect in vaginal epithelium [20,22]	Agonist	++antagonist	+ antagonist
Arzoxifene	Only in breast, no advantage over tamoxifen. Preclinical data showing atrophy in rat's endometrium [20].	Agonist	+antagonist	+antagonist
Fulvestran Steroidal antiestrogen	Use in tamoxifen-resistant breast cancer [18,20]. A powerful antiestrogen, binding with high affinity to the ER, without agonist effect [18].	N/A	++++antagonist	+++antagonist

Impact of SERM Agonists and Antagonists on Breast, Endometrium, and Bone

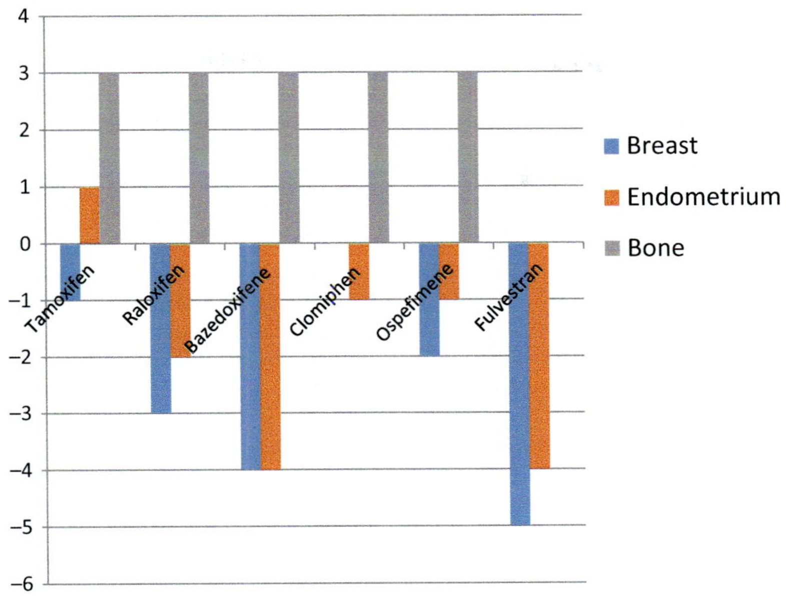

SERM agonist +/antagonist −

Clinical Evidence of the Use of SERMs in Uterine Leiomyoma

There is very limited experience in the use of SERMs as a treatment for uterine leiomyoma, with a few trials showing modest benefits and others not showing any additional advantages, either as a single agent or add-back therapy to a GnRH agonist.

Clomiphene citrate has not been fully studied for the treatment of uterine leiomyoma; in one case report, a significant growth of a single leiomyoma was observed during treatment with this particular SERM [23]. Tamoxifen has also been largely avoided owing to its known agonist effect on the uterus/leiomyomas. On the other hand, because of its biological effects and pharmacologic characteristics (please refer to Table 13.2), raloxifene has been the preferred choice among SERMs for the medical treatment of uterine leiomyoma.

In postmenopausal women, Palomba et al. conducted a pilot study in 2002 that included 90 asymptomatic postmenopausal patients with uterine leiomyoma and divided them into three different arms: one group was treated with 60 mg of raloxifene daily, a second group used 180 mg daily and the third groups was a placebo group. They were treated for a total of six 28-day cycles, without any significant statistical difference in leiomyoma size among the three groups [24]. In 2005, this same group conducted a prospective, randomized, double-blinded, placebo-controlled study that included 40 postmenopausal women selected for hysterectomy. They were randomized into two groups: one treated with raloxifene for a total of three cycles of 28 days each using a dose of 180 mg/day versus a placebo group. They concluded that after treatment, there was a statistically significant decrease in both uterine volume and leiomyoma size in the raloxifene group compared with baseline and placebo groups. After treatment, decrease in uterine and leiomyoma volumes were -11.8 ± 6.3 cm^3 and -17.4 ± 6.1 cm^3, respectively, in the raloxifene group, and 1.6 ± 0.9 cm^3 and 1.9 ± 1.1 cm^3, respectively, in the placebo group. In addition, after hysterectomy, they studied the proliferation and apoptotic indexes for the raloxifene and placebo groups. Leiomyoma cells and adjacent myometrial cells revealed evidence of antiproliferative and apoptotic effects in the raloxifene-treated group [22]. These studies summarize the limited experience in treating postmenopausal women with SERMs.

In premenopausal women, Jirecek et al., in 2004, performed a prospective, randomized, open, controlled trial with 25 premenopausal women with uterine leiomyomas, 13 of them treated with 180 mg of raloxifene a day for a total of 3 months versus a control group of 12 women with similar clinical characteristics without any medical intervention. They measured the volume of leiomyomas at 1 and 3 months via ultrasonography. In the raloxifene group, there was a statistically significant decrease in volume of 22.2% at the 3-month interval versus no significant changes in the control group [25]. In addition, Palomba et al., in 2002, performed a prospective, single-blind, randomized, placebo-controlled trial evaluating the role of raloxifene in combination with a GnRH analogue in 100 premenopausal women, utilizing leuprolide acetate in combination with 60 mg of raloxifene and a control group using only leuprolide acetate with a placebo tablet. After six 28-day cycles, a statistically significant difference in leiomyoma volume and size between the groups was observed compared with baseline; however, there was not any significant difference in GnRH vasomotor-related symptoms [26].

In conclusion, the data on the use of SERMs in both premenopausal and postmenopausal women with uterine leiomyoma are scant, and more studies are needed to establish a clear role of these agents in the medical management of uterine leiomyomas, perhaps utilizing the new-generation SERMs. It appears that there may be a significant improvement in leiomyoma size with the use of raloxifene; however, the evidence suggests the use of higher doses (180 mg/day) in order to be effective. Although significant adverse reactions were not reported in any of these studies, it is important to be aware of the potential serious side effects of this medication at this dosage, such as thromboembolic phenomena specifically in postmenopausal patients. Furthermore, the use of raloxifene in combination with a GnRH analogue did not reveal improvement in symptomatology associated with hypoestrogenism during treatment.

REFERENCES

1. Yin P, Lin Z, Cheng YH et al. Progesterone receptor regulates Bcl-2 gene expression through direct binding to its promoter region in uterine leiomyoma cells. *J Clin Endocrinol Metab.* 2007;92(11):4459–66.
2. Matsuo H, Maruo T, Samoto T. Increased expression of Bcl-2 protein in human uterine leiomyoma and its up-regulation by progesterone. *J Clin Endocrinol Metab.* 1997;82(1):293–9.
3. Xu Q, Takekida S, Ohara N et al. Progesterone receptor modulator CDB-2914 down-regulates proliferative cell nuclear antigen and Bcl-2 protein expression and up-regulates caspase-3 and poly(adenosine 5′-diphosphate-ribose) polymerase expression in cultured human uterine leiomyoma cells. *J Clin Endocrinol Metab.* 2005;90(2):953–61.
4. Bulun SE, Simpson ER, and Word RA. Expression of the CYP19 gene and its product aromatase cytochrome P450 in human uterine leiomyoma tissues and cells in culture. *J Clin Endocrinol Metab.* 1994;78(3):736–43.
5. Noble LS, Simpson ER, Johns A, and Bulun SE. Aromatase expression in endometriosis. *J Clin Endocrinol Metab.* 1996;81(1):174–9.
6. Bulun SE, Zeitoun KM, Takayama K, and Sasano H. Molecular basis for treating endometriosis with aromatase inhibitors. *Hum Reprod Update.* 2000;6(5):413–8.
7. Noble LS, Takayama K, Zeitoun KM et al. Prostaglandin E2 stimulates aromatase expression in endometriosis-derived stromal cells. *J Clin Endocrinol Metab.* 1997;82(2):600–6.
8. Brandon DD, Bethea CL, Strawn EY et al. Progesterone receptor messenger ribonucleic acid and protein are overexpressed in human uterine leiomyomas. *Am J Obstet Gynecol.* 1993;169(1):78–85.
9. Brandon DD, Erickson TE, Keenan EJ et al. Estrogen receptor gene expression in human uterine leiomyomata. *J Clin Endocrinol Metab.* 1995;80(6):1876–81.
10. Viville B, Charnock-Jones DS, Sharkey AM, Wetzka B, and Smith SK. Distribution of the A and B forms of the progesterone receptor messenger ribonucleic acid and protein in uterine leiomyomata and adjacent myometrium. *Hum Reprod.* 1997;12(4):815–22.
11. Song H, Lu D, Navaratnam K, and Shi G. Aromatase inhibitors for uterine fibroids. *Cochrane Database Syst Rev.* 2013(10):CD009505.
12. Hilario SG, Bozzini N, Borsari R, and Baracat EC. Action of aromatase inhibitor for treatment of uterine leiomyoma in perimenopausal patients. *Fertil Steril.* 2009;91(1):240–3.
13. Parsanezhad ME, Azmoon M, Alborzi S et al. A randomized, controlled clinical trial comparing the effects of aromatase inhibitor (letrozole) and gonadotropin-releasing hormone agonist (triptorelin) on uterine leiomyoma volume and hormonal status. *Fertil Steril.* 2010;93(1):192–8.
14. Gurates B, Parmaksiz C, Kilic G, Celik H, Kumru S, and Simsek M. Treatment of symptomatic uterine leiomyoma with letrozole. *Reprod Biomed Online.* 2008;17(4):569–74.
15. Shozu M, Murakami K, Segawa T, Kasai T, and Inoue M. Successful treatment of a symptomatic uterine leiomyoma in a perimenopausal woman with a nonsteroidal aromatase inhibitor. *Fertil Steril.* 2003;79(3):628–31.
16. Carr BR, Marshburn PB, Weatherall PT et al. An evaluation of the effect of gonadotropin-releasing hormone analogs and medroxyprogesterone acetate on uterine leiomyomata volume by magnetic resonance imaging: A prospective, randomized, double blind, placebo-controlled, crossover trial. *J Clin Endocrinol Metab.* 1993;76(5):1217–23.
17. Dutertre M and Smith CL. Molecular mechanisms of selective estrogen receptor modulator (SERM) action. *J Pharmacol Exp Ther.* 2000;295(2):431–7.
18. Shelly W, Draper MW, Krishnan V, Wong M, and Jaffe RB. Selective estrogen receptor modulators: An update on recent clinical findings. *Obstet Gynecol Surv.* 2008;63(3):163–81.
19. Goldstein SR, Siddhanti S, Ciaccia AV, and Plouffe L. A pharmacological review of selective oestrogen receptor modulators. *Hum Reprod Update.* 2000;6(3):212–24.
20. Komm BS, and Mirkin S. An overview of current and emerging SERMs. *J Steroid Biochem Mol Biol.* 2014;143:207–22.
21. Santen RJ, Kagan R, Altomare CJ, Komm B, Mirkin S, and Taylor HS. Current and evolving approaches to individualizing estrogen receptor-based therapy for menopausal women. *J Clin Endocrinol Metab.* 2014;99(3):733–47.
22. Wurz GT, Kao CJ, and DeGregorio MW. Safety and efficacy of ospemifene for the treatment of dyspareunia associated with vulvar and vaginal atrophy due to menopause. *Clin Interv Aging.* 2014;9:1939–50.
23. Frankel T and Benjamin F. Rapid enlargement of a uterine fibroid after clomiphene therapy. *J Obstet Gynaecol Br Commonw.* 1973;80(8):764.
24. Palomba S, Orio F, Morelli M et al. Raloxifene administration in premenopausal women with uterine leiomyomas: A pilot study. *J Clin Endocrinol Metab.* 2002;87(8):3603–8.
25. Jirecek S, Lee A, Pavo I, Crans G, Eppel W, and Wenzl R. Raloxifene prevents the growth of uterine leiomyomas in premenopausal women. *Fertil Steril.* 2004;81(1):132–6.
26. Palomba S, Russo T, Orio F et al. Effectiveness of combined GnRH analogue plus raloxifene administration in the treatment of uterine leiomyomas: A prospective, randomized, single-blind, placebo-controlled clinical trial. *Hum Reprod.* 2002;17(12):3213–9.

14

Tranexamic Acid (TA)

John Storment and Camille Storment

Introduction

There are several options for the treatment of fibroids, including surgery (hysterectomy or myomectomy) and medical management. Medical management includes hormonal therapies such as gonadotropin-releasing hormone (GnRH) agonists, and nonhormonal therapies (nonsteroidal anti-inflammatory drugs and tranexamic acid) [1].

Choosing the best option of medical management should be based on the patient's medical history, symptoms and reproductive plans. The goals of treatment include symptom relief, reduction of fibroid size and the improvement or maintenance of fertility. Because fibroids are most often benign, the most conservative treatment approach should be considered. Treatment should be used to maximize symptom relief with the fewest side effects.

Medical management may be used in women wishing to preserve their fertility or for women approaching menopause who wish to avoid surgical intervention. For women requiring surgery, medical therapy may still be recommended preoperatively to minimize blood loss. In general, medical management can be classified into hormonal and nonhormonal treatment. Hormonal therapies reduce fibroid growth and symptoms by blocking the hormonal receptors in fibroid cells and reducing the levels of estrogen and progesterone circulating throughout the fibroid tissue [1]. Nonhormonal therapies, such as nonsteroidal anti-inflammatory drugs and tranexamic acid, have also demonstrated effectiveness in decreasing menstrual blood loss (MBL).

Data show the presence of extensive fibrinolysis in the menstrual blood of women with heavy menstrual bleeding [3]. This has prompted investigation into the use of antifibrinolytic agents to decrease menorrhagia by increasing clot formation [4,5]. Activation of the clotting cascade occurs at the site of tissue injury. It involves the formation of thrombin, which cleaves fibrinogen to fibrin and produces hemostasis. Dissolution of this clot is then activated by fibrin in an effort to keep the vessel open. Fibrinolysis occurs when plasminogen (trapped within the clot) binds to lysine, resulting in a degradation of the fibrin clot. Excessive fibrinolysis can be prevented by tranexamic acid (TA) keeping the clot more stable [6]. TA, a synthetic derivative of the amino acid lysine, binds to plasminogen and blocks the interaction of plasmin with fibrin, thereby preventing clot dissolution [6]. Although its mechanism of action raises concern about an increased risk of thrombosis, this association has not been seen in clinical trials [7].

Management of Heavy Menstrual Bleeding

TA is available in the United States in oral or injectable form. The modified release oral form (Lysteda, Ferring Pharmaceuticals Inc., NJ), is approved by the US FDA for the treatment of cyclic heavy menstrual bleeding [8]. The injectable form, Cyklokapron, is indicated in patients with hemophilia for short-term use (2–8 days) to reduce or prevent hemorrhage and reduce the need for replacement therapy during and following tooth extraction [9]. Outside of the US, TA has been used to decrease bleeding in other surgical specialties. This chapter will focus primarily on the use of oral TA for heavy menstrual bleeding (HMB) due to fibroids.

The primary cause of HMB in patients with fibroids is a change in the venous structure of the myometrium and endometrium, whereby the fibroids cause venule dilation [10]. This leads to venous compression and local release of vasoactive growth factors, which contribute to increased vascularity of the leiomyomatous uterus. As vessel caliber increases, the normal hemostatic actions of platelets and the fibrin plug decreases [11].

TA has been shown to decrease mean menstrual blood loss (MBL) in women with and without uterine fibroids, in theory due to its impact on the coagulation cascade as a competitive plasmin inhibitor [5]. Eder et al. evaluated 371 women with HMB (including 147 with fibroids) over 3 months. They demonstrated a significant reduction in MBL compared with placebo, with the greatest reduction in MBL among women with fibroids. TA was well tolerated with minimal side effects.

It is unclear whether TA also decreases menorrhagia in patients with fibroids by other mechanisms. Lakhani et al. evaluated the effect of TA on vascular resistance in women with fibroids. The control group (women with DUB but without fibroids) demonstrated reduced impedance (measured via resistance index and pulsatility index with ultrasound) with TA, but the women with fibroids showed no drop in impedance. This may indicate that TA does not directly affect uterine vascular resistance but, rather, impacts the fibroid by its antifibrinolytic activity [7]. Further, myomas in women treated with TA demonstrate increased necrosis. Ip et al. [18] assessed the histologic features of fibroids in women receiving TA. They concluded that TA induced necrosis of fibroids, with larger fibroids being more prone to necrosis. This may contribute to an increase in posttreatment pain or low-grade fever, but this has not been consistently seen in clinical trials.

Perioperative Management

TA has also been evaluated as a means to decrease perioperative blood loss in different types of surgery. Reduction in blood loss has been demonstrated in cardiac surgery, liver transplant surgery and oral surgery, as well as some gynecologic surgeries (such as cold knife conization) [19]. However, for women undergoing abdominal myomectomies, the benefit of preoperative TA has not been as evident [20]. In a prospective, randomized, double-blind, placebo-controlled trial, Caglar et al demonstrated no reduction in perioperative blood loss or hemoglobin levels. In a subgroup analysis of these data, they showed that TA may decrease blood loss in women with fibroids >6 cm, but this warrants further study. A more recent study evaluated intravenous TA as an adjunct to vasopressin in a randomized, double-blind, placebo-controlled trial and confirmed that although a decrease in blood loss was seen, it was not statistically significant [21].

In women with symptomatic fibroids who are attempting pregnancy, it is often recommended to proceed with surgical intervention because of the impact the fibroid may have on the pregnancy itself. For those patients with small fibroids or in patients where surgery is contraindicated, it is reasonable to recommend TA to help control their symptoms of menorrhagia while still attempting conception. Although it has not been studied, oral TA should be safe to take even for patients undergoing fertility treatments given its short half-life and mechanism of action. Regardless of the exact mechanism, it is clear that TA decreases the hyperfibrinolysis seen in women with HMB [22]. This results in a more stable and prolonged fibrin-based clot, thereby decreasing menstrual volume. It offers a safe, well-tolerated, nonhormonal option to decrease MBL for patients with or without fibroids.

Pharmacology

The most commonly prescribed and studied regimen for oral TA (in women with normal renal function) is two 650 mg tablets taken three times daily (3900 mg/day) for a maximum of 5 days during monthly menstruation [8]. TA may be administered without regard to meals. In women with impaired renal function, dosing adjustments should be made [16]. TA is contraindicated in women with active thrombosis or a history of thrombosis. Concomitant use with oral contraceptives should be avoided [14,17]. Most studies on the effect of TA on reducing menstrual blood loss have led to good results in patients with and without leiomyomas [1]. Compared with placebo, TA has much better success in reducing menstrual blood loss with minimal side effects, such as headaches, allergies and discomfort, in only a small percentage of patients [2].

The innovative, modified-release TA formulation results in controlled dissolution of the drug, which reduces the gastrointestinal side effects. Phase I studies show both formulations (immediate release and modified release) to be bioequivalent [12]. It is available as a 650 mg oral tablet. Two studies have demonstrated TA to be an effective nonhormonal treatment for HMB [7,13], and long-term data have demonstrated the tolerability of TA, with the most frequent side effects being headache, nasal and sinus symptoms and back pain [15].

Summary

Tranexamic acid is a safe treatment for heavy menstrual bleeding in patients with uterine fibroids. It is a reasonable option for patients planning hysterectomy or myomectomy to allow time to improve preoperative anemia. Tranexamic acid may prevent the need for surgical removal of leiomyomas by controlling heavy menstrual bleeding associated with fibroids without negatively affecting fertility.

REFERENCES

1. Kashani BN, Centini G, Morelli SS, Weiss G, and Petraglia F. Role of medical management for uterine Leiomyomas. *Best Pract Res Clin Obstet Gynaecol.* 2015; 34:85–103.
2. Peitsidis P and Koukoulomati A. Tranexamic acid for the management of uterine fibroid tumors: A systematic review of the current evidence. *World J Clin Cases* 2014.
3. Dockeray CJ, Sheppard BL, and Bonnar J. The fibrinolytic system in normal menstruation and excessive uterine bleeding and the effect of tranexamic acid. *Eur J Obstet Gynecol Reprod Biol.* April 1987;24(4):309–318.
4. Peitsidis P and Koukoulomati A. Tranexamic acid for the management of uterine fibroid tumors: A systematic review of the current evidence. *World J Clin Cases* 2014 December 16;2(12):893–898.
5. Eder S, Baker J, Gersten,J, Mabey RG, and Adomako T. Efficacy and safety of oral tranexamic acid in women with heavy menstrual bleeding and fibroids. *Womens Health.* 2013;9(4):397–403.
6. McCormack PL. Tranexamic acid. A review of its use in the treatment of Hyperfibrinolysis. *Drugs.* 2012:72(5);585–617.
7. Lukes AS, Moore KA, Muse KN, et al. Tranexamic acid treatment for heavy menstrual bleeding: A randomized controlled trial. *Obstet Gynecol.* 2010;116:865–75.
8. Ferring USA. *Full Prescribing Information.* Available at http://www.ferringusa.com/wp-content/uploads/2016/07/LystedaPI_3.2016.pdf. (Accessed on 15 January 2017)
9. Pfizer. *Full Prescribing Information.* Available at https://www.pfizer.com/products/product-detail/cyklokapron. (Accessed on 20 January 2017)
10. Farrer-Brown G, Beilby JO, and Tarbit MH. Venous changes in the endometrium of myomatous uteri. *Obstet Gynecol.* 1971; 38(5): 743–51.
11. Stewart EA and Nowak RA. Leiomyoma-related bleeding: a classic hypothesis updated for the molecular era. *Hum Reprod Update.* 1996;2(4):295–306.
12. Moore K, Morin I, Marenco T, Lavigne JR, and Morelli G. Pharmacokinetic studies of 2 novel oral formulations of tranexamic acid therapy. *Am J Ther.* 2012;19(3):190–198.
13. Freeman EW, Lukes A, VanDrie R, Mabey RB, Gersten J, and Adomako TL. A dose-response study of a novel, oral tranexamic acid formulation for heavy menstrual bleeding. *Am J Obstet Gynecol.* 2011;205(4):319.e1–319 e7.
14. ACOG *Committee Opinion Management of Acute Abnormal Uterine Bleeding*; Number 557 April 2013.

15. Muse K, Lukes AS, Gersten J, Waldbaum A, Mabey RG, and Trott E. Long-term evaluation of safety and health related quality of life in women with heavy menstrual bleeding treated with oral tranexamic acid. *Womens Health.* 2011;7(6):699–707.
16. RxList. Lysteda: Drug description. Available at: https://www.rxlist.com/lysteda-drug.htm#description. (Accessed on 10 January 2017)
17. Stewart EA. Uterine fibroids. *N Engl J Med.* 2015;372:1646–55.
18. Ip PP, Lam KW, Cheung CL, Yeung MC, Pun TC, Chan QK, and Cheung AN. Tranexamic acid-associated necrosis and intralesional thrombosis of uterine leiomyomas: A clinicpathologic study of 147 cases emphasizing the importance of drug induced necrosis and early infarcts in leiomyomas. *Am J Surg Pathol.* 2007;31;1215–1224 (PMID: 17667546)
19. Dunn CJ and Goa KL. Tranexamic Acid: a review of its use in surgery and other indications. *Drugs.* 1999;57:1005–1032 (PMID 10400410)
20. Caglar GS, Tasci Y, Kayikcioglu F, and Haberal A. Intravenous tranexamic acid use in myomectomy; a prospective randomized double blind placebo controlled study. *Eur J OBstet Gynecol Reprod Biol.* 2008;137:227–231 (PMID 17499419]
21. Ngichabe S, Obura T, and Stones W. Intravenous tranexamic acid as an adjunct haemostat to ornipressin during open myomectomy. A randomized double blind placebo controlled trial. *Ann Surg Innov Res.* 2015;9:10.
22. Dockeray CJ, Sheppard BL, Daly L et al. The fibrinolytic enzyme system in normal menstruation and excessive uterine bleeding and the effect of tranexamic acid. *Eur J Obstet Gynecol Reprod Biol.* 1987 April;24:309–18.

15

Alternative Therapies in the Treatment of Uterine Leiomyoma

Anatte E. Karmon

Despite the high prevalence of uterine fibroids in reproductive-age women, surgery remains the mainstay of treatment while medical and alternative therapies are less well described in the literature [1,2]. Although hysterectomy and myomectomy are common and highly effective treatments for fibroid disease, both can be morbid procedures and, in the case of hysterectomy, preclude future childbearing.

Data on the use of "complementary," "alternative" or "holistic" treatments for fibroid disease are extremely scant. However, it behooves all clinicians caring for women with fibroids to familiarize themselves with such therapies and their possible mechanisms of action, as their use is not uncommon. Among a cohort of 933 women with symptomatic uterine fibroids, 34% of women reported using diet as a treatment, 37% reported using herbs and 16% reported using acupuncture [1]. A summary of alternative treatments is provided in Table 15.1. The purpose of this chapter is to familiarize the reader with the availability of alternative therapies and limited data supporting the use of alternative therapies for the treatment of fibroid disease.

Vitamin D and Fibroid Disease

The biologically active form of vitamin D (1α,25-dihydroxyvitamin D) is a lipid-soluble hormone with both genomic and nongenomic effects [3]. Its steroid-like activity regulates the expression of a variety of genes, including some that are classically involved with malignant transformation. By inhibiting cellular proliferation, differentiation and growth, vitamin D may reduce cancer risk [3–5]. Numerous studies have suggested that vitamin D deficiency is a risk factor for fibroids [6–8], and it is hypothesized that higher prevalence of vitamin D deficiency in African Americans may be part of the reason as to why these women are two to three times more likely to have fibroids as compared with Caucasian women [9]. Several polymorphisms associated with vitamin D levels on genome-wide association studies (GWASs) have been identified, and a recent study related the presence of such polymorphisms to risk of uterine leiomyoma among women who self-identify as black [9].

Given that vitamin D is most likely involved in fibroid pathogenesis, it follows that supplementation with vitamin D or its analogues may be a promising treatment for fibroid disease. Vitamin D has been shown to inhibit cell proliferation in an *in vitro* leiomyoma cell line [10] and has also been demonstrated to reduce fibroid size in the Eker rat model [11]. Maintenance treatment of vitamin D deficiency with 1500–2000 IU of vitamin D daily is low cost and carries little risk of toxicity [12,13]. Randomized controlled trials investigating the efficacy of vitamin D therapy for human uterine leiomyoma are needed before any clinical recommendations can be made.

Dietary Exposures in Fibroid Pathobiology and Treatment

Although little is known about the impact of diet on uterine leiomyoma, the use of supplements and dietary modifications to treat fibroids and their symptoms is not uncommon [1]. Dietary fat is positively correlated with plasma estrone [14], and studies investigating the role of dietary fat in hormone-sensitive conditions (i.e., endometriosis and endometrial cancer) have generally shown a positive association between high dietary fat and disease risk [15,16]. However, few studies have investigated the relationship between uterine leiomyomas, which are hormone-sensitive tumors, and dietary fat [17–19]. A prospective study on fat intake and risk of fibroids demonstrated an increased incidence of uterine fibroids among women with higher intakes of long-chain omega-3 fatty acids, although no association with total fat intake was seen [19]. The authors suggested that the relationship between omega-3 fatty acids and fibroids might be explained by chance, omega-3 fatty acids in general or the endocrine-disrupting chemicals found in some fish [19]. Other studies have not demonstrated a consistent association between fat and uterine leiomyoma [17,18].

On the other hand, low dairy intake may be associated with increased risk for uterine leiomyoma [20,21]. The physiologic mechanism behind this relationship is unknown but could be related to the high levels of vitamin D and calcium in dairy products, both of which reduce cellular proliferation [3,20,22]. Although black women are more likely to report lactose intolerance, avoid dairy products and suffer from fibroids compared with women with European ancestry [23,24], controlling for ancestry does not appreciably change the relationship between dairy intake and uterine leiomyoma. Moreover, a dose–response relationship between dairy intake and leiomyoma risk has been described [20]. Caffeine and alcohol have been shown to affect hormone profiles and reproductive outcomes in both men and women [25–28], although data regarding their impact on fibroids are limited. In terms of alcohol consumption, both positive [29,30] and null associations [17] with uterine leiomyoma have been reported in the literature. The mechanism for a positive association could involve alcohol's relation with higher levels of estrogen [27], a hormone known to promote fibroid growth. Interestingly, beer was shown to have a stronger association with leiomyoma risk compared with wine or liquor [30]. The authors hypothesized that this could be related to the presence of a phytoestrogen in beer,

TABLE 15.1

Select Alternative Therapies in the Treatment of Fibroid Disease

Therapy or Intervention	Possible Mechanism of Action	References
Vitamin D	Inhibition of cellular proliferation, differentiation and growth	Baird et al. [6], Paffoni et al. [7], Sabry et al. [8], Wise et al. [9], Blauer et al. [10], Halder et al. [11]
Decreased fat intake	Decreased estrone level	Chiaffarino et al. [17], Nagata et al. [18], Wise et al. [19]
Increased dairy intake	Increased vitamin D and calcium intakes	Wise et al. 2010 [21], Wise et al. 2013 [20]
Decreased alcohol intake	Decreased estradiol levels, decreased 8-prenylnarigenin (a phytoestrogen)	Wise et al. [30], Marshall et al. [29], Chiaffarino et al. [17]
Curcumin	Induction of apoptosis, promotion of wound healing, regulation of cellular growth	Malik et al. [38]
Lycopene	Regulation of the cell cycle, modulation of oxidative DNA damage	Sahin et al. 2007 [40], Sahin et al. 2004 [42]
Chinese herbs—Guizhi Fuling formula	Unknown	Liu et al. [51], Chen et al. [32]
Acupuncture	Immune system and neurohormone modulation	Zhang et al. [54], Cakmak et al. [56], Habek et al. [55]

8-prenylnarigenin, which has been demonstrated to stimulate the growth of *in vitro* breast cancer cell lines [30,31]. Although few studies have been conducted on the topic, overall caffeine consumption does not appear to be related to fibroid risk [17,30]. One study reported a positive association between leiomyoma risk and caffeine intake ≥500mg/day among women <35 years old, although overall association with caffeine was null [30].

Supplements and Treatment of Fibroid Disease

The use of supplements for the treatment of uterine leiomyoma or its symptoms is not uncommon in North America. In a recent study conducted in the San Francisco Bay area, 37% of participants with symptomatic uterine fibroids reported using herbs to treat their symptoms, and of these women, 38% reported feeling "a lot better" after their use and <5% reported bothersome side effects [1]. In other parts of the world, traditional medicines are often used alone or in conjunction with Western medicines to treat symptomatic uterine fibroids. Numerous such alternative treatments have been described in the literature, ranging from various herbal mixtures used in Chinese medicine [32,33] to the utilization of pangolin carcasses in traditional Yorubic medicine [34].

Curcumin, a food additive that has been used as a spice and a medicine, may hold antiproliferative properties, making it potentially useful as a treatment for fibroid disease. Through its impact on a number of molecular signaling pathways, curcumin has been shown to induce apoptosis, promote wound healing and regulate cellular growth [35–37]. The prevalence of its use and the *in vivo* effectiveness of curcumin in treating uterine leiomyoma are not known, although *in vitro* studies suggest it could be a promising therapy. In their study utilizing human fibroid cell lines, Malik et al. demonstrated that curcumin exposure inhibited cellular proliferation and also upregulated total caspase activity, enzymes that are key players in apoptosis initiation [38]. The expression of fibronectin, an extracellular matrix protein upregulated in fibroid tissue compared to myometrium [39], was decreased among fibroid cells exposed to curcumin [38].

Lycopene, a carotene found in certain red fruits and vegetables including tomatoes, is an antioxidant with antineoplastic properties [40]. Higher intake of tomato products is negatively associated with certain cancers, including those of the prostate, cervix and ovary [41]. The tumor-suppressive mechanisms of action for lycopene and tomato products are unclear but may involve an impact on cell cycle regulatory proteins and/or modulation of oxidative DNA damage [40]. Studies done in the Japanese quail, an animal model for uterine fibroids, demonstrate decreased incidence of leiomyoma among quails supplemented with lycopene [42] and tomato powder [40]. Whether lycopene or tomato powder supplementation will prove an effective treatment for fibroids in humans has yet to be elucidated.

Aromatase inhibitors, such as letrozole and anastrozole, are currently used as adjunctive treatments for estrogen-sensitive conditions such as breast cancer, endometriosis and uterine fibroids. As potent inhibitors of estrogen in a variety of tissues, aromatase inhibitors are excellent medical therapies for those patients in whom gonadotropin-inhibiting agents are less than ideal, such as postmenopausal patients with minimal ovarian estrogen production. They can also be used in combination with gonadotropin-inhibiting agents to magnify their estrogen-suppressing effects or eliminate the estrogen "flare" accompanying gonadotropin-releasing hormone agonists at initiation of treatment [43]. Owing to their undeniable success at inducing a hypoestrogenic state, aromatase inhibitors often elicit bothersome, as well as serious, side effects such as bone loss and hot flashes [44,45]. Natural compounds with aromatase inhibition activity offer the possibility of suppressing estrogen with fewer side effects [46], although data on their clinical use are limited. One such compound reported in the literature is grape seed extract. Through the inhibition of aromatase activity and expression, grape seed extract has been shown to reduce tumor growth in a breast cancer xenograft model [47]. However, a study evaluating the impact of freeze-dried grape powder supplementation on the hormone levels of 18 postmenopausal women did not demonstrate a significant difference in levels pre- and post-treatment [48]. As with other supplements of interest, clinical trials are needed to determine the utility of grape seed extract as a treatment specifically for uterine leiomyoma.

Treatment of Fibroid Disease and Symptoms with Acupuncture and Traditional Chinese Medicine

Traditional Chinese medicine (TCM) therapies and acupuncture are reportedly commonly used as treatments for symptomatic uterine fibroids, although the exact prevalence in the Western world is unknown [49]. In Taiwan, a study of 35,786 women with newly diagnosed fibroids reported that the majority of their subjects (87.1%) had visited TCM clinics. Among those who utilized TCM, 61.8% used herbal remedies [50].

Descriptions on the usage and effectiveness of TCM on fibroid disease are present mainly in Chinese literature. However, quality clinical trials are few in number. In addition, because TCM tailors herb combinations to the symptoms of a specific individual [49], designing randomized controlled trials true to TCM principles can be challenging. Nonetheless, practitioners should be aware of the more common TCM therapies and the data supporting their use.

A Cochrane review published in 2013 evaluated 21 randomized trials investigating Chinese herbal preparations for the treatment of uterine fibroids [51]. Because of the limited data and high possibility of bias in most of the included trials, there is not enough evidence to draw any firm conclusions on the safety and efficacy of treatment. Of note, compared to mifepristone treatment, *Tripterygium wilfordii* extract supplementation was associated with a greater reduction in fibroid volume and uterine size, and the Guizhi Fuling herbal formula plus mifepristone was associated with a greater reduction in fibroid volume compared with mifepristone alone [51].

The Guizhi Fuling herbal formula is one of the most common TCM treatments for uterine fibroids [32,50] and consists *of Ramulus Cinnamomi, Poria, Semen Persicae, Radix Paeoniae Rubra* or *Radix Paeoniae Alba* and *Cortex Moutan* [32]. A systematic review of randomized clinical trials (all conducted in China and published in Chinese) suggested that the Guizhi Fuling formula may be of benefit in reducing fibroid volume and treating dysmenorrhea, although, again, the included trials are of poor quality. No trial reported serious adverse events [32]. The TCM-described mechanisms of action of the Guizhi Fuling formula include blood invigoration, stasis dissolution and resolution of masses [32]. The potential molecular mechanisms of action are unknown.

Acupuncture, having been practiced in Asia for more than 4000 years, is primarily a TCM treatment, involving needling particular points of the body. Variations of this practice have arisen and include acupressure (applying pressure on acupuncture points with fingers or devices) and electroacupuncture (utilizing electrical current to enhance the effects of traditional acupuncture) [52]. In TCM terms, acupuncture works by normalizing energy flow through the body's meridians. According to this theory, symptoms arise from obstruction of these energy pathways [53]. In terms of Western science-based mechanisms, it has been proposed that acupuncture may modulate immune system activity through an impact on cytokines. In addition, acupuncture may affect the release of neurohormones such as endorphins [52]. Although the use of acupuncture to treat fibroid disease may not be uncommon (16% of surveyed subjects in one study [1]), very limited data exist on its effectiveness. A Cochrane review published in 2010 sought to include all randomized controlled trials on the topic. After reviewing available literature, no trials met the inclusion criteria [54]. A few case reports have demonstrated beneficial results of acupuncture on fibroid size and bleeding [55,56]; however, clinical trials are needed to confirm these findings.

Despite the lack of quality data regarding the utilization of alternative therapies to treat fibroid disease, their use is common in North America and abroad [1,49,50]. Although numerous proven therapies for uterine leiomyoma exist, there is clearly a place for these less-well-studied alternative treatments. Future investigations should focus on elucidating the efficacy and safety of these therapies.

REFERENCES

1. Jacoby VL, Jacoby A, Learman LA et al. Use of medical, surgical and complementary treatments among women with fibroids. *Eur J Obstet Gynecol Reprod Biol.* 2014;182:220–5.
2. Patel A, Malik M, Britten J, Cox J, and Catherino WH. Alternative therapies in management of leiomyomas. *Fertil Steril.* 2014;102(3):649–55.
3. Brakta S, Diamond JS, Al-Hendy A, Diamond MP, and Halder SK. Role of vitamin D in uterine fibroid biology. *Fertil Steril.* 2015;104(3):698–706.
4. Holick MF. Sunlight and vitamin D for bone health and prevention of autoimmune diseases, cancers, and cardiovascular disease. *Am J Clin Nutr.* 2004;80(6 Suppl):1678S–88S. doi:10.1093/ajcn/80.6.1678S
5. Chen TC and Holick MF. Vitamin D and prostate cancer prevention and treatment. *Trends Endocrinol Metab.* 2003;14(9):423–30.
6. Baird DD, Hill MC, Schectman JM, and Hollis BW. Vitamin d and the risk of uterine fibroids. *Epidemiology.* 2013;24(3):447–53.
7. Paffoni A, Somigliana E, Vigano P et al. Vitamin D status in women with uterine leiomyomas. *J Clin Endocrinol Metab.* 2013;98(8):E1374–8.
8. Sabry M, Halder SK, Allah AS, Roshdy E, Rajaratnam V, and Al-Hendy A. Serum vitamin D3 level inversely correlates with uterine fibroid volume in different ethnic groups: A cross-sectional observational study. *Int J Womens Health.* 2013;5:93–100.
9. Wise LA, Ruiz-Narvaez EA, Haddad SA, Rosenberg L, and Palmer JR. Polymorphisms in vitamin D-related genes and risk of uterine leiomyomata. *Fertil Steril.* 2014;102(2):503–10 e1.
10. Blauer M, Rovio PH, Ylikomi T, and Heinonen PK. Vitamin D inhibits myometrial and leiomyoma cell proliferation *in vitro. Fertil Steril.* 2009;91(5):1919–25.
11. Halder SK, Sharan C, and Al-Hendy A. 1,25-dihydroxyvitamin D3 treatment shrinks uterine leiomyoma tumors in the Eker rat model. *Biol Reprod.* 2012;86(4):116.
12. Wu JL and Segars JH. Is vitamin D the answer for prevention of uterine fibroids? *Fertil Steril.* 2015;104(3):559–60.
13. Holick MF. Vitamin D deficiency. *N Engl J Med.* 2007;357(3):266–81.
14. Aubertin-Leheudre M, Gorbach S, Woods M, Dwyer JT, Goldin B, and Adlercreutz H. Fat/fiber intakes and sex hormones in healthy premenopausal women in USA. *J Steroid Biochem Mol Biol.* 2008;112(1–3):32–9.
15. Missmer SA, Chavarro JE, Malspeis S et al. A prospective study of dietary fat consumption and endometriosis risk. *Hum Reprod.* 2010;25(6):1528–35.
16. Littman AJ, Beresford SA, and White E. The association of dietary fat and plant foods with endometrial cancer (United States). *Cancer Causes Control.* 2001;12(8):691–702.
17. Chiaffarino F, Parazzini F, La Vecchia C, Chatenoud L, Di Cintio E, and Marsico S. Diet and uterine myomas. *Obstet Gynecol.* 1999;94(3):395–8.
18. Nagata C, Nakamura K, Oba S, Hayashi M, Takeda N, and Yasuda K. Association of intakes of fat, dietary fibre, soya isoflavones and alcohol with uterine fibroids in Japanese women. *Br J Nutr.* 2009;101(10):1427–31.
19. Wise LA, Radin RG, Kumanyika SK, Ruiz-Narvaez EA, Palmer JR, and Rosenberg L. Prospective study of dietary fat and risk of uterine leiomyomata. *Am J Clin Nutr.* 2014;99(5):1105–16.

20. Wise LA, Palmer JR, Ruiz-Narvaez E, Reich DE, and Rosenberg L. Is the observed association between dairy intake and fibroids in African Americans explained by genetic ancestry? *Am J Epidemiol.* 2013;178(7):1114–9.
21. Wise LA, Radin RG, Palmer JR, Kumanyika SK, and Rosenberg L. A prospective study of dairy intake and risk of uterine leiomyomata. *Am J Epidemiol.* 2010;171(2):221–32.
22. Jacobson EA, James KA, Newmark HL, and Carroll KK. Effects of dietary fat, calcium, and vitamin D on growth and mammary tumorigenesis induced by 7,12-dimethylbenz(a) anthracene in female Sprague-Dawley rats. *Cancer Res.* 1989;49(22):6300–3.
23. Jackson KA, and Savaiano DA. Lactose maldigestion, calcium intake and osteoporosis in African-, Asian-, and Hispanic-Americans. *J Am Coll Nutr.* 2001;20(2 Suppl):198S–207S.
24. Baird DD, Dunson DB, Hill MC, Cousins D, and Schectman JM. High cumulative incidence of uterine leiomyoma in black and white women: Ultrasound evidence. *Am J Obstet Gynecol.* 2003;188(1):100–7.
25. Muthusami KR and Chinnaswamy P. Effect of chronic alcoholism on male fertility hormones and semen quality. *Fertil Steril.* 2005;84(4):919–24.
26. Gaskins AJ, Rich-Edwards JW, Williams PL, Toth TL, Missmer SA, and Chavarro JE. Pre-pregnancy caffeine and caffeinated beverage intake and risk of spontaneous abortion. *Eur J Nutr.* 2018;57(1):107–17. doi:10.1007/s00394-016-1301-2.
27. Katsouyanni K, Boyle P, and Trichopoulos D. Diet and urine estrogens among postmenopausal women. *Oncology.* 1991;48(6):490–4.
28. Lucero J, Harlow BL, Barbieri RL, Sluss P, and Cramer DW. Early follicular phase hormone levels in relation to patterns of alcohol, tobacco, and coffee use. *Fertil Steril.* 2001; 76(4):723–9.
29. Marshall LM, Spiegelman D, Barbieri RL et al. Variation in the incidence of uterine leiomyoma among premenopausal women by age and race. *Obstet Gynecol.* 1997;90(6):967–73.
30. Wise LA, Palmer JR, Harlow BL et al. Risk of uterine leiomyomata in relation to tobacco, alcohol and caffeine consumption in the Black Women's Health Study. *Hum Reprod.* 2004;19(8):1746–54.
31. Rong H, Boterberg T, Maubach J et al. 8-Prenylnaringenin, the phytoestrogen in hops and beer, upregulates the function of the E-cadherin/catenin complex in human mammary carcinoma cells. *Eur J Cell Biol.* 2001;80(9):580–5.
32. Chen NN, Han M, Yang H et al. Chinese herbal medicine Guizhi Fuling Formula for treatment of uterine fibroids: A systematic review of randomised clinical trials. *BMC Complement Altern Med.* 2014;14:2.
33. Sang H. Clinical and experimental research into treatment of hysteromyoma with promoting qi flow and blood circulation, softening and resolving hard lump. *J Tradit Chin Med.* 2004;24(4):274–9.
34. Soewu DA and Ayodele IA. Utilisation of pangolin (*Manis* sps) in traditional Yorubic medicine in Ijebu province, Ogun State, Nigeria. *J Ethnobiol Ethnomed.* 2009;5:39.
35. Sidhu GS, Singh AK, Thaloor D et al. Enhancement of wound healing by curcumin in animals. *Wound Repair Regen.* 1998;6(2):167–77.
36. Shishodia S, Singh T, and Chaturvedi MM. Modulation of transcription factors by curcumin. *Adv Exp Med Biol.* 2007;595:127–48.
37. Shishodia S, Amin HM, Lai R, and Aggarwal BB. Curcumin (diferuloylmethane) inhibits constitutive NF-kappaB activation, induces G1/S arrest, suppresses proliferation, and induces apoptosis in mantle cell lymphoma. *Biochem Pharmacol.* 2005;70(5):700–13.
38. Malik M, Mendoza M, Payson M, and Catherino WH. Curcumin, a nutritional supplement with antineoplastic activity, enhances leiomyoma cell apoptosis and decreases fibronectin expression. *Fertil Steril.* 2009;91(5 Suppl):2177–84.
39. Malik M, Webb J, and Catherino WH. Retinoic acid treatment of human leiomyoma cells transformed the cell phenotype to one strongly resembling myometrial cells. *Clin Endocrinol (Oxf).* 2008;69(3):462–70.
40. Sahin K, Ozercan R, Onderci M et al. Dietary tomato powder supplementation in the prevention of leiomyoma of the oviduct in the Japanese quail. *Nutr Cancer.* 2007;59(1):70–5.
41. Giovannucci E. Tomatoes, tomato-based products, lycopene, and cancer: Review of the epidemiologic literature. *J Natl Cancer Inst.* 1999;91(4):317–31.
42. Sahin K, Ozercan R, Onderci M et al. Lycopene supplementation prevents the development of spontaneous smooth muscle tumors of the oviduct in Japanese quail. *Nutr Cancer.* 2004;50(2):181–9.
43. Bedaiwy MA, Mousa NA, Casper RF. Aromatase inhibitors: Potential reproductive implications. *J Minim Invasive Gynecol.* 2009;16(5):533–9.
44. Fontaine C, Meulemans A, Huizing M et al. Tolerance of adjuvant letrozole outside of clinical trials. *Breast.* 2008;17(4):376–81.
45. Eastell R and Hannon R. Long-term effects of aromatase inhibitors on bone. *J Steroid Biochem Mol Biol.* 2005;95(1–5):151–4.
46. Khan SI, Zhao J, Khan IA, Walker LA, and Dasmahapatra AK. Potential utility of natural products as regulators of breast cancer-associated aromatase promoters. *Reprod Biol Endocrinol.* 2011;9:91.
47. Kijima I, Phung S, Hur G, Kwok SL, Chen S. Grape seed extract is an aromatase inhibitor and a suppressor of aromatase expression. *Cancer Res.* 2006;66(11):5960–7.
48. Allen SV, Pruthi S, Suman VJ et al. Evaluation of the aromatase inhibition potential of freeze-dried grape powder. *J Diet Suppl.* 2015;12(4):373-382. doi:10.3109/19390211.2014.952863.
49. Mehl-Madrona L. Complementary medicine treatment of uterine fibroids: A pilot study. *Altern Ther Health Med.* 2002;8(2):34–6, 8–40, 2, 4–6.
50. Yen HR, Chen YY, Huang TP et al. Prescription patterns of Chinese herbal products for patients with uterine fibroid in Taiwan: A nationwide population-based study. *J Ethnopharmacol.* 2015;171:223–30.
51. Liu JP, Yang H, Xia Y, and Cardini F. Herbal preparations for uterine fibroids. *Cochrane Database Syst Rev.* 2013(4):CD005292.
52. Acupuncture (PDQ(R)): Health Professional Version. PDQ Cancer Information Summaries. Bethesda (MD); 2002.
53. Lao L. Acupuncture techniques and devices. *J Altern Complement Med.* 1996;2(1):23–5.
54. Zhang Y, Peng W, Clarke J, and Liu Z. Acupuncture for uterine fibroids. *Cochrane Database Syst Rev.* 2010(1):CD007221.
55. Habek D and Aksamija A. Successful acupuncture treatment of uterine myoma. *Acta Clin Croat.* 2014;53(4):487–9.
56. Cakmak YO, Akpinar IN, Yoldemir T, and Cavdar S. Decreasing bleeding due to uterine fibroid with electroacupuncture. *Fertil Steril.* 2011;96(1):e13–5.

16

Laparotomy for Surgical Treatment of Uterine Fibroids

Jeffrey M. Goldberg and Zaraq Khan

Just three decades ago, the therapeutic options available to women with symptomatic uterine fibroids were limited to hysterectomy and abdominal myomectomy (performed via laparotomy; also referred to as open myomectomy). Currently, there are several uterine-sparing treatment modalities available, including medical treatments for uterine fibroids, conventional and robot-assisted laparoscopic myomectomies [1,2], vaginal and hysteroscopic myomectomies [3], uterine artery embolization (UAE) [4] and magnetic resonance-guided focused ultrasound surgery (MRgFUS) [5]. However, each of these treatment options have limitations precluding universal application in all patients with myomas. The size and number of fibroids dictate the surgical approach to myomectomies in most cases. Additionally, skilled surgeons are required for most laparoscopic and vaginal myomectomies. Likewise, even though UAE is widely used in the US and Western Europe, it is associated with a range of complications, including abnormal placentation in subsequent pregnancies. Since data regarding fertility outcomes after the procedure are still limited, UAE is not currently recommended for women who may desire to conceive [6]. Similarly, even though MRgFUS is noninvasive, it requires sophisticated technology that is provided in few medical centers and outcome data, including pregnancy, are lacking.

Hence, with all its perceived potential drawbacks that include surgical invasiveness, excessive perioperative blood loss, risk of infection and adhesion formation, conventional abdominal myomectomy still remains the primary method for conservative treatment for symptomatic uterine fibroids. Moreover, because of the recent safety concerns regarding the use of laparoscopic power morcellation [7], larger abdominal wall incisions are required for the delivery of intact myomas, making conventional abdominal myomectomy relevant again.

Preoperative Assessment

Abdominal myomectomy is typically performed in women with intramural or subserosal fibroids. Intracavitary fibroids may also be removed during abdominal myomectomy. However, a hysteroscopic approach is the procedure of choice for such lesions, given that it is a very minimally invasive procedure with a faster recovery and less perioperative morbidity, as well as no compromise of myometrial integrity which could potentially increase the risk of uterine rupture during pregnancy. Appropriate candidates for abdominal myomectomy are women with the following characteristics:

1. Very large symptomatic fibroid(s) where conventional or robot-assisted laparoscopic myomectomy is not feasible.
2. Submucosal fibroids where the majority of the fibroid is intramural and not amenable to hysteroscopic resection.
3. Where a laparotomy is required to treat other intra-abdominal pathology other than the fibroid.

In cases where an abdominal myomectomy has been deemed the best option, it is important that the woman is counseled appropriately and the reason for choosing a non-minimally invasive procedure is explained.

Imaging

Aside from a thorough history and physical examination, women who are planning to undergo myomectomy should undergo imaging to help determine the best surgical approach, including ruling out other incidental findings that may impact surgical planning. Imaging with pelvic ultrasonography is typically sufficient for women undergoing abdominal myomectomy [8]. Magnetic resonance imaging (MRI), however, is considered the best modality for visualizing the number, size and location of all fibroids when a minimally invasive procedure is planned as it may be difficult or impossible to locate the presence of small and/or deep myomas by palpation. Furthermore, MRI may help distinguish myomas from uterine sarcomas and adenomyomas [9].

Laboratory Evaluation

Since myomectomy carries a risk for significant blood loss, a baseline complete blood count is suggested for all patients. Given that abnormal uterine bleeding is one of the most common symptoms of uterine cancer, as well as benign myomas, endometrial sampling should be considered, especially in women >35 years or those who have risk factors for uterine cancer. Serum lactate dehydrogenase (LDH) levels and its isoenzymes may also aid in the diagnosis of leiomyosarcoma when a high suspicion exists [10].

Prophylactic Antibiotics

Abdominal myomectomy is considered a clean procedure since it does not involve a vaginal or intestinal incision. The American College of Obstetricians and Gynecologists (ACOG) has advised that prophylactic antibiotics not be used for such procedures [11]. Others, including the authors, disagree based on the rationale that the surgical-site infection risk is similar to hysterectomy, for which antibiotics are universally recommended [12,13]. Also, the blood-filled myometrial dead spaces following excision of myomas provide an excellent environment for bacterial growth. Finally, it may reduce the urge to consider antibiotic treatment for the self-limited postoperative fever so common after myomectomy.

Preoperative Anemia

Women with symptomatic fibroids often have heavy menstrual bleeding leading to chronic blood loss anemia. Any preexisting anemia should be corrected prior to surgery by iron therapy. Amenorrhea may also be induced with leuprolide acetate or continuous oral contraceptives to facilitate correction of anemia. Women at high risk should have their blood cross-matched for the procedure.

Surgical Measures and Techniques

Abdominal myomectomies are typically performed under general anesthesia, though some may be performed under regional anesthesia. The basic principles involved in the procedure are:

1. Decision of appropriate skin and fascia incision for adequate exposure
2. Application of measures to reduce blood loss (discussed in Chapter 24)
3. Appropriate uterine incision(s)
4. Removal of the fibroid
5. Closure of defect
6. Application of measures to reduce postoperative adhesions (discussed in Chapter 25)

The patient is placed in the dorsal lithotomy position with no hip flexion. This allows access to the uterine manipulator, which is inserted in order to manipulate the uterus, perform transcervical chromotubation for documentation of tubal patency and to help delineate the endometrial cavity for preventing inadvertent entry.

Decision of Appropriate Skin and Fascia Incision for Adequate Exposure

The type and size of the skin incision is paramount for optimizing surgical exposure during an abdominal myomectomy. Traditionally, transverse suprapubic skin incisions are made for smaller uteri while vertical midline incisions (infraumbilical or those extending more cephalad to the umbilicus) are reserved for larger uteri. The fascial incision is equally important. The fascia is always incised vertically with vertical midline skin incisions to provide maximum exposure (Figure 16.1). There are, however, several options for incising the fascia in cases where a transverse suprapubic skin incision is made.

The most common incision is the classic Pfannenstiel incision (Figure 16.2). A transverse skin incision 2–5 cm above the pubic symphysis, usually around 8–15 cm in length, is made. After the skin is entered, the incision is carried through the subcutaneous tissue to the anterior rectus sheath, which is incised transversely. The upper and lower fascial edges are grasped with a clamp, elevated and dissected bluntly and sharply off of the underlying rectus muscles. The rectus muscles are separated along the midline raphe. The peritoneum is next incised vertically.

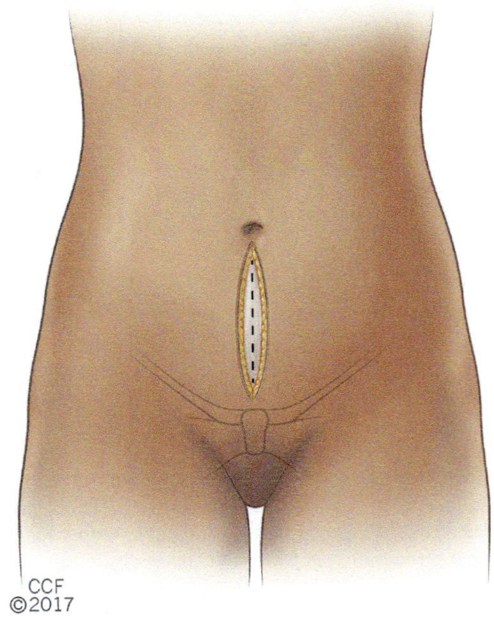

FIGURE 16.1 A midline incision with vertical skin and fascial incision. This type of incision is usually reserved for extremely large fibroids and women with a prior midline incision.

A Maylard incision (also known as the Mackenrodt incision) is also a transverse incision through the skin and fascia but the fascia is NOT separated from the rectus muscles (Figures 16.3 and 16.4). The deep inferior epigastric vessels are identified at the lateral undersurface of the muscles, clamped, transected and suture ligated. The rectus muscles are then incised transversely

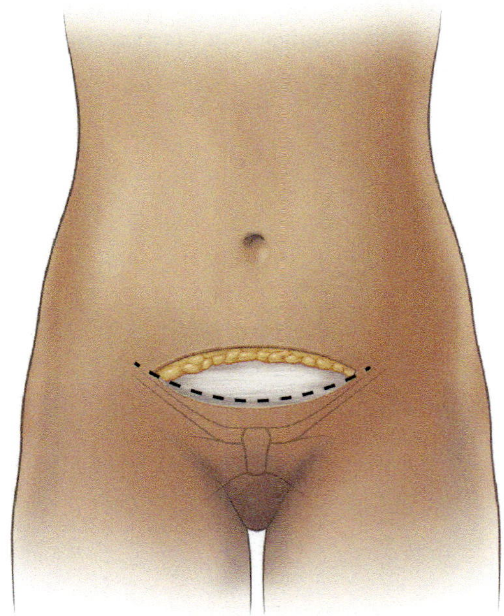

FIGURE 16.2 Pfannenstiel incision is the most commonly used incision for pelvic surgery. The skin and fascia are incised transversely. The fascia is dissected off of the rectus muscles and the muscle bellies are separated in the midline. The peritoneum is incised vertically.

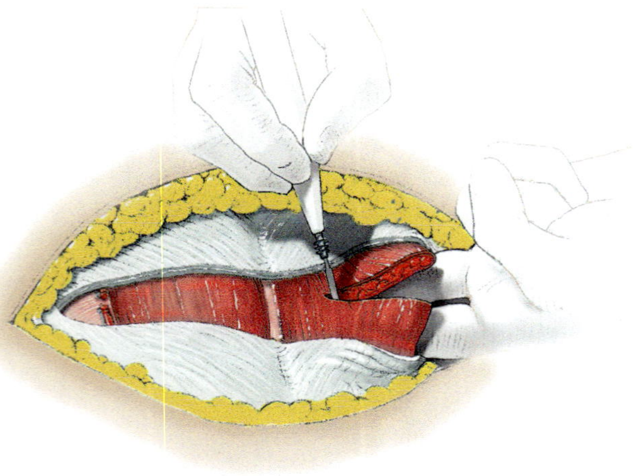

FIGURES 16.3 Maylard incision gives more exposure than a Pfannenstiel incision. The skin and fascia are incised transversely. The epigastric vessels are identified, clamped, cut and ligated. The rectus muscles are cut transversely and the peritoneum is also incised transversely.

with electrocautery. The peritoneum is also incised transversely. The skin, fascia and peritoneum can all be extended from one anterior iliac spine to the other, affording outstanding exposure enabling even the largest myomas to be removed without having to resort to a vertical incision.

A Küstner incision also begins with a transverse suprapubic skin incision. Subcutaneous tissue is separated from the rectus sheath in a vertical plane to reveal the linea alba (Figure 16.5). The fascia and peritoneum are both incised vertically in the midline. The authors prefer to use this incision for minilaparotomy (~4–6 cm) as it provides optimal exposure with the disposable round self-retaining wound retractors; Mobius (CooperSurgical, Inc, Trumbull, CT) and Alexis (Applied Medical, Rancho Santa Margarita, CA).(Figure 16.6). Like the Maylard incision, it is a good choice in patients with a prior Pfannenstiel incision since it avoids the difficulty that is often encountered when trying to dissect the adhesions between the rectus fascia and muscles.

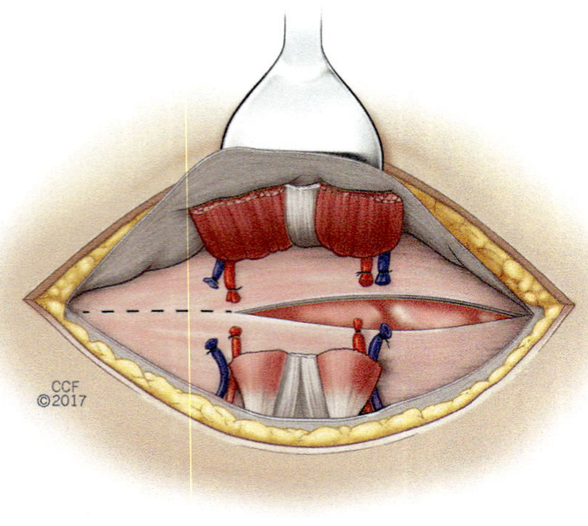

FIGURES 16.4 The peritoneum is also incised transversely. The incision may be extended laterally to the iliac spines to provide excellent access for large uteri through a low transverse incision.

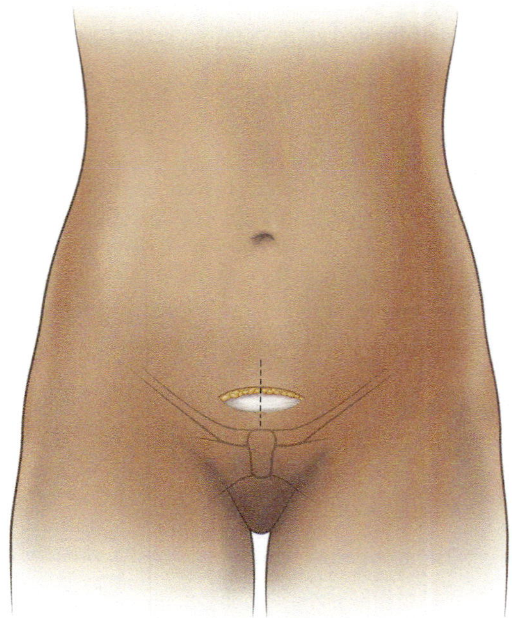

FIGURE 16.5 The Küstner incision utilizes a transverse skin incision but the fascia and peritoneum are incised vertically. The authors use this incision for minilaparotomies.

Despite the small incision, large myomas can be removed (Figure 16.7).

In order to reduce the risk of organ injury with peritoneal entry, a 5 mm laparoscope may be inserted in the right upper quadrant (Palmer's point) in cases in which significant pelvic adhesions are anticipated. Additionally, laparoscopic lysis of adhesions is often easier, especially with a minilaparotomy incision.

Applications of Measures to Reduce Blood Loss

Various modalities can be used to decrease blood loss at the time of myomectomy. These are discussed in detailed Chapter 24.

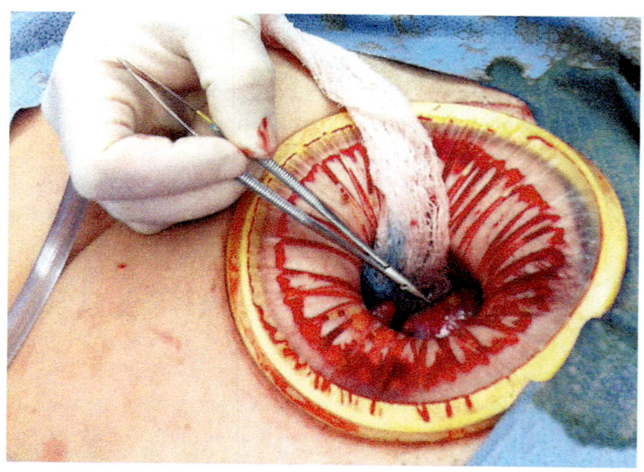

FIGURE 16.6 The round self-retaining wound retractor provides good exposure with the Kustner incision.

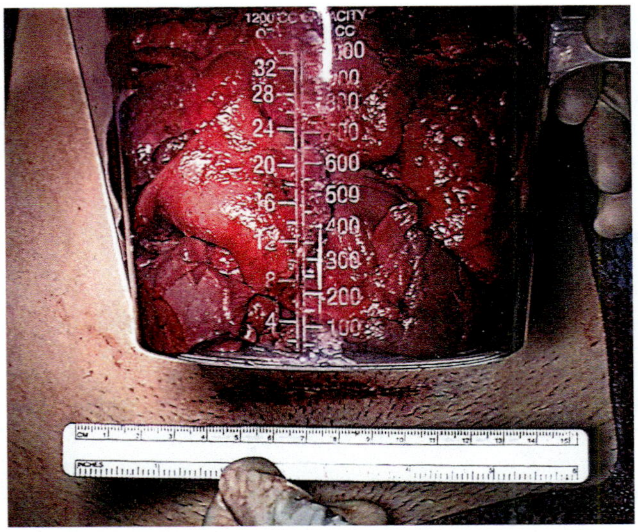

FIGURE 16.7 Large myomas can be removed though a minilaparotomy incision. The patient had a 20-week-gestational-size uterus with multiple fibroids. A 5 cm suprapubic transverse skin incision can be noted here. Note the large volume of morcellated myomas removed through this small incision.

Appropriate Uterine Incision(s)

The uterine incisions are dependent on the number, location and size of the fibroids and their proximity to the fallopian tube and the uterine vasculature. The incision should be placed to enable the removal of as many myomas as possible without causing excessive myometrial damage. The authors prefer transverse incisions which run parallel to the myometrial vasculature to diminish bleeding. Vertical uterine incisions may be selected in cases where lateral extention may damage the fallopian tubes or uterine vessels. Multiple incisions are sometimes needed but should be kept to a minimum. Anterior incisions are generally preferred to posterior ones based on limited evidence that they may reduce postoperative adhesion [14]. The incision is carried through the myoma capsule and into the myoma itself (Figure 16.8).

Removal of Fibroid

The fibroid is gently elevated with a single tooth tenaculum, myoma screw or perforating towel clamps while pushing the

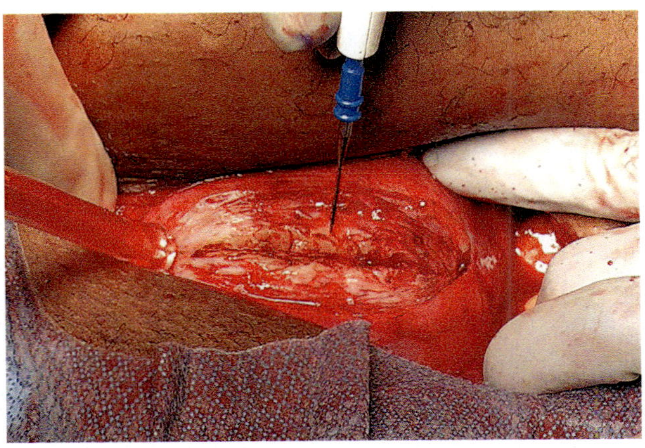

FIGURE 16.8 A transverse uterine incision is made through the serosa, myometrium and myoma capsule and into the myoma itself.

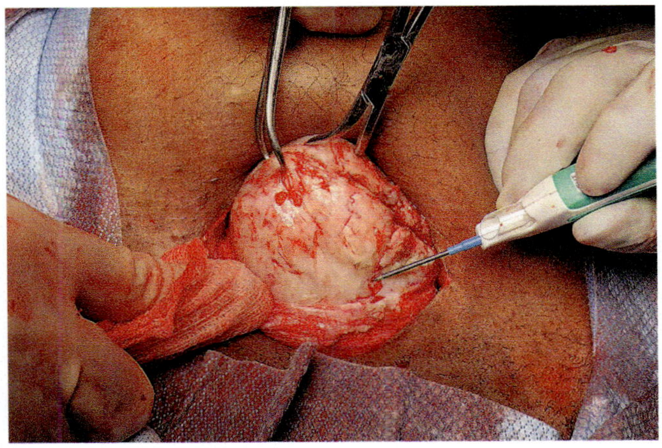

FIGURES 16.9 A single tooth tenaculum or perforating towel clamp is used to elevate the myoma as the plane between the myoma and its capsule is established. The myoma is progressively enucleated.

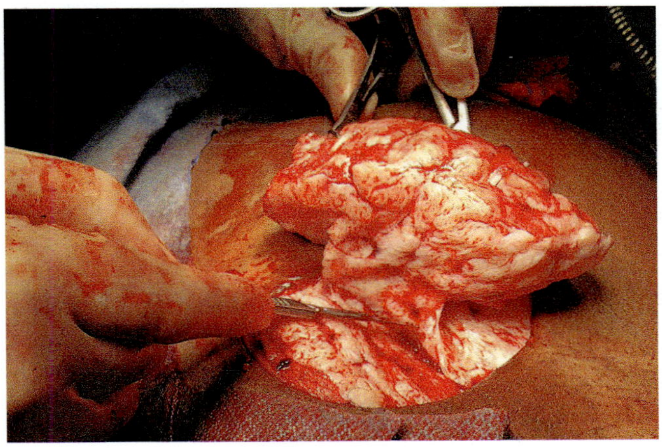

FIGURES 16.10 Large myomas may be morcellated in-situ with a scalpel to facilitate completion of the excision.

myoma capsule down off of the lesion. A scalpel or unipolar electrode may also be used to divide adherent capsule fibers to help enucleate the myoma (Figure 16.9). As more of the myoma is exposed, the clamps are advanced toward the myoma base and the dissection continues until the specimen is completely excised. Depending on the size of the myoma, it can either be removed from the pelvis intact or morcellated above the skin incision if too large to be delivered through the minilaparotomy. Very large fibroids may be morcellated *in situ* within the myometrium using a scalpel to facilitate complete removal (Figure 16.10).

Closure of the Defect

Following the removal of the myomas, the myometrial defects are closed in layers with 1 or 0 delayed absorbable suture. The goals are to prevent an inherent weakness of the uterine wall, as well as to eliminate any dead spaces that may lead to hematomas. Deep myometrial defects are closed with interrupted figure of eight sutures, then imbricated with layers of running sutures (Figures 16.11 and 16.12). The serosa is then approximated using a running 3–0 delayed absorbable suture, locking only for hemostasis

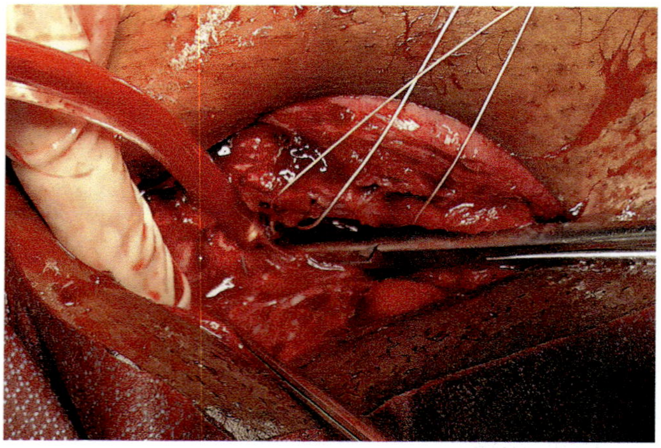

FIGURES 16.11 The myometrial defect is approximated using layers of 0-delayed absorbable suture to eliminate the dead space and reinforce the uterine wall.

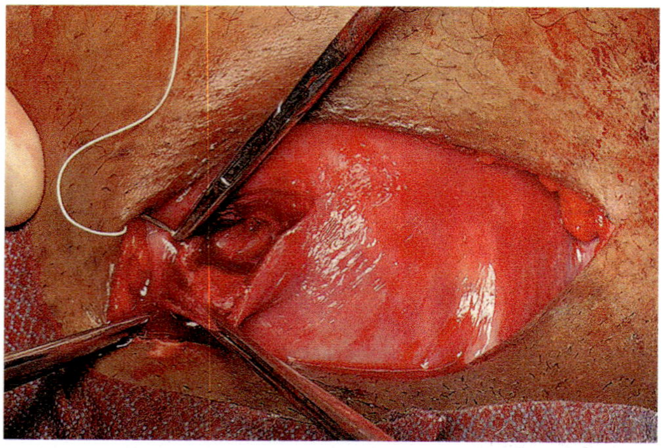

FIGURES 16.12 The superficial myometrial layers are repaired by imbrication over the deeper layers.

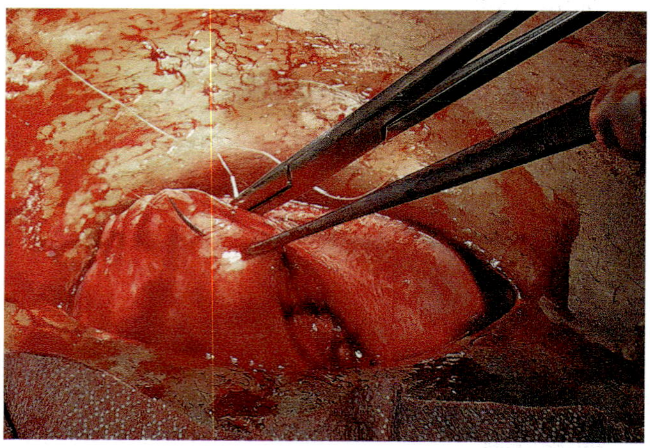

FIGURE 16.13 The uterine serosa is approximated using running 3–0 delayed absorbable suture.

(Figure 16.13). There is no evidence that a baseball stitch reduces adhesion formation. In cases where the endometrial cavity is breached, the endometrium is repaired as a separate layer using an interrupted or running 4–0 delayed absorbable suture.

Applications of Measures to Reduce Postoperative Adhesions

There are several different techniques that can be used to reduce the risk of postoperative adhesions. These are discussed in detail in Chapter 25.

Common Complications

Hemorrhage and Conversion to Hysterectomy

Bleeding is common during myomectomies, with average blood loss of around 200–800 mL [15–17]. The risk of a blood transfusion after myomectomy can vary from 2%–28% [15,16,18]. Larger size and higher number of fibroids, as well as endometrial cavity entry are associated with greater blood loss [19]. Approximately 1%–4% of all abdominal myomectomies are converted to hysterectomy, primarily owing to uncontrolled bleeding [20].

Postoperative Fevers

Fever occurs within 48 hours after surgery in approximately 12%–67% of women following myomectomy [18,20,21]. Proposed mechanisms for unexplained postmyomectomy fever include hematomas or inflammatory mediators at the myomectomy sites. The use of prophylactic antibiotics and meticulous hemostasis help to minimize postoperative fevers [13].

Postoperative Adhesions as a Long-Term Complication

Postoperative adhesions can be seen after abdominal myomectomies. See Chapter 25 for more details.

Outcomes after Abdominal Myomectomy

Improvement of Quality of Life and Symptoms

Even though abdominal myomectomy has been performed for over a century, outcome data are very limited. Older reports have shown improvement of symptoms in up to 80% of patients [22]; unfortunately, the large series of abdominal myomectomies do not comment on relief of symptoms, patient satisfaction or quality of life following surgery [18,23–25].

Persistence or Recurrence of Fibroids

A substantially large number of women after abdominal myomectomy will have fibroids on subsequent evaluation; however, most will not require any additional treatment for fibroid-related symptoms. Approximately 27%–62% of women will have evidence of fibroids 5–10 years after myomectomy [26–28]. Younger women, those with multiple fibroids at time of myomectomy [29] and those who did not conceive after surgery [27] are more likely to have new or persistent lesions. Additionally, women who received preoperative gonadotropin-releasing hormone analogues (GnRH analogs) are more likely to have persistent fibroids after surgery. Risk factors for women requiring subsequent surgery for fibroid-related symptoms are not well studied. In one report, 34% of women needed a second surgery within 7 years of follow-up [30].

Conclusion

Even with the advent of newer treatment modalities, abdominal myomectomy remains an important treatment for uterine myomas in women desiring future fertility, or those who just wish to avoid a hysterectomy. It does not have the limitations of size and number of myomas, which is an issue with the newer therapeutic options. It is making a resurgence now that power morcellators have been removed from many operating rooms, requiring a laparotomy incision to remove the myomas after laparoscopic or robotic myomectomy.

REFERENCES

1. Tinelli A, Hurst BS, Hudelist G et al. Laparoscopic myomectomy focusing on the myoma pseudocapsule: Technical and outcome reports. *Hum Reprod (Oxford, England).* 2012;27(2):427–35.
2. Moawad GN, Samuel D, Abi Khalil ED. Tips and Tricks: Single-Site Robotic-Assisted Myomectomy. *J Minim Invasive Gynecol.* 2016;23(6):861.
3. Plotti G, Plotti F, Di Giovanni A, Battaglia F, and Nagar G. Feasibility and safety of vaginal myomectomy: A prospective pilot study. *J Minim Invasive Gynecol.* 2008;15(2):166–71.
4. Marshburn PB, Matthews ML, and Hurst BS. Uterine artery embolization as a treatment option for uterine myomas. *Obstet Gynecol Clin North Am.* 2006;33(1):125–44.
5. Zupi E, Centini G, Sabbioni L, Lazzeri L, Argay IM, and Petraglia F. Nonsurgical alternatives for uterine fibroids. *Best Pract Res Clin Obstet Gynaecol.* 2015;34:122–31.
6. Kaump GR and Spies JB. The impact of uterine artery embolization on ovarian function. *Journal of Vascular and Interventional Radiology : JVIR.* 2013;24(4):459–67.
7. Rosenbaum L. N-of-1 Policymaking--Tragedy, trade-offs, and the demise of morcellation. *N Engl J Med.* 2016;374(10):986–90.
8. Dueholm M, Lundorf E, Hansen ES, Ledertoug S, and Olesen F. Accuracy of magnetic resonance imaging and transvaginal ultrasonography in the diagnosis, mapping, and measurement of uterine myomas. *Am J Obstet Gynecol.* 2002;186(3):409–15.
9. Testa DA, Di Legge A, Bonatti M, Manfredi DR, and Scambia DG. Imaging techniques for evaluation of uterine myomas. *Best Pract Res Clin Obstet Gynaecol.* 2015;34:37–53.
10. Goto A, Takeuchi S, Sugimura K, and Maruo T. Usefulness of Gd-DTPA contrast-enhanced dynamic MRI and serum determination of LDH and its isozymes in the differential diagnosis of leiomyosarcoma from degenerated leiomyoma of the uterus. *Int J Gynecol Cancer.* 2002;12(4):354–61.
11. ACOG practice bulletin No. 104: Antibiotic prophylaxis for gynecologic procedures. *Obstet Gynecol.* 2009;113(5):1180–9.
12. Rodriguez JF, Trobo AR, Garcia MV et al. The effect of performance feedback on wound infection rate in abdominal hysterectomy. *Am J Infect Control.* 2006;34(4):182–7.
13. Mukhopadhaya N, De Silva C, and Manyonda IT. Conventional myomectomy. *Best Pract Res Clin Obstet Gynaecol.* 2008;22(4):677–705.
14. Tulandi T, Murray C, and Guralnick M. Adhesion formation and reproductive outcome after myomectomy and second-look laparoscopy. *Obstet Gynecol.* 1993;82(2):213–5.
15. Sawin SW, Pilevsky ND, Berlin JA, and Barnhart KT. Comparability of perioperative morbidity between abdominal myomectomy and hysterectomy for women with uterine leiomyomas. *Am J Obstet Gynecol.* 2000;183(6):1448–55.
16. Iverson RE, Jr., Chelmow D, Strohbehn K, Waldman L, and Evantash EG. Relative morbidity of abdominal hysterectomy and myomectomy for management of uterine leiomyomas. *Obstet Gynecol.* 1996;88(3):415–9.
17. West S, Ruiz R, and Parker WH. Abdominal myomectomy in women with very large uterine size. *Fertil Steril.* 2006;85(1):36–9.
18. LaMorte AI, Lalwani S, and Diamond MP. Morbidity associated with abdominal myomectomy. *Obstet Gynecol.* 1993;82(6):897–900.
19. Schuring AN, Garcia-Rocha GJ, Schlosser HW, Greb RR, Kiesel L, and Schippert C. Perioperative complications in conventional and microsurgical abdominal myomectomy. *Arch Gynecol Obstet.* 2011;284(1):137–44.
20. Olufowobi O, Sharif K, Papaionnou S, Neelakantan D, Mohammed H, and Afnan M. Are the anticipated benefits of myomectomy achieved in women of reproductive age? A 5-year review of the results at a UK tertiary hospital. *J Obstet Gynaecol.* 2004;24(4):434–40.
21. Rybak EA, Polotsky AJ, Woreta T, Hailpern SM, and Bristow RE. Explained compared with unexplained fever in postoperative myomectomy and hysterectomy patients. *Obstet Gynecol.* 2008;111(5):1137–42.
22. Buttram VC, Jr. and Reiter RC. Uterine leiomyomata: Etiology, symptomatology, and management. *Fertil Steril.* 1981;36(4):433–45.
23. Ikpeze OC and Nwosu OB. Features of uterine fibroids treated by abdominal myomectomy at Nnewi, *Nigeria. J Obstet Gynaecol.* 1998;18(6):569–71.
24. Sirjusingh A, Bassaw B, and Roopnarinesingh S. The results of abdominal myomectomy. *West Indian Med J.* 1994;43(4): 138–9.
25. Vercellini P, Maddalena S, De Giorgi O, Pesole A, Ferrari L, and Crosignani PG. Determinants of reproductive outcome after abdominal myomectomy for infertility. *Fertil Steril.* 1999;72(1):109–14.
26. Acien P and Quereda F. Abdominal myomectomy: Results of a simple operative technique. *Fertil Steril.* 1996;65(1):41–51.
27. Candiani GB, Fedele L, Parazzini F, and Villa L. Risk of recurrence after myomectomy. *Br J Obstet Gynaecol.* 1991;98(4):385–9.
28. Fedele L, Parazzini F, Luchini L, Mezzopane R, Tozzi L, and Villa L. Recurrence of fibroids after myomectomy: A transvaginal ultrasonographic study. *Hum Reprod (Oxford, England).* 1995;10(7):1795–6.
29. Hanafi M. Predictors of leiomyoma recurrence after myomectomy. *Obstet Gynecol.* 2005;105(4):877–81.
30. Stewart EA, Faur AV, Wise LA, Reilly RJ, and Harlow BL. Predictors of subsequent surgery for uterine leiomyomata after abdominal myomectomy. *Obstet Gynecol.*2002;99(3):426–32.

17

Laparoscopic Myomectomy

Anthony N. Imudia and Erika Parker New

Introduction

When fibroids (leiomyomas or myomas) cause intolerable symptoms such as heavy uterine bleeding, pelvic pressure with urinary tract dysfunction or infertility, surgical management may be performed with myomectomy or hysterectomy. For those women who desire future fertility, myomectomy is an excellent management option. Fibroids may impact fertility by distorting the uterine cavity or even by obstructing the fallopian tubes.

As compared to open myomectomy via laparotomy, laparoscopic myomectomy is associated with less postoperative pain and a shorter hospital stay [1]. Other benefits include a greater number of patients that fully recover 2 weeks following surgery, less drop in patient hemoglobin and fewer overall complications. While laparoscopic myomectomy often results in longer operating times due to the complexity of the procedure and skill involved, surgeon experience and advances in surgical tools may save time in the operating room [2]. When comparing future outcomes after laparoscopic versus open myomectomy, there is no difference in recurrence of fibroids, return for repeat myomectomy or in hysterectomy at a later date [1].

Comparative studies of robot-assisted laparoscopic myomectomy with standard laparoscopic myomectomy show that robot-assisted cases involve even longer operative times, with one study showing an adjusted mean increase of 76 minutes. While robotic cases were also associated with a greater estimated blood loss, postoperative complications were not significantly different between the two [3]. For more information on robotic-assisted myomectomy, please refer to Chapter 18.

Patient Selection and Preoperative Planning

The ideal candidate for laparoscopic myomectomy is a woman who is symptomatic from her fibroids and desires future fertility. When considering surgical approach, both the location and size of the fibroids are critical factors to consider. Both intramural and subserosal fibroids can be removed by laparoscopic myomectomy; however, submucosal myomas are better served through hysteroscopic resection. Performing a hysteroscopy prior to laparoscopic myomectomy will assist in establishing the optimal approach and identifying submucosal myomas [4].

There is no maximum limit for how many or how large fibroids must be for safe removal by laparoscopic myomectomy. A meta-analysis showed anywhere from one to seven fibroids may be amenable to laparoscopic removal, even those as large as 10 cm in diameter [2]. Each surgeon must consider his or her own skill and experience to create individualized criteria for patient selection [5].

Certain preoperative conditions are helpful to consider in selecting candidates for laparoscopic myomectomy. Dubuisson et al. examined factors that were associated with conversion to an open procedure during laparoscopic myomectomy. Those factors associated with conversion were an estimated myoma size $\geq$5 cm by ultrasound, intramural type, anterior location and preoperative GnRH use [6]. Use of GnRH agonists prior to surgery is controversial. In theory, shrinking the size of myomas would make for an easier surgery; however, experience shows a higher risk of myoma recurrence, as well as greater difficulty in enucleating the softer tissue [7].

Appropriate preoperative preparation can assist in proper patient selection. In addition to a bimanual pelvic exam and imaging with transvaginal ultrasound (TVUS), magnetic resonance imaging (MRI) should be performed to map the number, location and depth of extension of myomas. Although both imaging modalities accurately detect the presence of fibroids, MRI is superior for determining the position and depth of extension into the uterine wall [8].

Surgical Procedure

Owing to the risk of entering the uterine cavity, as well as the use of chromopertubation, the patient should be given preoperative antibiotics, first-line being cefazolin [9]. After induction of general anesthesia, the patient should be positioned on the operating room table in the dorsal lithotomy position with her feet in stirrups and with Trendelenburg tilt as needed. Uterine manipulation is essential for adequate visualization of myomas, and a Pelosi Uterine Manipulator (Apple Medical Corporation, Marlborough, MA), for example, allows for uterine anteversion. In addition, this device allows for injection of methylene blue or indigo Carmine to perform chromopertubation during surgery, to determine whether or not the endometrium has been compromised.

Port placement consists of a 5–12 mm umbilical port primarily for the camera as well as three accessory ports forming an arc on the superior aspect of the abdomen (Figure 17.1). Occasionally, the camera port is placed few centimeters above the umbilicus (supra-umbilical) to ensure adequate distance between the fundus of the uterus or myoma and the camera (Figure 17.2). It is important to have the ports placed sufficiently high to ergonomically access the myomas. For example, the further the fibroid

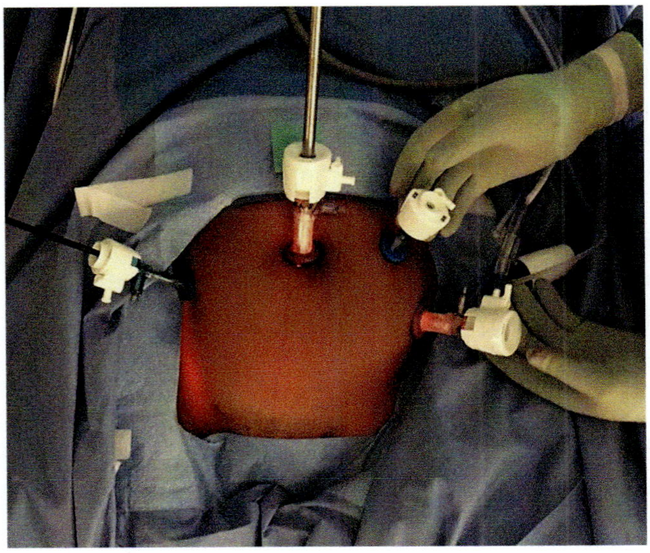

FIGURE 17.1 Laparoscopic port configuration for uterus with small myomas (<16 weeks gestation size).

uterus rises above the pelvic brim, the higher the ports must be placed [7]. In order to reduce blood loss, vasopressin may be injected into the plane between the myometrium and the myoma's capsule (Video 17.1), resulting in a characteristic blanching effect (Figure 17.3) [7]. Vasopressin can be administered concentrated (20 units in 60 mL of normal saline) or diluted (20 units in 400 mL of normal saline) without reported differences in estimated blood loss during surgery [10].

VIDEO 17.1 https://youtu.be/x4H3xIhaxDg
Injection of vasopressin prior to initial uterine incision.

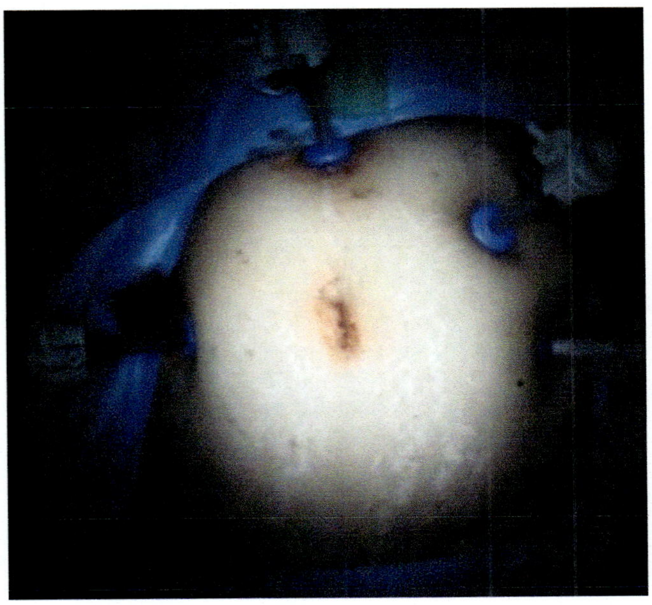

FIGURE 17.2 Laparoscopic port configuration for uterus with large myomas (usually ≥16 weeks gestation size).

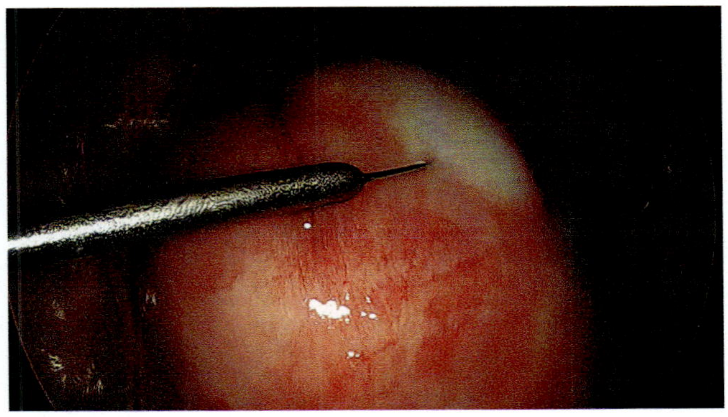

FIGURE 17.3 Injection of diluted vasopressin between the myoma and subserosal layer of the uterus to decrease blood loss.

Surgical Technique

It is recommended that the initial uterine incision is made transverse or horizontally directly over the site of the myoma (Figure 17.4). This horizontal incision allows for easier laparoscopic suturing than a vertical incision [11]. For this incision, the Sonicision cordless ultrasonic device (Coviden) is the instrument of choice at our institution; however, another capable device is the Harmonic Scalpel (Ethicon) [11], monopolar scissors or laser. Enucleation of the fibroid is achieved by grasping the fibroid with a single-toothed tenaculum and providing counter-traction while using both blunt and sharp dissection to develop the plane around the capsule, allowing for extraction of the fibroid (Video 17.2) [5].

VIDEO 17.2 https://youtu.be/0yhfMZo4YtQ
Enucleation of uterine fibroid laparoscopically.

Once the myoma has been removed, the resulting hysterotomy requires double-layer closure of the myometrium and serosal closure with or without the baseball-stitch technique. There are two methods of suturing that allow adequate closure of the uterine incision after myomectomy. The traditional method is to use interrupted sutures. A newer technique involves use of a continuous barbed suture, namely the V-Loc (Covidien). A loop on

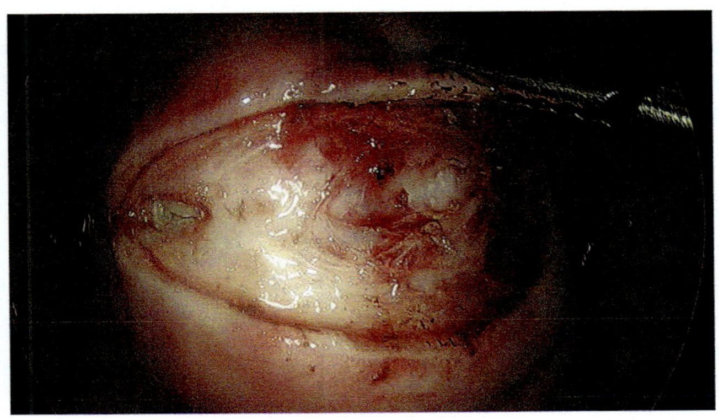

FIGURE 17.4 Initial horizontal or transverse uterine incision directly on top of the myoma.

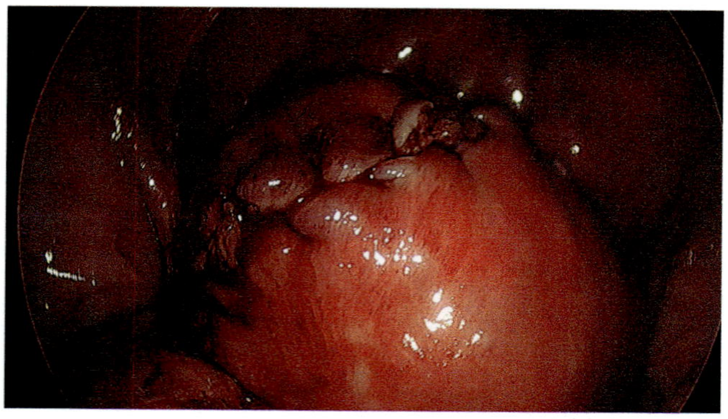

FIGURE 17.5 Hysterotomy closed laparoscopically following myomectomy.

the end of the suture allows for the needle to be thread through, with no knots required (Videos 17.3 and 17.4). A single-site study showed that using an absorbable barbed suture not only saved time in the operating room, but resulted in less blood loss [12]. A multicenter retrospective study that compared postoperative healing after traditional interrupted sutures versus continuous barbed suture found no significant difference in healing, complications, hematoma formation or reduction in scar on ultrasound during the 6 months after surgery. With the positive intraoperative benefits of shorter operative time and less blood loss, barbed suture appears to be the preferable method for closing the uterus (Figure 17.5) [13].

VIDEO 17.3 https://youtu.be/yq41thi23kU
Two-layer myometrial closure using barbed suture (V-Loc).

VIDEO 17.4 https://youtu.be/sARNxLEiRBA
Laparoscopic closure of the serosal layer using a baseball-stitch technique.

Interceed (Ethicon) may be placed over the hysterotomy site to help prevent adhesion formation. A Cochrane review on the use of barrier agents to prevent formation of adhesions gives low-level evidence to support the effectiveness in decreasing adhesions after a "second look" laparoscopy [14]. Overall however, adhesions after laparoscopic myomectomy are significantly less than in abdominal myomectomy based on a study that performed postoperative diagnostic laparoscopy to evaluate for adhesion formation [15] (see Video 17.5).

VIDEO 17.5 https://youtu.be/usjntHO5iqs
Conventional laparoscopic myomectomy.

Performing minimally invasive surgery such as laparoscopic myomectomy leaves the question of how to remove the enucleated fibroid tissue. Power morcellation, which uses a rotating knife to slice the tissue into small pieces that could be removed without making a larger incision, was the gold standard until 2014 before the FDA recommended against this practice. Different methods for specimen retrieval are now being utilized following minimally invasive myomectomy. All these are discussed in detail in Chapter 22.

Complications

When counseling and obtaining informed consent prior to surgery, it is critical to address potential complications. Major complications include blood loss requiring transfusion; hematoma formation; return to the operating room for unplanned surgery; urinary, bladder or bowel injury and conversion to laparotomy. Minor complications include postoperative fever, wound infection and cystitis. A large multicenter study of over 2000 patients, as well as one surgeon's case study of over 1000 patients, showed a 7.1%–11.1% risk of any complication during laparoscopic myomectomy, with the majority of complications being minor [4]. The most common reason for converting to a laparotomy is in cases of heavy blood loss with need to obtain swift hemostasis [2]. This often occurs while closing the hysterotomy, and faster closure helps to reduce blood loss and potentially decrease conversion rate [4].

Postoperative Management

One benefit of this minimally invasive surgical technique is that patients may be discharged home the same day, and a majority of patients will return to normal daily activities within 2 weeks after surgery [11]. Patients should be counseled on how long to wait before conceiving and implications on future method of delivery.

Conclusion

Laparoscopic myomectomy has many benefits over open myomectomy, most notably shorter hospital stay and fewer overall complications. While this procedure requires a longer operating time, this may be decreased with increasing surgeon experience. Success lies in proper patient selection and thorough preoperative evaluation and planning.

REFERENCES

1. Bhave Chittawar P, Franik S, Pouwer AW, and Farquhar C. Minimally invasive surgical techniques versus open myomectomy for uterine fibroids. *Cochrane Database Syst Rev.* 2014;10:CD004638.
2. Jin C, Hu Y, Chen XC et al. Laparoscopic versus open myomectomy--a meta-analysis of randomized controlled trials. *Eur J Obstet Gynecol Reprod Biol.* 2009;145(1):14–21.
3. Gargiulo AR, Srouji SS, Missmer SA, Correia KF, Vellinga TT, and Einarsson JI. Robot-assisted laparoscopic myomectomy compared with standard laparoscopic myomectomy. *Obstet Gynecol.* 2012;120(2 Pt 1):284–91.

4. Paul GP, Naik SA, Madhu KN, and Thomas T. Complications of laparoscopic myomectomy: A single surgeon's series of 1001 cases. *Aust N Z J Obstet Gynaecol*. 2010;50(4):385–90.
5. Mattei A, Cioni R, Bargelli G, and Scarselli G. Techniques of laparoscopic myomectomy. *Reprod Biomed Online*. 2011; 23(1):34–9.
6. Dubuisson JB, Fauconnier A, Fourchotte V, Babaki-Fard K, Coste J, and Chapron C. Laparoscopic myomectomy: Predicting the risk of conversion to an open procedure. *Hum Reprod*. 2001;16(8):1726–31.
7. Rossetii A, Sizzi O, Chiarotti F, and Florio G. Developments in techniques for laparoscopic myomectomy. *J Soc Laparoendoscopic Surg*. 2007;11:34–40.
8. Dueholm M, Lundorf E, Hansen ES, Ledertoug S, and Olesen F. Accuracy of magnetic resonance imaging and transvaginal ultrasonography in the diagnosis, mapping, and measurement of uterine myomas. *Am J Obstet Gynecol*. 2002;186(3):409–15.
9. ACOG practice bulletin No. 104: Antibiotic prophylaxis for gynecologic procedures. *Obstet Gynecol*. 2009:113(5):1180–9.
10. Cohen SL, Senapati S, Gargiulo AR et al. Dilute versus concentrated vasopressin administration during laparoscopic myomectomy: A randomised controlled trial. *BJOG: An Int J Obstet Gynaecol*. 2017;124(2):262–268.
11. Hurst BS, Matthews ML, and Marshburn PB. Laparoscopic myomectomy for symptomatic uterine myomas. *Fertil Steril*. 2005;83(1):1–23.
12. Angioli R, Plotti F, Montera R et al. A new type of absorbable barbed suture for use in laparoscopic myomectomy. *Int J Gynaecol Obstet*. 2012;117(3):220–3.
13. Tinelli R, Litta P, Angioni S et al. A multicenter study comparing surgical outcomes and ultrasonographic evaluation of scarring after laparoscopic myomectomy with conventional versus barbed sutures. *Int J Gynaecol Obstet*. 2016;134.
14. Ahmad G, O'Flynn H, Hindocha A, and Watson A. Barrier agents for adhesion prevention after gynaecological surgery. *Cochrane Database Syst Rev*. 2015(4):CD000475.
15. Bulletti C, Polli V, Negrini V, Giacomucci E, and Flamigni C. Adhesion formation after laparoscopic myomectomy. *J Am Assoc Gyn Lap*. 1996;3(4):533–6.

18

Computer-Assisted Laparoscopic Myomectomy

Randi H. Goldman and Antonio R. Gargiulo

The approval by the European Commission (CE) and the United States Food and Drug Administration (FDA) of the Intuitive Surgical da Vinci(R) surgical system for gynecologic surgery in 1999 and 2005 has provided a complementary technique to traditional laparoscopic surgery [1,2]. To date, at more than 20 years from its formal introduction, the da Vinci(R) surgical system remains the only commercially available platform for computer-assisted gynecologic surgery (another FDA-approved robotic surgical platform, the Senhance by Transenterix, has been FDA approved for over two years but has not been able to sell units and is practically a nonentity in the current clinical scenario). For the purpose of this chapter, we will use the terms "computer-assisted surgery" and "robotic surgery" interchangeably, with the understanding that the former is scientifically correct, and the latter has become the one of common use. Indeed, while the da Vinci(R) surgical system is not a robot but rather a computer-assisted teleoperator, there is little doubt that the field of computer-assisted surgery will evolve into that of bona fide robotics in the near future. Computer-assisted surgery is now a well-established, next-generation laparoscopic technique that has enhanced the types of minimally invasive approaches we can offer, while broadening the patient base for which minimally invasive surgery is an option. The technical advantages of robotic surgery are vast and include, perhaps most importantly, superior instrumentation. Surgeons using the da Vinci system enjoy seven degrees of freedom per instrument arm: four from the wristed instruments (pitch, yaw, roll and grip) and another three from the robotic arm itself (insertion, pitch and yaw) [3]. Furthermore, the robotic system has the advantages of filtering natural tremor; providing a magnified, high-definition, three-dimensional image and improving surgeon comfort. These technological advantages translate in actual operative advantages, including a faster learning curve and virtual ambidexterity [4,5,6]. The dexterity enjoyed with robotic surgery remains unmatched and allows for improved precision in the operating room. Last, but most definitely not least, the entire technical skill set for safe advanced robotic surgery can be acquired on dedicated virtual simulators, avoiding the unnecessary exposure of patients to the early phase of the surgeons' learning curve [7,8]. Such de-coupling of technical proficiency from direct on-patient learning is one of the hidden gems of computer-assisted surgery, that is destined to become more and more relevant as patient-centered medicine grows as an important new concept. A recommended list of instruments to use during a robotic myomectomy can be found in Table 18.1 [9].

It has been well established that in every surgical field, laparoscopic surgeries are superior to open (laparotomy) procedures [10–17]. Multiple randomized controlled trials have demonstrated that minimally invasive laparoscopic myomectomy can be offered as a same-day procedure and, compared to open myomectomy, is typically associated with less blood loss and postoperative pain, a faster return to activity, smaller scars and fewer overall complications [17,18].

Many patients who choose to undergo myomectomy do so in consideration of future reproductive goals. For these patients, laparoscopic approaches have yielded equivalent or better cumulative pregnancy and live birth rates in multiple clinical trials [13–15]. Regarding obstetric risk, however, pregnancies following laparoscopic myomectomy are less likely to result in uterine rupture (0%–1.1%) [15,19–21] compared with an open approach (0%–4%) [22,23]. In fact, the uterine rupture rate following laparoscopic myomectomy approximates the risk to a subsequent pregnancy following a prior low transverse cesarean section (0.32%) [23]. Furthermore, adhesion formation is significantly lower following a laparoscopic myomectomy (29%–35%) than an open myomectomy (55%–94%), as seen during second-look laparoscopy [24,25]. This is of prime importance for reproductive-aged women, as adhesions make future abdominal procedures, including cesarean sections, more difficult. Adhesions may also cause chronic pain and infertility [26–28]. As a result of the aforementioned considerations, the American Society of Reproductive Medicine (ASRM) recommends a minimally invasive approach to myomectomy for appropriate patients, with the use of adhesion barriers to minimize the likelihood of adhesion formation [29]. Sadly, this is one of the least observed ASRM recommendations, as it remains accepted practice for gynecologic surgeons worldwide to perform abdominal myomectomies in women for whom the minimally invasive route would most definitely be considered "appropriate" by better-trained and/or better-equipped surgical teams. In the age of patient-centered medicine and computer-assisted surgery, such a surgeon-centered approach to care (i.e., defining the appropriateness for minimally invasive surgery based on a surgeon's manual skills rather than the type of pathology) should no longer be tolerated. The fact that this surgeon-centered approach is accepted in women's health but not in men's health adds insult to injury. To be specific, when it became clear that laparoscopic prostatectomy provided significant

TABLE 18.1

Surgical Steps and Recommended Instruments for Computer-Assisted Laparoscopic Myomectomy

Surgical Steps	Recommended Instruments	Additional EndoWrist Instrument Options
Hysterotomy Fibroid enucleation and management	Monopolar: Hot Shears (Monopolar curved scissors) Bipolar: PK Dissecting Forceps 3rd instrument arm: Tenaculum forceps	Monopolar: • Permanent cautery hook • Permanent cautery spatula Bipolar: • Maryland bipolar forceps 3rd instrument arm: • ProGrasp forceps • Cobra grasper or Cadiere forceps Suction & irrigation: • EndoWrist One suction/irrigator
Multilayer suture closure of defect (deep layers) Multilayer suture closure of defect (serosal layer)	Suturing: Mega SutureCut Needle driver Long-tip forceps	Suturing: • Mega needle driver • Large needle driver • Mega SutureCut needle driver

Source: Adapted from Gargiulo AR, and Nezhat C. Robot-Assisted Myomectomy: Broadening the Laparoscopist's Armamentarium. In: *Uterine Myoma, Myomectomy and Minimally Invasive Treatments* Cham: Springer International Publishing; 2015, pp. 193–202.

advantages over open prostatectomy, but that only a handful of surgeons could perform them, the entire field of urology embraced robotic prostatectomy, reducing open prostatectomy in developed countries to a niche surgery for nostalgic surgeons (and poorly informed patients). Not so for gynecologic procedures, where a veritable ideological war based on the false pretense of cost containment has been waged against robotic surgery in spite of the evidence pointing to an unjustifiably low adoption of minimally invasive myomectomy and other advanced gynecologic surgeries [30–32].

The main merit of robot-assisted laparoscopic myomectomy is that it allows women to undergo a minimally invasive surgical approach in the setting of large or deeply seated myomas that would otherwise be removed routinely via laparotomy. A recent study by Barakat et al. found that even in the setting of a larger fibroid burden in a robot-assisted myomectomy group (compared with a traditional laparoscopic myomectomy group), there were no differences in blood loss, operative time or hospital stay [33]. In this same study, patients who underwent a robot-assisted procedure had the same tumor load removed as those patients who underwent a laparotomy. The superior instrumentation provided by the robotic system allows large fibroids to be enucleated in a controlled, precise fashion and the myoma bed to be sutured layer by layer, ensuring a proper closure.

Laparoscopic myomectomy is a "suture-heavy" procedure, and computer-assisted surgery enables laparoscopic suturing (arguably the most time-consuming, challenging, yet vital part of the procedure) to be completed in a facile and controlled fashion. Importantly, the faster a wound is closed, the less blood loss a patient suffers. However, an effective myomectomy technique is not defined by how fast one sutures, but rather by how fast one sutures well. A recent study has evaluated the importance of proper wound closure with respect to adhesion formation using a second-look laparoscopy performed 6 months after laparoscopic myomectomy, finding that the presence of postsurgical adhesions was associated with the quality of myoma bed closure; if a protruding wound was detected, the patient was 2.5 times more likely to have concurrent adhesive disease [34]. This is more likely to occur following a single-layer closure, that is the closure most often performed in traditional laparoscopic myomectomy [35]. Instead, with robot-assisted myoma bed closure, protruding wounds can be eliminated with a multilayer closure technique [36,37].

There have been concerns regarding the longer operative time in some studies for robot-assisted laparoscopic myomectomy. In a study by Gargiulo et al. that compared operative time between robotic myomectomy and laparoscopic myomectomy, it was found that robotic procedures took, on average, 76 minutes longer [38]. However, the vast majority of wound approximations were being executed with conventional suture (requiring extensive knot tying) in the robotic group and with barbed suture (requiring no knot tying) in the laparoscopic group. In retrospect, we now know that barbed suture shortens operative time and decreases blood loss and should be the gold standard for use in any minimally invasive myomectomy [38,39]. It is very likely that the lack of barbed suture in the robotic group contributed to the longer operative time observed in this study.

As with any surgery, careful patient selection is the key to success and to avoiding unanticipated conversion to laparotomy. Each surgeon has his or her own comfort level regarding which patients are appropriate candidates for computer-assisted surgery based on the anticipated difficulty of the procedure. To improve patient selection, we strongly recommend preoperative imaging with magnetic resonance imaging (MRI) [9]. MRI is essential in helping surgeons plan out a procedure by detailing the size and location of each myoma. Furthermore, the images can be displayed throughout the procedure and used intraoperatively as a guide. As a general rule, based on the first 750 such operations performed by our team (with a 0.1% reported conversion to open surgery), patients with fewer than 15 total myomas, with a leading myoma of less than 15 cm in size, are appropriate candidates for robotic myomectomy [3].

Proper port placement at the time of a robotic myomectomy is essential to the success and ease of the procedure (Figure 18.1) [40]. The central camera port must be a sufficient distance away from the working area to allow for optimal visualization and operating space. For a majority of cases, the camera port is placed intra-umbilically; however, for patients with large myomas or short torsos, the camera port can be placed in a midline supra-umbilical location. Recent evidence shows that a high placement of the primary port has no chance of injuring the falciform ligament of the liver (even in the smallest patients) if it falls within the first 6.5 cm cephalad to the umbilicus [41]. Each additional port should be at least 8 cm away from the other ports so that the robotic arms can enjoy full mobility with a minimum of external collisions of the robotic arms. Depending on the anticipated difficulty of the case, the size and location of the myomas and the patient's preferred cosmetic results, we use a total of three or four robotic ports (including the camera arm port) in addition to an assistant port [9]. More recently, following the FDA advisory

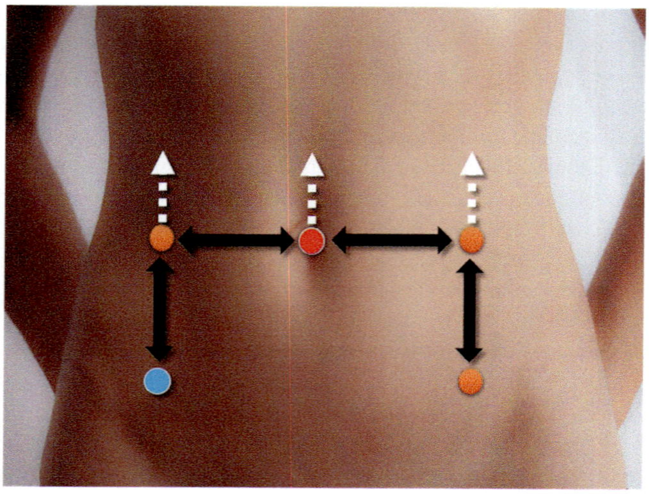

FIGURE 18.1 Robotic port placement. Our robotic port placement for myomectomy is depicted in this figure. The red circle represents the location of the camera port, which must be a sufficient distance away from the working area to allow for optimal visualization and operating space (due to the hourglass effect of the myoma over the uterine corpus which occurs during enucleation). Typically, the camera port is placed intra-umbilically. For patients with large myomas (or short torsos), the camera port can be placed in a midline supra-umbilical location up to 6.5 cm cephalad to the umbilicus without risking injury to the falciform ligament. The robotic operative ports are denoted by orange circles and should be at least 8 cm away from all other ports to maximize mobility and to minimize external collisions of the robotic arms. The assistant port is represented by the blue circle, which we typically place in the right lower quadrant.

on uterine tissue morcellation and the consequent removal of laparoscopic morcellators from the operating rooms of many hospitals, we have had to adopt a contained myoma extraction through a modified open laparoscopy incision in order to keep offering minimally invasive myomectomy (Figure 18.2). As a natural evolution of this requirement, we have developed and published a novel single-site robotic technique that allows us to perform the entire minimally invasive myomectomy through the same incision that we use to extract the specimen (Figure 18.3). Single-site robotic myomectomy is currently routinely offered to our patients with fibroids under 6 cm [42–44].

Effective enucleation of a fibroid is the fundamental step of any myomectomy. Myomectomy is rigorously intracapsular, and preservation of the neurovascular bundle is thought to be essential for adequate functional repair of the myometrium (Figure 18.4) [45–47]. The hysterotomy must be large enough to allow delivery of the myoma: a hysterotomy that is too large will generally bleed more during enucleation and will require more suturing to repair. Robotic myomectomy is a delicate affair: the tenaculum stabilizes the tumor, the uterine manipulator stabilizes the uterus and the operator second (or second and third) instrument will push away the surrounding myometrium (in the form of the myoma pseudocapsule) until the tumor is delivered. Steady, three-dimensional, magnified visualization assists with careful dissection in the appropriate tissue planes [9,48]. Ideally, a surgeon should attempt to enucleate all fibroids safely through the smallest number of hysterotomies needed and should avoid

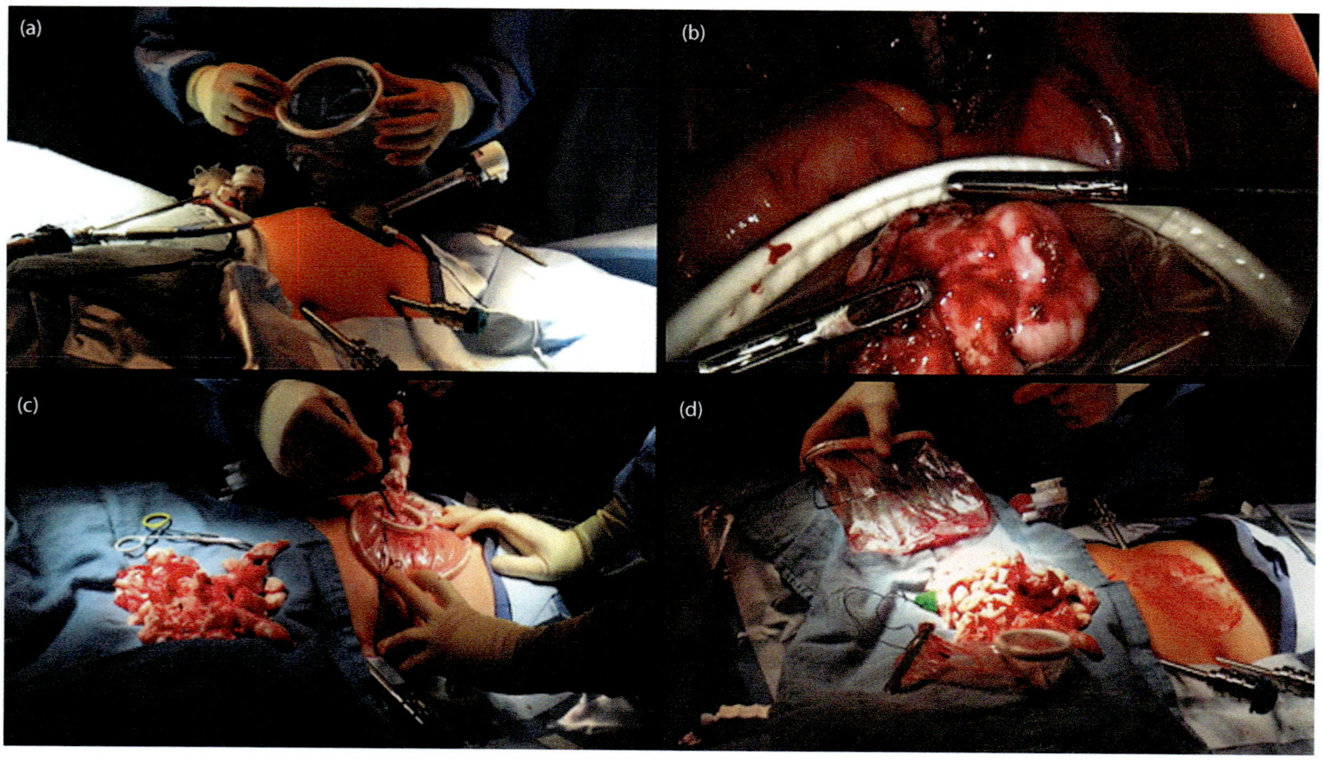

FIGURE 18.2 Contained myoma extraction. Following the 2014 FDA advisory on uterine tissue morcellation, we have adopted a contained myoma extraction technique. (a) Following fibroid enucleation, the umbilical incision is extended to approximately 2–2.5 cm (i.e., to a classic open laparoscopy sagittal incision), and a bag is placed intraabdominally. (b) The surgical specimen is laparoscopically placed inside the bag. (c) The edge of the bag is exteriorized through the umbilical incision and the specimen contained in the bag is pulled in direct contact with the modified open laparoscopic umbilical site, undermined with a surgical knife and extracted by hand. (d) At the completion of morcellation, the bag is removed through the umbilical incision and checked for damage or evidence of spill.

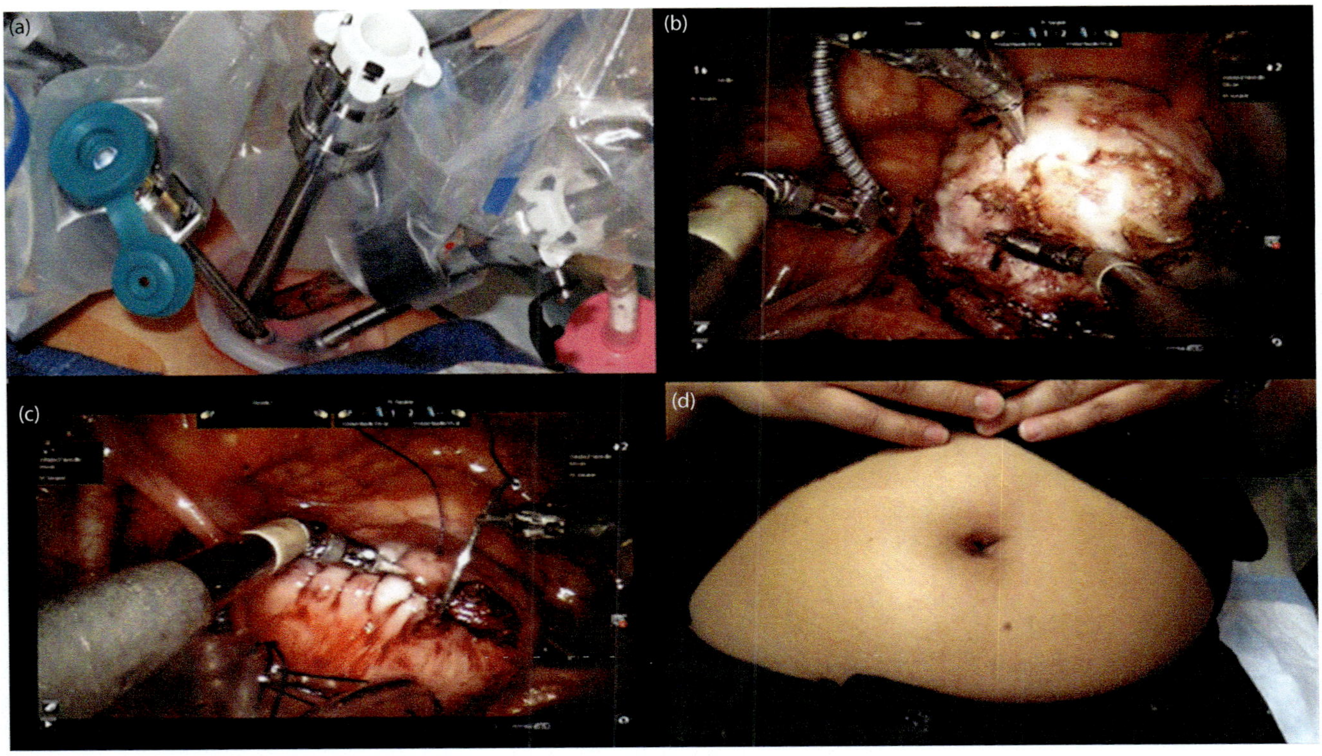

FIGURE 18.3 Single-site robotic myomectomy. (a) With our novel single-site robotic technique, an entire myomectomy can be performed through the same 2.5 cm umbilical incision needed for tissue extraction. (b) Special curved instruments are placed through a dedicated single-site port. (c) Robotic suturing with wristed instruments through the single-site port allows for accurate layer-by-layer closure of the myoma bed. (d) This ultra-minimally invasive single surgical site allows for minimal to no visible scarring and, in the context of a procedure that currently requires a 2.5 cm incision for contained tissue extraction, it saves the patient three additional entry wounds.

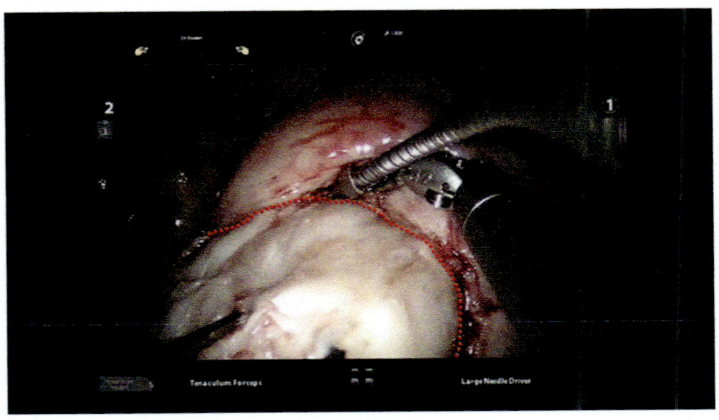

FIGURE 18.4 Intracapsular fibroid enucleation. The fundamental step of any myomectomy is the enucleation of the fibroid(s), which should occur exclusively at the level of the pseudocapsule (red dotted line). Intracapsular enucleation allows for preservation of the neurovascular bundle surrounding the tumor, which is thought to be essential for adequate functional repair of the myometrium. Once a hysterotomy is made and the tumor is stabilized, the surrounding myometrium (including the myoma pseudocapsule) is purposefully pushed aside and the tumor delivered.

injuring the endometrial cavity and the fallopian tubes. While the hysterotomy is best made with an instrument connected to an energy source, in order to limit blood loss and keep a clear operative field, the remainder of the enucleation is mostly achieved through blunt dissection and traction-countertraction. Chromopertubation can be performed during myomectomy in select cases, to assess for entrance into the endometrial cavity. Because the enucleation and the repair portions of the procedure may be time-consuming, they are often responsible for a majority of the blood loss. To reduce intraoperative blood loss (and the associated need for transfusion), we recommend several techniques [9]. Gonadotropin-releasing hormone (GnRH) agonists have routinely been used to reduce the size of large myomas prior to surgery and may be used for a few months prior to a planned procedure. However, their use has the potential to distort tissue planes and could make enucleation more difficult [48,49]. It is our standard to use both intraoperative rectal misoprostol (400 mcg) as well as diluted vasopressin injected into the myometrium to reduce the amount of intraoperative blood loss. Vasopressin must be used cautiously, as it can cause severe cardiac disturbances. However, one must remember that adverse outcomes with vasopressin are very rare. Vasopressin has a plasma half-life of about 10–20 minutes and cardiac events (including cardiovascular arrest) have not been reported with doses smaller than 10 units. Because of this, we use repeated doses of 5 units of vasopressin at 60–120 minute intervals during our procedure. Because vasopressin affects diuresis and can affect blood pressure, communication with the anesthesiologist is critical at this point in the procedure [50–52]. Tranexamic acid has recently entered the armamentarium of the gynecologic surgeon for this type of operation [53]. We employ this antifibrinolytic agent liberally in our practice, for patients in which the blood loss is expected to be substantial, or the starting hematocrit is less than ideal.

As mentioned bove, of the greatest benefits that robot-assisted myomectomy provides is the quality of the hysterotomy closure. The gold standard for hysterotomy repair is a multilayer closure with no exposed suture; this microsurgical standard applies to all myomectomies, independently of whether they are performed through an invasive or with a minimally invasive approach. Single-layer closures cause hematoma formation and healing by second intention, while exposed sutures cause pelvic adhesions: both of these have no place in modern reproductive surgery. A proper wound approximation will decrease blood loss, the chances of adhesion formation and the risk of future uterine rupture [9,34,36,37]. It is important to make an open statement of what represents adequate microsurgical technique for the myomectomy operation, because it is a sad reality that minimally invasive myomectomy has become synonymous with "simplified" techniques in many cases. This is not an ethically acceptable logical step, because patients are completely unaware of such "shortcuts", and therefore cannot make an informed decision regarding which surgical team to trust. The rule is simple, the basic tenets of myomectomy are constant and independent of technique used: (1) intracapsular myomectomy, (2) closure in layers, (3) no exposed sutures. These can be achieved via laparotomy or laparoscopy, but the operation does not change based on the access modality. When the rules of engagement are clear, the role of the robot in making the laparoscopic transition possible for many surgeons becomes much more clear.

Barbed suture is now routinely used to close the deep myometrial and even the serosal layers. Barbed suture provides appropriate tissue tension and re-approximation of surgical planes and allows for a faster closure (and less blood loss) [38,39,54,55]. Once hemostasis is confirmed, we routinely apply an adhesion barrier such as Interceed to hysterotomy sites, to further reduce the risk of postoperative adhesion formation [56].

Concerns regarding unintended laparoscopic morcellation of malignant uterine tumors have been prevalent in the medical community and in the media. As a result, tissue extraction following minimally invasive procedures has become significantly more challenging for gynecologists [57–60]. Following recent FDA recommendations against electromechanical morcellation of uterine tissue, many more patients and physicians have opted to undergo laparotomy as opposed to a minimally invasive approach, in an attempt to mitigate a potential upstaging of cancer not detected during a preoperative work-up. In theory, this would decrease mortality associated with hysterectomy or myomectomy. In contrast to this presumption, however, a recent decision analysis using 100,000 hypothetical premenopausal women predicted that more deaths would actually result from the increased adoption of open hysterectomies than from the spread of a malignant leiomyosarcoma via laparoscopy with morcellation in the rare patients affected [61]. The projected increase in number of deaths following an open procedure is explained by the higher chance of postoperative complications such as blood clots. Nevertheless, because leiomyosarcomas are not often diagnosed until surgical pathology returns, concerns about disseminating a potential cancer intraoperatively must be taken seriously. Techniques have been proposed wherein a specimen such as a myoma or uterus is placed in a bag laparoscopically following enucleation [62]. The bag is then brought up to the patient's skin through one of the port sites, which has been enlarged to approximately 25 mm. The specimen can then be carefully hand-morcellated and removed from the patient's body without dissemination of myoma fragments. This technique has allowed all of our patients who make the standard inclusion criteria for a robot-assisted laparoscopic approach to continue to receive minimally invasive surgery despite restrictions on morcellation [63]. However, in the spirit of providing a chapter that is both practical and scientifically honest, we should recognize that our current efforts to limit the potential spread of malignant cells in the setting of minimally invasive myomectomy has no rationale whatsoever, because the uterine serosa has already been breached, and uterine tumors have already had a chance to shed thousands of cells around the abdomen before being contained.

Learning surgical techniques, such as robot-assisted myomectomy, can be challenging. In medicine, we have traditionally used the "see one, do one, teach one" mantra. This has been a "necessary evil" of surgery in the twentieth century and the only way to perpetuate surgical knowledge for future generations. Because of this, this philosophy of surgical teaching is still widely accepted, in spite of all evidence pointing to a higher chance of complications during the surgeon's learning curve. Ultimately, patents are expected to relinquish a small part of their safety during surgery, a sort of token to pay to assure that future generations of patients will still have access to well-trained surgeons. This is a true ethical conundrum, which is evolving as new technology becomes available.

Robotic training consoles have enabled the teaching and learning of robotic surgical techniques to be simulated and thus have largely separated technical training from direct patient care. Instead of learning on an actual patient during a live procedure, physicians and trainees can spend time perfecting robotic simulations, from basic suturing to performing hysterectomies, on a training console well before they attempt to replicate that surgery on a live patient. This is beneficial for all involved. The operator learning curve with the robotic system is relatively fast and can be enhanced with the use of training consoles [7,64,65]. Virtual simulation training has allowed many providers to learn computer-assisted surgery techniques efficiently, allowing for a switch from laparotomy to a minimally invasive approach.

Robot-assisted myomectomy has expanded the patient base for whom laparoscopic surgery is possible. Patients who previously only had the option of an open myomectomy can now enjoy the benefits of a minimally invasive approach via computer-assisted surgery. The visualization and precision afforded by robot-assisted surgery remains unmatched and is particularly useful in myomectomy. While perfecting robotic techniques demands time and practice, learning the requisite skills to perform robotic surgery can be decoupled from direct patient care by use of virtual reality simulators, with potentially dramatic impact on overall quality of surgical care in a teaching hospital setting.

Disclaimer

Dr. Gargiulo reports being a consultant to Medicaroid, Inc., and Lumenis, Inc.

REFERENCES

1. Advincula AP, Song A, Burke W, and Reynolds RK. Preliminary experience with robot-assisted laparoscopic myomectomy. *J Am Assoc Gynecol Laparosc*. 2004 November; 11(4):511–8.

2. O'Sullivan OE and O'Reilly BA. *Gynecological Surgery and the Robot*. 2014;6:59–70.
3. Quaas AM, Einarsson JI, Srouji S, and Gargiulo AR. Robotic myomectomy: A review of indications and techniques. *Rev Obstet Gynecol*. 2010;3(4):185–91.
4. Mucksavage P, Kerbl DC, and Lee JY. The da Vinci(®) surgical system overcomes innate hand dominance. *J Endourol*. 2011 August;25(8):1385–8.
5. Moorthy K, Munz Y, Dosis A et al. Dexterity enhancement with robotic surgery. *Surg Endosc*. 2004 May;18(5):790–5.
6. Choussein, S Srouji SS, Farland LV, Wietsma A et al. Robotic assistance confers ambidexterity to laparoscopic surgeons. *J Minim Invasive Gynecol*. 2018;25(1):76–83.
7. Culligan P, Gurshumov E, Lewis C, Priestley J, Komar J, and Salamon C. Predictive validity of a training protocol using a robotic surgery simulator. *Female Pelvic Med Reconstr Surg*. 2014 January–February;20(1):48–51.
8. Gargiulo AR. Will computer-assisted surgery shake the foundations of surgical ethics in the age of patient-centered medicine? *OBG Manag Suppl*. 2015;S20–4.
9. Gargiulo AR and Nezhat C. Robot-Assisted Myomectomy: Broadening the Laparoscopist's Armamentarium. In: A. Tinelli and A. Malvasi (eds.) *Uterine Myoma, Myomectomy and Minimally Invasive Treatments* Cham: Springer International Publishing; 2015, pp. 193–202.
10. Alessandri F, Lijoi D, Mistrangelo E, Ferrero S, and Ragni N. Randomized study of laparoscopic versus minilaparotomic myomectomy for uterine myomas. *J Minim Invasive Gynecol*. 2006;13(2):92–7.
11. Cicinelli E, Tinelli R, Colafiglio G, and Saliani N. Laparoscopy vs minilaparotomy in women with symptomatic uterine myomas: A prospective randomized study. *J Minim Invasive Gynecol*. 2009;16(4):422–6.
12. Fanfani F, Fagotti A, Bifulco G, Ercoli A, Malzoni M, and Scambia G. A prospective study of laparoscopy versus minilaparotomy in the treatment of uterine myomas. *J Minim Invasive Gynecol*. 2005;12(6):470–4.
13. Palomba S, Zupi E, Russo T et al. A multicenter randomized, controlled study comparing laparoscopic versus minilaparotomic myomectomy: Short-term outcomes. *Fertil Steril*. 2007 October;88(4):942–51.
14. Palomba S, Zupi E, Falbo A et al. A multicenter randomized, controlled study comparing laparoscopic versus minilaparotomic myomectomy: Reproductive outcomes. *Fertil Steril*. 2007 October;88(4):933–41.
15. Seracchioli R, Manuzzi L, Vianello F et al. Obstetric and delivery outcome of pregnancies achieved after laparoscopic myomectomy. *Fertil Steril*. 2006 July;86(1):159–65.
16. Mais V, Ajossa S, Guerriero S, Mascia M, Solla E, and Melis GB. Laparoscopic versus abdominal myomectomy: A prospective, randomized trial to evaluate benefits in early outcome. *Am J Obstet Gynecol*. 1996 February;174(2):654–8.
17. Jin C, Hu Y, Chen X et al. Laparoscopic versus open myomectomy--A meta-analysis of randomized controlled trials. *Eur J Obstet Gynecol Reprod Biol*. 2009 July;145(1):14–21.
18. Moustafa S, Duke C, Sood A, Dun E, and Dabaja A. 30-Day postoperative outcomes of minimally invasive versus abdominal myomectomy: An analysis of the National Surgical Quality Improvement Program (NSQIP) Database 2005–2013. *Fertil Steril*. 2015;104:e179–80.
19. Sizzi O, Rossetti A, Malzoni M et al. Italian multicenter study on complications of laparoscopic myomectomy. *J Minim Invasive Gynecol*. 1979;14(4):453–62.
20. Pitter MC, Gargiulo AR, Bonaventura LM, Lehman JS, and Srouji SS. Pregnancy outcomes following robot-assisted myomectomy. *Hum Reprod*. 2013 January;28(1):99–108.
21. Parker WH, Einarsson J, Istre O, and Dubuisson J-B. Risk factors for uterine rupture after laparoscopic myomectomy. *J Minim Invasive Gynecol*. 2009;17(5):551–4.
22. Garnet JD. Uterine rupture during pregnancy. An analysis of 133 patients. *Obstet Gynecol*. 1964 June;23:898–905.
23. Spong CY, Landon MB, Gilbert S et al. Risk of uterine rupture and adverse perinatal outcome at term after cesarean delivery. *Obstet Gynecol*. 2007 October;110(4):801–7.
24. Takeuchi H and Kinoshita K. Evaluation of adhesion formation after laparoscopic myomectomy by systematic second-look microlaparoscopy. *J Am Assoc Gynecol Laparosc*. 2002 November;9(4):442–6.
25. Dubuisson JB, Fauconnier A, Chapron C, Kreiker G, and Nörgaard C. Second look after laparoscopic myomectomy. *Hum Reprod*. 1998 August;13(8):2102–6.
26. Awonuga AO, Fletcher NM, Saed GM, and Diamond MP. Postoperative adhesion development following cesarean and open intra-abdominal gynecological operations: A review. *Reprod Sci*. 2011 December;18(12):1166–85.
27. Vrijland WW, Jeekel J, van Geldorp HJ, Swank DJ, and Bonjer HJ. Abdominal adhesions: Intestinal obstruction, pain, and infertility. *Surg Endosc*. 2003 July;17(7):1017–22.
28. Duffy DM, diZerega GS. Adhesion controversies: Pelvic pain as a cause of adhesions, crystalloids in preventing them. *J Reprod Med*. 1996 January;41(1):19–26.
29. Surgeons PC of AS for RM in collaboration with S of R. Pathogenesis, consequences, and control of peritoneal adhesions in gynecologic surgery: A committee opinion. *Fertil Steril*. 2013 May;99(6):1550–5.
30. Liu G, Zolis L, Kung R, Melchior M, Singh S, and Cook EF. The laparoscopic myomectomy: A survey of Canadian gynaecologists. *J Obstet Gynaecol Canada*. 2010;32(2):139–48.
31. Wright JD, Ananth CV, Tergas AI et al. An economic analysis of robotically assisted hysterectomy. *Obstet Gynecol*. 2014 May;123(5):1038–48.
32. Wright JD, Ananth CV, Lewin SN et al. Robotically assisted vs laparoscopic hysterectomy among women with benign gynecologic disease. *JAMA*. 2013 February 20; 309(7):689–98.
33. Barakat EE, Bedaiwy MA, Zimberg S, Nutter B, Nosseir M, and Falcone T. Robotic-assisted, laparoscopic, and abdominal myomectomy: A comparison of surgical outcomes. *Obstet Gynecol*. 2011 February;117(2 Pt 1):256–65.
34. Kumakiri J, Kikuchi I, Kitade M et al. Association between uterine repair at laparoscopic myomectomy and postoperative adhesions. *Acta Obstet Gynecol Scand*. 2012 March; 91(3):331–7.
35. Pluchino N, Litta P, Freschi L et al. Comparison of the initial surgical experience with robotic and laparoscopic myomectomy. *Int J Med Robot*. 2014 June;10(2):208–12.
36. Gargiulo AR, Srouji SS, Missmer SA et al. Robot-assisted laparoscopic myomectomy compared with standard laparoscopic myomectomy. *Obstet Gynecol*. 2012 August;120(2 Pt 1):284–91.

37. Einarsson JI, Vellinga TT, Twijnstra AR, Chavan NR, Suzuki Y, and Greenberg JA. Bidirectional barbed suture: An evaluation of safety and clinical outcomes. *JSLS*. 2010 July–September;14(3):381–5.
38. Alessandri F, Remorgida V, Venturini PL, and Ferrero S. Unidirectional barbed suture versus continuous suture with intracorporeal knots in laparoscopic myomectomy: A randomized study. *J Minim Invasive Gynecol*. 1996;17(6):725–9.
39. Angioli R, Plotti F, Montera R et al. A new type of absorbable barbed suture for use in laparoscopic myomectomy. *Int J Gynaecol Obstet*. 2012 June;117(3):220–3.
40. Cela V, Freschi L, Simi G et al. Fertility and endocrine outcome after robot-assisted laparoscopic myomectomy (RALM). *Gynecol Endocrinol*. 2013 January;29(1):79–82.
41. Bedaiwy MA, Zhang A, Henry D, Falcone T, and Soto E. Surgical anatomy of supraumbilical port placement: Implications for robotic and advanced laparoscopic surgery. *Fertil Steril*. 2015;103(4:e33).
42. Gargiulo AR, Bailey AP, and Srouji SS. Robot-assisted single-incision laparoscopic myomectomy: Initial report and technique. *J Robot Surg*. 2013 June;7(2):137–42.
43. Lewis EI, Srouji SS, and Gargiulo AR. Robotic single-site myomectomy: Initial report and technique. *Fertil Steril*. 2015 May;103(5):1370–7.e1.
44. Moawad GN, Tyan P, Paek J et al. Comparison Between Single-Site and Multiport Robot-Assisted Myomectomy. *J Robot Surg* 2019;13(6):757–64.
45. Tinelli A, Mynbaev OA, Sparic R et al. Angiogenesis and vascularization of uterine leiomyoma: Clinical value of pseudocapsule containing peptides and neurotransmitters. *Curr Protein Pept Sci*. 2016 March 22;17.
46. Tinelli A, Malvasi A, Hurst BS et al. Surgical management of neurovascular bundle in uterine fibroid pseudocapsule. *JSLS*. 2012 January–March;16(1):119–29.
47. Malvasi A, Cavallotti C, Nicolardi G et al. NT, NPY and PGP 9.5 presence in myomeytrium and in fibroid pseudocapsule and their possible impact on muscular physiology. *Gynecol Endocrinol*. 2013 February;29(2):177–81.
48. Lewis EI and Gargiulo AR. The Role of Hysteroscopic and Robot-assisted Laparoscopic Myomectomy in the Setting of Infertility. *Clin Obstet Gynecol*. 2016 March;59(1):53–65.
49. Muzii L, Boni T, Bellati F et al. GnRH analogue treatment before hysteroscopic resection of submucous myomas: A prospective, randomized, multicenter study. *Fertil Steril*. 2010 September;94(4):1496–9.
50. Hobo R, Netsu S, Koyasu Y, and Tsutsumi O. Bradycardia and cardiac arrest caused by intramyometrial injection of vasopressin during a laparoscopically assisted myomectomy. *Obstet Gynecol*. 2009 February;113(2 Pt 2):484–6.
51. Nezhat F, Admon D, Nezhat CH, Dicorpo JE, and Nezhat C. Life-threatening hypotension after vasopressin injection during operative laparoscopy, followed by uneventful repeat laparoscopy. *J Am Assoc Gynecol Laparosc*. 1994 November;2(1):83–6.
52. Tulandi T, Béique F, and Kimia M. Pulmonary edema: A complication of local injection of vasopressin at laparoscopy. *Fertil Steril*. 1996 September;66(3):478–80.
53. Fusca L, Perelman I, Fergusson D et al. The Effectiveness of Tranexamic Acid at Reducing Blood Loss and Transfusion Requirement for Women Undergoing Myomectomy: A Systematic Review and Meta-analysis. *J Obstet Gynaecol Can*. 2019;41(8):1185–92.e1.
54. Zhang Y, Ma D, Li X, and Zhang Q. Role of barbed sutures in repairing uterine wall defects in laparoscopic myomectomy: A systemic review and meta-analysis. *J Minim Invasive Gynecol*. 2016;23(5):684–91.
55. Greenberg JA and Goldman RH. Barbed suture: A review of the technology and clinical uses in obstetrics and gynecology. *Rev Obstet Gynecol*. 2013;6(3–4):107–15.
56. Tinelli A, Malvasi A, Guido M et al. Adhesion formation after intracapsular myomectomy with or without adhesion barrier. *Fertil Steril*. 2011;95(5):1780–5.
57. U.S. Food and Drugs Administration. *Safety Communications - Updated Laparoscopic Uterine Power Morcellation in Hysterectomy and Myomectomy*. FDA Safety Communication Center for Devices and Radiological Health. Available from: http://www.fda.gov/MedicalDevices/Safety/AlertsandNotices/ucm424443.htm
58. AAGL Advancing Minimally Invasive Gynecology Worldwide. AAGL practice report: Morcellation during uterine tissue extraction. *J Minim Invasive Gynecol*. 2009;21(4):517–30.
59. Brown J. AAGL advancing minimally invasive gynecology worldwide: Statement to the FDA on power morcellation. *J Minim Invasive Gynecol*. 2014;21(6):970–1.
60. Executive Summary Power Morcellation and Occult Malignancy in Gynecologic Surgery 2014. Available from: https://www.acog.org/~/media/TaskForceandWorkGroupReports/Public/MorcellationSpecialReport.pdf
61. Siedhoff MT, Wheeler SB, Rutstein SE et al. Laparoscopic hysterectomy with morcellation vs abdominal hysterectomy for presumed fibroid tumors in premenopausal women: A decision analysis. *Am J Obstet Gynecol*. 2015 May;212(5):591.e1–8.
62. Srouji SS, Kaser DJ, and Gargiulo AR. Techniques for contained morcellation in gynecologic surgery. *Fertil Steril*. 2015 April;103(4):e34.
63. Cohen SL, Clark NV, Ajao MO et al. Prospective Evaluation of Manual Morcellation Techniques: Minilaparotomy Versus Vaginal Approach. *J Minim Invasive Gynecol*. 2019;26(4):702–8.
64. Lenihan JP, Kovanda C, and Seshadri-Kreaden U. What is the learning curve for robotic assisted gynecologic surgery? *J Minim Invasive Gynecol*. 1989;15(5):589–94.
65. Lim PC, Kang E, and Park DH. Learning curve and surgical outcome for robotic-assisted hysterectomy with lymphadenectomy: Case-matched controlled comparison with laparoscopy and laparotomy for treatment of endometrial cancer. *J Minim Invasive Gynecol*. 2009;17(6):739–48.

19

Hysteroscopic Vaporization of Uterine Myoma

Annie Leung and Togas Tulandi

Introduction

Hysteroscopic approach has changed the management of intrauterine pathologies, including submucous myoma. The standard treatment of submucous myoma is by using a resectoscopic loop-electrode under direct hysteroscopic vision [1,2]. However, myoma resection is associated with accumulation of tissue fragments obscuring the visualization. Also, it might require repeated withdrawal of the resectoscope to remove those fragments, resulting in prolongation of the procedure and increased risk of infection. Bleeding during the procedure could obscure the operator's view, requiring increased pressure of the distension medium to clear the operative field, thus increasing the risks of fluid overload.

In order to overcome those technical difficulties, a vaporization technique was developed in urology [3]. In a meta-analysis, transurethral electrovaporization was associated with a significant reduction in bleeding, duration of surgery and morbidity, as well as short hospital stay and recovery [4]. The efficacy was similar to that of conventional transurethral prostatectomy, with a lower cost. Vaporization has since been adapted in gynecology [5]. In this chapter, we review the physical properties of electrovaporization, operative technique, its application in gynecology and general recommendations in clinical use (see also Table 19.1).

Electrovaporization Electrode: Physical Properties

One commercially available vaporizing electrode is the VaporTrode (Circon ACMI, Stamford, CT). It produces synchronous vaporization and coagulation of tissue using a high-frequency cutting current. The configuration of thin ridges and large contact areas between the grooves that separate the ridges utilizes the edge density property of electricity. Edge density is the concentration of electrons producing an area of high current density at the point of contact and a consequent thermal reaction, which causes the tissue temperature to rise rapidly until vaporization (100°C) [6].

The instrument is powered by an electrosurgical generator with radiofrequencies between 400,000 and 1,000,000 Hz. Depending on the settings, various actions could be achieved, including cutting, fulguration, dissection, or vaporization. In electrosurgical *cutting*, continuous radiofrequency sine waves alternating frequency from positive to negative at the operating frequency of the electrical current generator results in high heat for cutting action. In electrosurgical *fulguration*, the coagulation waveform is composed of short bursts of radiofrequency sine waves with a pause between each burst. Although the waveforms may have the same peak voltage, the average power delivered per unit time is less in the coagulation mode because the current in the coagulation mode is in the pause mode most of the time.

In electrosurgical *desiccation*, current is passed through the electrical resistance of the tissue, and heat is generated in the tissue. As the tissue gets hot, water is slowly driven out of the tissue, and this tissue becomes desiccated. Visually, the color of the tissue turns into a light brown color, which steams and bubbles as the water is driven out.

In electrovaporization, the current utilized in the electrode is set at a higher power than that utilized in standard cutting. Therefore, as the electrode contacts fresh tissue cells, it provides a high enough current density to vaporize the contacted tissue cells. However, if the contact on the same spot is maintained, the underlying tissue cells start to desiccate instead of vaporizing because of the increasing resistance generated by the dried-out tissue. The degree of desiccation is governed by the quality of the contact to the tissue and the time spent on that spot by the electrode. The longer the contact, the deeper the desiccation effect. Since the procedure is performed using glycine as a distending medium, the desiccated tissue is constantly rehydrated, making it available for vaporization on a subsequent pass. In short, electrovaporization vaporizes the unwanted tissue, provides hemostasis and prevents water reabsorption by the development of a zone of desiccation below the vaporized tissue. The heat that is generated produces a zone of coagulation in the adjoining layer of tissue, and the depth of vaporization depends on duration of contact, resistance (debris on the electrode) and wattage of the generator.

Operative Technique

Operative Setup

Preoperative preparation may include insertion of laminaria stents the night before surgery [6]. Operators should be familiar with the capabilities of the generator and adjust the current according to the observed tissue effect. Power curves of the generator can be chosen to maintain power output over the widest

TABLE 19.1

Summary of Hysteroscopic Vaporization Studies

	System	Procedure	Preoperative Preparation	Median Operative Time (minutes)	Median Fluid Deficit (mL)	Complications
Glasser [6]	AccuBar	44 (29 EA+MYO, 6 MYO, 9 EA)	Laminaria GnRH agonist	NR	163 (0–62)	
Vercellini [13]	VaporTrode	40 (26 EA+MYO, 14 EA)	GnRH agonist	10 (7–12)	90 (0–200)	
Vercellini [14]	VaporTrode	47 EA	None	8 (7–11)	70 (0–175)	
Vilos [16]	VersaPoint	9 cases (3 uterine septums, 1 synechiae, 2 polyps, 3 myoma)	None	NR	NR	
Kung [17]	VersaPoint	10 cases (7 polyps, 6 MYO, 3 uterine septums, 1 synechiae)	None	41 (6–115)	0–900	
Garry [22]	Laser	600 EA	Danazol or GnRH agonist	25 (5–105)	603 (0–6700)	2 postoperative endometritis
Philips [23]	Laser	58 EA±MYO	Danazol, medroxyprogesterone acetate or GnRH agonist	36	872	1 fluid overload 1 uterine perforation

Abbreviations: EA, endometrial ablation; MYO, myomectomy; NR, not reported.

range of impedance: 160–300 W of pure cut current to vaporize and 60–70 W to fulgurate bleeding points. Glasser et al. described the use of a 27F continuous-flow resectoscope with a 12° lens (Olympus, Lake Success, NY) [6]. The cervix is dilated to 10 mm or 11 mm, and the uterus is distended with 1.5% glycine or 3% sorbitol solution. Guidelines regarding the use of hysteroscopic distension media should be followed with close monitoring of fluid balance [7].

Risk of Malignancy

It is important to obtain tissue from the myoma prior to vaporization for pathologic analysis using a wire loop. In a series of 92 patients, two leiomyosarcomas were found, underscoring the value of tissue sampling [8].

Approaches to Various Myoma Configurations

A variety of surgical approaches to remove a submucous myoma has been advocated. Type 0 submucous myoma can be resected using a wire loop using pure cutting current, and the myoma fragments are then removed from the uterine cavity. Compared to resection, electrovaporization leads to tissue desiccation and is associated with minimal fluid absorption and blood loss. It is a preferable technique for a large submucous myoma. A large myoma can be first bivalved to the level of the endomyometrial junction, followed by vaporization from the periphery to the center [6]. Pieces of tissue can be extracted with a forceps or morcellated. With the use of both techniques, the wattage should be decreased to 110 W pure cutting current for the wire loop. Once a specimen is severed from its uterine attachment, the energy pathway to the return electrode or "ground plate" is lost. Further electrical morcellation or vaporization of the detached tissue becomes almost impossible.

Depth of Tissue Vaporization and Coagulation and Electrodesiccation

Immediate contact vaporization is governed by the initial contact current density delivered to the myoma surface. The device generally vaporizes tissue to a depth of 3–4 mm, with an additional coagulation zone of 1–3 mm. If the electrode becomes coated with char or tissue debris, it can be cleaned by switching to 70 W coagulation current and rapidly rolling it over the surface of the cavity that was previously vaporized.

Leaving the electrode stationary could lead to diminished vaporization secondary to the phenomenon of "electrodesiccation." Electrodesiccation occurs when the electrode is held stationary and the surface tissue dries out and resistance increases in tissue. As resistance increases, the heat created will desiccate the adjacent tissue (i.e., drying out rather than vaporizing the tissue). The depth of desiccation depends on the amount of time spent on that area and the power of the current delivered to overcome electrical tissue resistance. Accordingly, it is important to avoid coagulating intact tissue before vaporization since the devitalized surface tissue will create high resistance, preventing deep vaporization.

Risk of Perforation

The electrode should be moved slowly across tissue, applying current only when moving in the direction toward the operator. Prolonged pressure in one spot could result in uterine perforation. In order to avoid perforation at thin areas, such as the cornua, the power should be reduced to 80 W or 90 W so that the surface is desiccated only.

Dispersive Electrode Injury

Dispersive electrode is usually applied to the buttock or strapped around the leg. If the power setting is too high, it increases the current delivered through the electrodes, including the dispersive electrode, increasing the risk of dispersive pad skin burns [9]. This risk can be reduced with generators that measure tissue impedance, and the vaporization technique should be used with the lowest power setting necessary (below 200 W) [10].

Electrovaporization Versus Other Electrosurgical Techniques

Initial reports comparing myoma vaporization and conventional techniques showed that vaporization was associated with decreased operative time, minimal myoma chips and reduced intraoperative bleeding and intravasation of distending fluid [11].

Intravascular Fluid Absorption

In vivo studies showed that the vaporizing electrode produces furrows of similar depth to those of a standard cutting loop, but the depth of coagulation beneath the ablated area by the electrode is significantly greater compared with the loop [12]. The median amount of fluid deficit in a clinical pilot study on endometrial vaporization with a normal uterine cavity was 50 mL. This is due to the greater coaptation of myometrial vessels by thermal effect reducing fluid intravasation [13].

In a randomized study comparing vaporizing electrode and cutting loop for endometrial ablation [14], the authors reported that the mean fluid deficit was 70% less in women who had endometrial vaporization than in those with endometrial resection (difference of about 258 mL). Only one woman absorbed more than 500 mL in the endometrial vaporization group compared with 14 others in the resection group. No subjects developed signs or symptoms of fluid overload. The decreased systemic absorption of distension medium [14] was attributed to the greater degree of adjacent thermal injury [12]. There has been a suggestion that this advantage is also found in hysteroscopic myomectomy as well [15].

Operative Time

Vercellini et al. reported that endometrial vaporization was one and a half minutes faster than endometrial resection [14].

VersaPoint System

One of the electrosurgical vaporization systems is the co-axial bipolar electrode VersaPoint (Gynecare Inc., Somerville, NJ). It is designed to cut, desiccate and vaporize [16–19]. The 1.6-mm-diameter (5F), 36-cm-long, flexible bipolar electrode can be used through any operating hysteroscope. There are three electrode tips available: a spring to vaporize, a "twizzle" to cut and a ball to coagulate tissue. Since it is a bipolar electrode, it can be used with normal saline as a distending medium. In the vaporizing mode, the generator controls the creation of a vapor pocket or steam bubble, which upon contact with tissue, causes instantaneous vaporization of cellular water content. The energy follows the path of least resistance through the saline distention medium and returns to the generator through a parallel electrode, thus eliminating the need for a dispersive return pad electrode. The vaporizing electrode is 4 mm wide and 4 mm in diameter, while the corresponding cutting loop electrode has a diameter of 2.5 mm.

Laser Vaporization

The first report of laser vaporization of the prostate appeared in the urologic literature in 1992 [20]. The reported advantages include less blood loss compared with conventional resection techniques, particularly for patients on anticoagulants, but it may have higher re-retreatment rates [21]. Another technique is endometrial ablation using the neodymium:yttrium-aluminum-garnet laser (Nd:YAG). The reported success rate is over 90% [22]. Yet, a retrospective study comparing laser vaporization and the use of rollerball or wire loop electrodes showed comparable long-term outcomes at 4-year follow-up [23]. One significant disadvantage of the use of laser was the cost of the machine and fibers. Today, this technology is rarely used.

Plasma Energy

One of the novel emerging energy sources is plasma energy. The PlasmaJet system (Plasma Surgical Limited, Berkshire, UK) generates an electrically neutral stream of ionized argon gas by concentrating a low flow of inert argon gas between bipolar electrodes operating at a low voltage (30–60 V) [24]. The plasma jet possesses thermal, kinetic and light energies that penetrate tissue to a depth 0.5–2.0 mm, resulting in vaporization and coagulation. While it has yet to be adopted in hysteroscopic procedures, its application in gynecological conditions such as endometriosis [24–26] and peritoneal carcinoma [27] is expanding.

Conclusion

Electrovaporization for the treatment of uterine myoma and for endometrial ablation is associated with reduced blood loss and fluid deficit. The absence of tissue chips allows hysteroscopic myomectomy to be performed quickly and with few complications. Because of the very high currents, operators should be familiar with the generator settings.

REFERENCES

1. Murakami T, Tachibana M, Hoshiai T et al. Successful strategy for the hysteroscopic myomectomy of a submucous myoma arising from the uterine fundus. *Fertil Steril.* 2006;86:1513.e19–22.

2. Polena V, Mergui J-L, Perrot N et al. Long-term results of hysteroscopic myomectomy in 235 patients. *Eur J Obstet Gynecol Reprod Biol.* 2007;130:232–7.
3. Smith D, Khoubehi B, and Patel A. Bipolar electrosurgery for benign prostatic hyperplasia: Transurethral electrovaporization and resection of the prostate. *Curr Opin Urol.* 2005;15:95–100.
4. Poulakis V, Dahm P, Witzsch U et al. Transurethral electrovaporization vs transurethral resection for symptomatic prostatic obstruction: A meta-analysis. *BJU Int.* 2004; 94:89–95.
5. AAGL practice report: Practice guidelines for the diagnosis and management of submucous leiomyomas. *J Minim Invasive Gynecol.* 2012;19:152–71.
6. Glasser MH. Endometrial ablation and hysteroscopic myomectomy by electrosurgical vaporization. *J Am Assoc Gynecol Laparosc.* 1997;4:369–74.
7. Munro MG, Storz K, Abbott JA et al. AAGL practice report: Practice guidelines for the management of hysteroscopic distending media: (Replaces hysteroscopic fluid monitoring guidelines. *J Am Assoc Gynecol Laparosc.* 2000;7:167–168). *J Minim Invasive Gynecol.* 2013;20:137–48.
8. Corson SL and Brooks PG. Resectoscopic myomectomy. *Fertil Steril.* 1991;55:1041–4.
9. Vilos GA. Dispersive pad injuries associated with hysteroscopic surgery. *J Am Assoc Gynecol Laparosc.* 1999;6:364–7.
10. Raders JL. Dispersive pad injuries associated with hysteroscopic surgery. *J Am Assoc Gynecol Laparosc.* 1999;6:363–4.
11. Brooks PG. Resectoscopic myoma vaporizer. *J Reprod Med.* 1995;40:791–5.
12. Vercellini P, Oldani S, Milesi M et al. Endometrial ablation with a vaporizing electrode. I. Evaluation of *in vivo* effects. *Acta Obstet Gynecol Scand.* 1998;77:683–7.
13. Vercellini P, Oldani S, De Giorgi O et al. Endometrial ablation with a vaporizing electrode. II. Clinical outcome of a pilot study. *Acta Obstet Gynecol Scand.* 1998;77:688–93.
14. Vercellini P, Oldani S, Yaylayan L et al. Randomized comparison of vaporizing electrode and cutting loop for endometrial ablation. *Obstet Gynecol.* 1999;94:521–7.
15. Vercellini P, Oldani S, DeGiorgi O et al. Endometrial ablation with a vaporizing electrode in women with regular uterine cavity or submucous leiomyomas. *J Am Assoc Gynecol Laparosc.* 1996;3:S52.
16. Vilos GA. Intrauterine surgery using a new coaxial bipolar electrode in normal saline solution (Versapoint): A pilot study. *Fertil Steril.* 1999;72:740–3.
17. Kung RC, Vilos GA, Thomas B et al. A new bipolar system for performing operative hysteroscopy in normal saline. *J Am Assoc Gynecol Laparosc.* 1999;6:331–6.
18. Fernandez H, Gervaise A, and de Tayrac R. Operative hysteroscopy for infertility using normal saline solution and a coaxial bipolar electrode: A pilot study. *Hum Reprod.* 2000;15:1773–5.
19. Golan A, Sagiv R, Berar M et al. Bipolar electrical energy in physiologic solution--a revolution in operative hysteroscopy. *J Am Assoc Gynecol Laparosc.* 2001;8:252–8.
20. Costello AJ, Bowsher WG, Bolton DM et al. Laser ablation of the prostate in patients with benign prostatic hypertrophy. *Br J Urol.* 1992;69:603–8.
21. Tholomier C, Valdivieso R, Hueber PA et al. Photoselective laser ablation of the prostate: A review of the current 2015 tissue ablation options. *Can J Urol.* 2015;22(Suppl 1):45–52.
22. Garry R, Shelley-Jones D, Mooney P et al. Six hundred endometrial laser ablations. *Obstet Gynecol.* 1995;85:24–9.
23. Phillips DR. A comparison of endometrial ablation using the Nd:YAG laser or electrosurgical techniques. *J Am Assoc Gynecol Laparosc.* 1994;1:235–9.
24. Nezhat C, Kho KA, and Morozov V. Use of neutral argon plasma in the laparoscopic treatment of endometriosis. *JSLS.* 2009;13:479–83.
25. Roman H, Pura I, Tarta O et al. Vaporization of ovarian endometrioma using plasma energy: Histologic findings of a pilot study. *Fertil Steril.* 2011;95:1853–6.e1–4.
26. Deb S, Sahu B, Deen S et al. Comparison of tissue effects quantified histologically between PlasmaJet coagulator and Helica thermal coagulator. *Arch Gynecol Obstet.* 2012;286:399–402.
27. Sonoda Y, Olvera N, Chi DS et al. Pathologic analysis of ex vivo plasma energy tumor destruction in patients with ovarian or peritoneal cancer. *Int J Gynecol Cancer.* 2010;20:1326–30.

20

Hysteroscopic Myomectomy

Karissa Hammer and John C. Petrozza

Leiomyomas, also referred to as fibroids or myomas, are a common pathology encountered in gynecology. Patients with fibroid uteruses present with complaints such as heavy menstrual bleeding, cramping or pregnancy complications. There are medical and surgical options for treatment of these benign soft tissue tumors. A hysterectomy is the most definitive treatment for fibroids. However, many women have complaints related to fibroids during their reproductive years and desire future fertility. For fibroids located completely or partially within the uterine cavity, a hysteroscopic approach is the least invasive and most effective method that also maintains fertility.

This chapter will discuss the fibroid type best treated by the hysteroscopic approach, hysteroscopic myomectomy techniques, risks of the procedure, recovery and fertility impact of this surgery.

Fibroids Treated by Hysteroscopy

Fibroids can grow on any aspect of the uterus. The International Federation of Gynecology and Obstetrics (FIGO) classification system creates a standardized way of describing their location. The FIGO grades 0, 1 and 2 refer to submucosal fibroids that are those best suited for treatment with a hysteroscopic approach. FIGO grade 0 is a pedunculated myoma completely within the uterine cavity, grade 1 has less than half of the myoma within the myometrium and grade 2 has equal to or more than half of its volume within the myometrium and the remaining tissue within the uterine cavity. Each of these locations gives a surgeon access to the fibroid through the endometrial cavity, thus a hysteroscopic approach is the best surgical access for minimally invasive removal [1].

Preoperative Management

Prior to recommending a hysteroscopic myomectomy, a patient must have a thorough evaluation. A detailed history and physical is required, with specific concern for symptoms related to the fibroid such as excessive vaginal bleeding, anemia, pain, miscarriages or other fertility concerns. Understanding of the patient's other comorbidities and surgical history is also pertinent to assess readiness to undergo surgery with either local or general anesthesia. Patients must be medically optimized prior to the procedure. Physical exam should include an assessment of the uterine position and size, as well as the size and location of fibroid(s), if palpable. A pelvic ultrasound, at minimum, should be obtained to capture the location of the fibroid(s) and assess accessibility from the intracavitary approach [2]. If this image modality is not successful in delineating myoma location, a saline sonography and/or MRI can be performed [3]. Figure 20.1 illustrates a FIGO 0 fibroid and endometrial polyp within the uterine cavity by sonohysterogram.

In select cases, a provider may also consider laboratory assessment of normal electrolytes, hematocrit and blood type prior to proceeding for evaluation of anemia and any underlying electrolyte disturbances.

A few considerations prior to starting your hysteroscopic myomectomy include antibiotic prophylaxis, cervical dilation or preparation, pretreatment of the myomas and timing of procedure. Antibiotic prophylaxis is not recommended by the American College of Obstetricians and Gynecologists (ACOG). Postoperative infections are extremely rare, and use of antibiotic prophylaxis has not been shown to decrease the risk [4]. Cervical prep with ripening agents the night prior to procedure is controversial. Since a significant number of the complications associated with hysteroscopy occur during hysteroscope entry, some surgeons prefer prepping the cervix with misoprostol to soften the cervix and perhaps help with entry. However, there are mixed data with the success of this method and a best practice statement does not currently exist [2,3]. Intraoperative cervical preparation/dilation can be achieved with dilators up to the number correlating with the size of the hysteroscope to be used or, if in office, can consider hydrodilation with vaginoscopy. Some studies have recommended pretreatment of myomas with either ulipristal acetate or GnRH analogues to decrease the volume of the myoma prior to resection [5,6]. Pretreatment with these medications leads to a decrease in fibroid volume; however, the surgical planes are often compromised and become softer and more difficult to dissect [7,8]. These medications can also thin the endometrial lining, theoretically further improving visualization by decreased bleeding. Hysteroscopic myomectomy performed during the follicular phase is preferable for a thin endometrial lining (Table 20.1).

In cases in which the patient experiences excessive vaginal bleeding and does not desire fertility, a uterine artery embolization can be considered prior to hysteroscopy to improve visualization and decrease intraoperative blood loss [10]. A meta-analysis of uterine artery embolization (UAE) on pregnancy reported a decreased pregnancy rate and increased miscarriage rate after UAE [11]. For this reason, we recommend uterine myomectomy over embolization if future pregnancy is desired (Table 20.2).

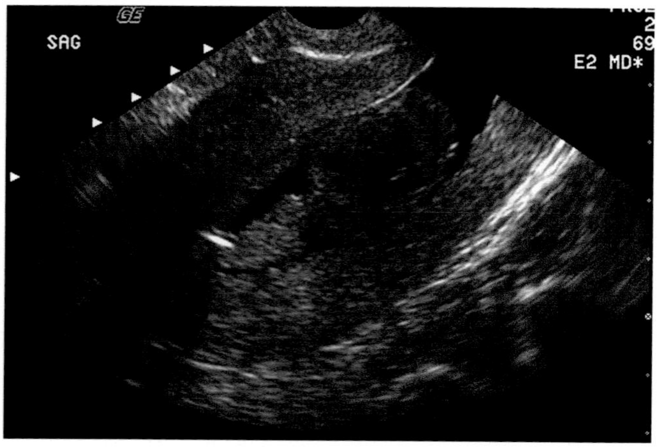

FIGURE 20.1 Sonohysterogram showing FIGO 0 fibroid and endometrial polyp.

Hysteroscopy Techniques

Since the first use of hysteroscopy, the technology has rapidly advanced to the point now where many of the procedures are done in the outpatient office setting. Techniques used for myomectomy must be chosen on a case-by-case basis and by surgeon skill to create a safe procedure for the individual patient. The techniques described in this chapter include monopolar resectoscope, bipolar resectoscope, cold loop, mechanical morcellation with tissue retrieval system and mass vaporization electrode.

TABLE 20.2

Impact of Uterine Fibroid Embolization (UFE) on Pregnancy

	Pregnancy (%)	Miscarriage (%)
RCTs	50	64
Cohort studies	69	56
Case series	29	25

Source: Karlsen K et al. *Arch Gynecol Obstet.* 2018;297:13–25 with permission.

The hysteroscope was adapted from the urologic resectoscope [2]. The resectoscope uses a handle with a spring technology to move a single looped wire within the uterine cavity. The wire loop can be considered "cold" without energy or energized with either monopolar or bipolar electric current [12]. The first energy devices were monopolar resectoscopes [13]. This improved coagulation and cutting intraoperatively; however, this energy type requires electrolyte-poor distending medium such as glycine 1.5% or sorbitol 3%. This distention media has a number of flaws, including a viscous nature that sticks and erodes the scope over time and potential for electrolyte imbalances for the patient such as hyponatremia [3,14]. Bipolar technology was later applied to the resectoscope device, allowing use of isotonic distention medium such as normal saline. Although the use of normal saline is more physiologic, there is still potential for electrolyte imbalances if the patient absorbs an excessive amount of the fluid intraoperatively. Regardless of the technology used, close monitoring of the fluid balances during this procedure is required [15] (Video 20.1).

TABLE 20.1

Hysteroscopic Myomectomy: Pre-Medication Effect on Endometrial Thinning, Fluid Deficits and Fibroid Shrinkage

	No Medication	Triptorelin	Letrozole	Ulipristal	*P* Value
	N = 23	N = 20	N = 11	N = 7	
Age (years)	35.0 +/− 4.7	36.3 +/− 5.4	36.8 +/− 5.1	38.4 +/− 4.3	0.419
Largest Myoma (cm)	2.7 +/− 0.5	2.8 +/− 0.4	3.0 +/− 0.4	2.9 +/− 0.3	0.254
Endometrium (mm)	3.9 +/− 1.0	2.3 +/− 0.6	4.1 +/− 1.0	6.9 +/− 3.3	<0.001
Fluid Deficit (mL)	457 +/− 139	340 +/− 112	366 +/− 111	371 +/− 103	0.003 (S vs. T) 0.048 (S vs. L) 0.110 (S vs. U)

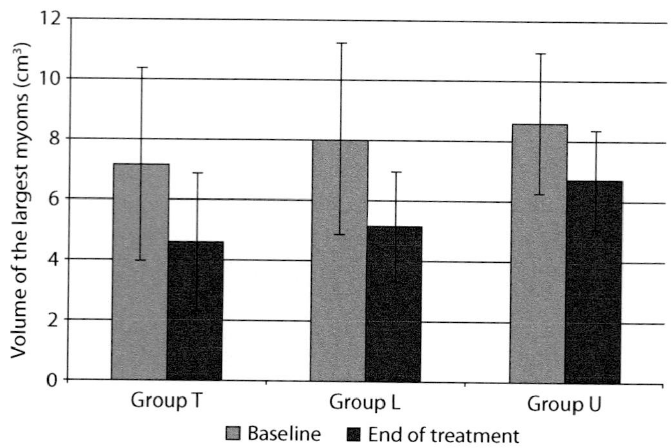

Source: Bizzarri N et al. *Eur J Obstet Gynecol Reprod Biol.* 2015;192:22–6, with permission.

VIDEO 20.1 https://youtu.be/0ZA1fRheSLM
Cold loop myomectomy.

The cold loop technique refers to use of a resectoscope without energy. Often, energy is originally used to make a cut at the base of the fibroid followed by cold wire loop passes to bluntly remove the fibroid from its capsulation within the myometrium, also referred to as enucleation. This technique is similarly used in abdominal myomectomies once a plane is identified to dissect the fibroid from normal myometrial tissue. This helps reduce cautery within the cavity [2,16,17].

A newer and very popular technology is a mechanical morcellator with tissue retrieval system such as Myosure, Truclear and Symphion devices. These systems include a window at the tip of the instrument which, when activated simultaneously, creates suction and cuts the pathology with a rotatory or up/down action. These devices are compatible with isotonic saline as a distention medium [3]. The suction created to remove pathology can also help clear blood-tinged fluid from the cavity for clearer visualization. There is not electric current for cutting or coagulation in the Myosure or Truclear devices; however, Symphion does have energy capabilities. They are most commonly used for type 0–1 fibroids. They are reported to have shortened operative times and decreased learning curves for surgeons [2,5]. Anecdotally, the more dense, calcified or larger the fibroid, the more difficult it is to remove with these devices (Video 20.2).

VIDEO 20.2 https://youtu.be/5VMlvB-7R9I
Symphion morcellator.

A less-common technology involves ablation of the uterine fibroid via radiofrequency ablation or thermal techniques. In this technique, an electrode is placed within the fibroid and causes tissue to desiccate [18]. The tissue often does not require additional removal, but if not completely desiccated, then may require removal with a wire loop. The tissue cannot be evaluated by histopathology [8].

Selecting a technique depends on surgeon training, fibroid location and size and available technology at the surgeon's facilities (Table 20.3).

TABLE 20.3

Pros and Cons of the Most Common Hysteroscopic Myomectomy Techniques

Technique	Pros	Cons
Monopolar resectoscope	• Energy coagulation and cutting capabilities • Decreased bleeding • Improved visualization	• Requires electrolyte-poor distention media • Evacuation of pathology requires removal of hysteroscope
Bipolar resectoscope	• Energy coagulation and cutting capabilities • Decreased bleeding • Improved visualization • Isotonic distention media	• Evacuation of pathology requires removal of hysteroscope
Cold wire loop	• Any distention media • No energy • Clean margins for pathologic evaluation • Can be used deep into the myometrium without fear of energy impacting tissue beyond the uterus	• No energy coagulation or cut capabilities • Decreased visualization with bleeding
Morcellator system	• System cuts and removes pathology • Can clear bleeding with vacuum suction on system • Does not require removing the hysteroscope to remove pathology • Shorter operative times • Single entry into uterine cavity with device	• No energy coagulation or cut • Decreased visualization with heavy bleeding • Limited by size and location of myoma
Radio frequency ablation	• Volume reduction • Preservation of surrounding myometrium • Single entry into uterine cavity with device	• Desiccates tissue so no histopathology can be performed • No energy coagulation or cut • Still under investigation • Reduces volume of myoma but not the entire fibroid

Postoperative Management

Depending on the location and depth of the removed fibroid, surgeons may choose to place a pediatric-sized Foley catheter within the uterine cavity. This practice is thought to decrease intrauterine adhesion formation. This practice is not associated with an increased infection risk, as demonstrated by Abuzeid et al. who evaluated over 1000 cases with postoperative uterine Foley placement and reported no infections [19]. Another common practice with little supportive research is the use of estrogen and progesterone supplementation postoperatively to support physiologic endometrial regeneration and possibly decrease risk of adhesion formation [20]. It may be beneficial to perform a diagnostic hysteroscopy 1–2 months after the procedure to ensure adequate healing and the absence of intrauterine adhesions.

Complications

Although hysteroscopic myomectomy is a relatively safe, minimally invasive surgery, there are still risks to be cognizant of and to discuss with your patient. First, electrolyte imbalances are the most common complication from prolonged hysteroscopic surgeries. These can vary from slight derangements in sodium levels to life-threatening alterations leading to arrhythmias and intensive care unit admissions [15,21,22]. For this reason, it is imperative to closely monitor hysteroscopic fluid going into the uterus, fluid retrieved through the hysteroscopic system and IV fluid being given by anesthesia [8,14].

Uterine procedures requiring dilation and instruments introduced into the uterus also have a risk of uterine perforation. This complication is reported at a rate of about 1% for operative hysteroscopy and less than 0.1% for diagnostic hysteroscopy [21,23]. Surgical planning includes a pelvic exam prior to instrumentation to gain an understanding of the position of the uterus and decrease this risk. If the cervical os is stenotic, an os finder can often be helpful to find a cervical pathway without creating a false passage or perforating.

Hemorrhage is a low risk with this procedure, but not zero. The bleeding from a myoma may obscure visualization and prohibit completion of the procedure in a single surgery. This can often be predicted and a two-step procedure can be planned in advance and the patient counseled appropriately [2,8,24]. Direct injection of vasopressin either into the paracervical junction or directly into the fibroid has been described to improve hemostasis and visualization during hysteroscopic myomectomy [25]. Patients must be counseled on postoperative warning signs of excessive blood loss and when to call their physician or come to the emergency room.

Adhesions from aggressive surgical technique or deep carving into the uterine myometrium below the endometrial lining can cause patients to return with abnormal uterine bleeding, infertility or pain [26]. Adhesive disease can be diagnosed with a diagnostic in-office hysteroscopy. If thin filmy adhesions are diagnosed, then these can be addressed with blunt dissection. When thick adhesions are encountered, more precise cutting with hysteroscopic scissors is required. Rates of reported adhesion formation after operative hysteroscopy range from <1% to 41% [26,27]. Anti-adhesion gels have not proved to prevent adhesion formation [8].

An unfortunate reality of this procedure is that the pathology may grow back over time, especially with those that have a large fibroid burden. If patients are near menopause, this risk decreases. For patients wishing to conceive, they should be encouraged to do so within a few years from this procedure to decrease the chances of regrowth and impact on the lining [8].

Rarely, a presumed uterine fibroid can be discovered to be a malignancy. If hysteroscopic surgery does identify a malignancy, the hysteroscopic fluid has a small risk of upstaging early endometrial cancers by disseminating cells within the peritoneal cavity, but this does not appear to influence disease prognosis [28]. This is a rare occurrence with an incidence reported as low as 0.86%, with increased risk over the age of 50 years old [29]. If found, prompt referral to a gynecologic oncologist is recommended.

Recovery

Hysteroscopic myomectomies are minimally invasive procedures that can be performed as an outpatient day procedure or in-office procedure. Patients generally have light to moderate vaginal bleeding that improves each postoperative day, until it stops and normal menses returns. If a pediatric Foley catheter is placed, removal 7–14 days postoperative is recommended. Postoperative pain should be managed with non-narcotic medications as feasible; nonsteroidal anti-inflammatory medications such as ibuprofen are very effective. Patients should have a follow-up with their surgeon within 2 weeks after the procedure to review the pathology report, assess recovery and discuss next steps in management.

Impact on Fertility

Fibroids that impact the endometrial lining, FIGO grades 0–2, may negatively impact embryo implantation and growth. Patients with fertility issues, prior poor obstetrical outcomes and symptoms related to fibroids should have their uterine cavity assessed and may be candidates for hysteroscopic myomectomy [30,31]. ASRM practice guidelines support hysteroscopic myomectomy for submucosal fibroids impacting the contour of the uterine cavity. The guidelines have the following conclusions: good evidence supporting improved pregnancy rates after hysteroscopic myomectomy (grade B), insufficient evidence to conclude that hysteroscopic myomectomy reduces likelihood of early pregnancy loss (grade C) and myomectomy is not recommended to improve fertility in asymptomatic women with non-cavity-distorting myomas [32].

Conclusion

Hysteroscopic myomectomy is a safe minimally invasive procedure that can effectively treat FIGO grade 0–2 fibroids. Preoperative management must be tailored to each patient and surgical technique picked based on surgeon's skill and patient's presentation. Postoperative recovery is quick and most patients successfully recover as outpatients. Fertility can be positively impacted by resection of submucosal fibroids impacting the endometrial lining.

REFERENCES

1. Wamsteker K, Emanuel MH, and de Kruif JH. Transcervical hysteroscopic resection of submucous fibroids for abnormal uterine bleeding: Results regarding the degree of intramural extension. *Obstet Gynecol.* 1993;82:736–40.
2. Pakrashi T. New hysteroscopic techniques for submucosal uterine fibroids. *Curr Opin Obstet Gynecol.* 2014;26:308–13.
3. Valentine LN and Bradley LD. Hysteroscopy for abnormal uterine bleeding and fibroids. *Clin Obstet Gynecol.* 2017;60:231–44.
4. ACOG practice bulletin No. 195: Prevention of infection after gynecologic procedures. *Obstet Gynecol.* 2018;131:e172–e89.
5. Friedman JA, Wong JMK, Chaudhari A, Tsai S, and Milad MP. Hysteroscopic myomectomy: A comparison of techniques and review of current evidence in the management of abnormal uterine bleeding. *Curr Opin Obstet Gynecol.* 2018;30:243–51.
6. Murji A, Wais M, Lee S, Pham A, Tai M, and Liu G. A multicenter study evaluating the effect of ulipristal acetate during myomectomy. *J Minim Invasive Gynecol.* 2018;25:514–21.

7. Favilli A, Mazzon I, Grasso M et al. Intraoperative effect of preoperative gonadotropin-releasing hormone analogue administration in women undergoing cold loop hysteroscopic myomectomy: A randomized controlled trial. *J Minim Invasive Gynecol.* 2018;25:706–14.
8. Thubert T, Foulot H, Vinchant M et al. Surgical treatment: Myomectomy and hysterectomy; Endoscopy: A major advancement. *Best Pract Res Clin Obstet Gynaecol.* 2016;34:104–21.
9. Bizzarri N, Ghirardi V, Remorgida V, Venturini PL, and Ferrero S. Three-month treatment with triptorelin, letrozole and ulipristal acetate before hysteroscopic resection of uterine myomas: Prospective comparative pilot study. *Eur J Obstet Gynecol Reprod Biol.* 2015;192:22–6.
10. Namkung J, Kang SY, Chung YJ, Cho HH, Kim JH, and Kim MR. Multidisciplinary approach in large-sized submucosal myoma: Hysteroscopic myomectomy after uterine artery embolization. *J Minim Invasive Gynecol.* 2019;26:643–7.
11. Karlsen K, Hrobjartsson A, Korsholm M, Mogensen O, Humaidan P, and Ravn P. Fertility after uterine artery embolization of fibroids: A systematic review. *Arch Gynecol Obstet.* 2018;297:13–25.
12. Deutsch A, Sasaki KJ, and Cholkeri-Singh A. Resectoscopic surgery for polyps and myomas: A review of the literature. *J Minim Invasive Gynecol.* 2017;24:1104–10.
13. Van Dijck C, Rex S, Verguts J, Timmerman D, Van de Velde M, and Teunkens A. Venous air embolism during hysteroscopic myomectomy: An analysis of 7 cases. *Gynecol Obstet Invest.* 2017;82:569–74.
14. Darwish AM, Hassan ZZ, Attia AM, Abdelraheem SS, and Ahmed YM. Biological effects of distension media in bipolar versus monopolar resectoscopic myomectomy: A randomized trial. *J Obstet Gynaecol Res.* 2010;36:810–7.
15. Litta P, Leggieri C, Conte L, Dalla Toffola A, Multinu F, and Angioni S. Monopolar versus bipolar device: Safety, feasibility, limits and perioperative complications in performing hysteroscopic myomectomy. *Clin Exp Obstet Gynecol.* 2014;41:335–8.
16. Mazzon I, Favilli A, Grasso M, Horvath S, Di Renzo GC, and Gerli S. Is cold loop hysteroscopic myomectomy a safe and effective technique for the treatment of submucous myomas with intramural development? A series of 1434 surgical procedures. *J Minim Invasive Gynecol.* 2015;22:792–8.
17. Mazzon I, Favilli A, Grasso M et al. Risk factors for the completion of the cold loop hysteroscopic myomectomy in a one-step procedure: A post hoc analysis. *Biomed Res Int.* 2018;2018:8429047.
18. Munro MG. Hysteroscopic myomectomy of FIGO type 2 leiomyomas under local anesthesia: Bipolar radiofrequency needle-based release followed by electromechanical morcellation. *J Minim Invasive Gynecol.* 2016;23:12–3.
19. Abuzeid OM, Hebert J, Ashraf M, Mitwally M, Diamond MP, and Abuzeid MI. Pediatric foley catheter placement after operative hysteroscopy does not cause ascending infection. *J Minim Invasive Gynecol.* 2018;25:133–8.
20. Conforti A, Alviggi C, Mollo A, De Placido G, and Magos A. The management of Asherman syndrome: A review of literature. *Reprod Biol Endocrinol.* 2013;11:118.
21. Haber K, Hawkins E, Levie M, and Chudnoff S. Hysteroscopic morcellation: Review of the manufacturer and user facility device experience (MAUDE) database. *J Minim Invasive Gynecol.* 2015;22:110–4.
22. Smith CC and Brown JPR. A case of cardiac arrhythmia from absorption of normal saline during hysteroscopic myomectomy. *J Minim Invasive Gynecol.* 2019;26:770–3.
23. Kayatas S, Meseci E, Tosun OA, Arinkan SA, Uygur L, and Api M. Experience of hysteroscopy indications and complications in 5,474 cases. *Clin Exp Obstet Gynecol.* 2014;41:451–4.
24. Bettocchi S, Di Spiezio Sardo A, Ceci O et al. A new hysteroscopic technique for the preparation of partially intramural myomas in office setting (OPPIuM technique): A pilot study. *J Minim Invasive Gynecol.* 2009;16:748–54.
25. Holloran-Schwartz MB, Harrison K, and Gimpelson R. Direct injection of vasopressin during hysteroscopic myomectomy: A case report. *J Reprod Med.* 2014;59:614–6.
26. Mazzon I, Favilli A, Cocco P et al. Does cold loop hysteroscopic myomectomy reduce intrauterine adhesions? A retrospective study. *Fertil Steril.* 2014;101:294–8 e3.
27. Shokeir TA, Fawzy M, and Tatongy M. The nature of intrauterine adhesions following reproductive hysteroscopic surgery as determined by early and late follow-up hysteroscopy: Clinical implications. *Arch Gynecol Obstet.* 2008;277:423–7.
28. Sainz de la Cuesta R, Espinosa JA, Crespo E, Granizo JJ, and Rivas F. Does fluid hysteroscopy increase the stage or worsen the prognosis in patients with endometrial cancer? A randomized controlled trial. *Eur J Obstet Gynecol Reprod Biol.* 2004;115:211–5.
29. Yuk JS, Shin JY, Moon HS, and Lee JH. The incidence of unexpected uterine malignancy in women undergoing hysteroscopic myomectomy or polypectomy: A national population-based study. *Eur J Obstet Gynecol Reprod Biol.* 2018;224:12–6.
30. Haimovich S, Mancebo G, Alameda F et al. Feasibility of a new two-step procedure for office hysteroscopic resection of submucous myomas: Results of a pilot study. *Eur J Obstet Gynecol Reprod Biol.* 2013;168:191–4.
31. Guo XC and Segars JH. The impact and management of fibroids for fertility: An evidence-based approach. *Obstet Gynecol Clin North Am.* 2012;39:521–33.
32. Practice Committee of the American Society for Reproductive Medicine. Removal of myomas in asymptomatic patients to improve fertility and/or reduce miscarriage rate: A guideline. *Fertil Steril.* 2017;108:416–25.

21

Fibroids: Location is (Almost) Everything

Emily A. Seidler and Louise P. King

Introduction

Uterine leiomyomas (fibroids or myomas) are the most common benign tumor in women. Fibroids are a leading cause of abnormal uterine bleeding (AUB) and subsequent anemia, pelvic pain and infertility. Although fibroids are the most common single reason for hysterectomy, most fibroids are asymptomatic. The prevalence and epidemiology of fibroids, therefore, is not well characterized and likely is underestimated. More recently, with the increased use of molecular profiling, it has been suggested that fibroids are not a single disease entity, but rather a common phenotype of multiple disease pathologies [1]. With this in mind, one must carefully approach the management of uterine fibroids, letting patient-specific symptomatology and goals guide treatment.

When to Intervene

Generally, we advise intervention only if the patient is symptomatic, whether secondary to pelvic pain or menorrhagia, for potential treatment of infertility or recurrent pregnancy loss or to potentially improve pregnancy outcomes. The evidence available to guide decision-making regarding fibroids in the setting of fertility and pregnancy is not robust. We will review here the evidence available.

Fertility

Fibroids likely decrease fertility and increase the risk of pregnancy loss, although definitive evidence of causation is not available.

The physical location of fibroids is key. Fibroids are typically characterized as serosal, intramural, submucosal, cervical or exophytic (see Figure 21.1). Fibroids in any location, with the possible exception of exophytic, may affect fertility. Intramural and submucosal fibroids may obstruct fallopian tubes/ostia/gamete transportation (fertilization) and/or may affect implantation and early pregnancy maintenance.

Submucosal fibroids are classically thought to be the most deleterious in the setting of desired fertility [2–4]. There are typically multiple other factors related to the presence of fibroids that affect fertility. Other than physical location, possible mechanisms affecting fertility include impaired uterine peristalsis, vascular changes and disruption of the endometrial biochemical milieu.

Assisted reproductive technologies can circumvent issues related to gamete transportation and fertilization. Yet, issues with abnormal endometrial receptivity and decreased implantation remain. This conclusion is supported by the finding that even non-cavity-distorting/intramural fibroids negatively affect IVF outcomes [5–10].

Obstetric Complications

Beyond the window of conception, leiomyoma—specifically intracavitary or submucosal myomata—can have significant obstetric implications. A recent series of meta-analyses by Jenabi et al. suggests that fibroids increase the risk of placenta previa [11], placental abruption [12] and fetal malpresentation and cesarean delivery at term [13], which are generally in line with common clinical belief. In contrast, another recent meta-analysis discredited the classic dogma that submucosal leiomyomas independently increase the risk of early spontaneous abortion. Sundermann et al. analyzed more than 20,000 pregnant women and found that presence of leiomyoma was not associated with increased risk of spontaneous abortion [14]. They hypothesize that failure of prior studies to adjust for confounders may have led to the opposite finding.

Jenabi et al. showed a significant association between uterine leiomyoma and placenta previa based on adjusted odds ratio estimates from case-control and cohort studies (2.21; 95% CI: 1.48, 2.94). Similarly, they found that the risk of placental abruption is higher in pregnant patients with existing uterine leiomyoma (2.63; 95% CI: 1.38, 3.88). The pathophysiology of these associations is unclear, but the presence of fibroids seems to increase the risk of abnormal placentation. In addition to the endometrial effect, the anatomical disruption of fibroids can affect an ongoing pregnancy, potentially resulting in malpresentation (2.65; 95% CI: 1.60, 3.70) and increased risk of cesarean delivery (2.60; 95% CI: 2.02, 3.18) at term. Given the clinical significance of these associations, further study is clearly warranted.

Pelvic Pain/Bulk Symptoms

In contrast to issues with fertility, pelvic pain and bulk symptoms can be caused by large and/or subserosal fibroids exerting pressure on surrounding pelvic structures. Such fibroids can cause bladder symptoms (frequency, incontinence, incomplete voiding) and bowel symptoms (rectal pressure).

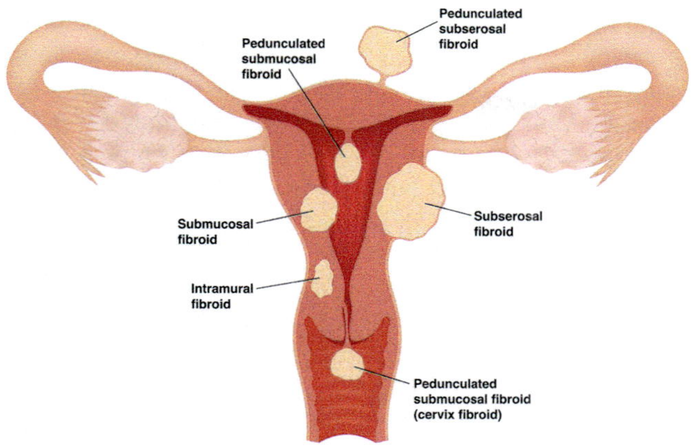

FIGURE 21.1 Locations of fibroids. (From https://www.health.harvard.edu/womens-health/what_to_do_about_fibroids, with permission.)

Treatment should always be offered if the patient reports symptoms, especially pain that is significant enough to disrupt her life choices. Such intervention should be fertility-sparing if the patient desires future fertility.

Bleeding

Fibroids in submucosal and intramural locations can cause heavy menstrual bleeding, which can be significant enough to lead to profound anemia. Treatment should be offered even if the patient reports bleeding that is merely bothersome to her despite no objective findings of anemia. As with pelvic pain and bulk symptoms, the type of treatment offered should be guided by fertility desires.

How to Intervene

Medical Options

Medical interventions include most hormonal methods such as progestins, most commonly Depo-Provera, long-acting intrauterine devices secreting progestins, and oral contraceptives. Nonhormonal alternatives include nonsteroidal anti-inflammatories and tranexamic acid. All these options improve a patient's bleeding profile, at least temporarily, but likely don't affect fibroid volume.

By contrast, GnRH agonists (GnRHa) can result in a temporary decrease in fibroid volume and bleeding profile. Short-term use of GnRHa pre-myomectomy can be helpful to decrease fibroid volume, preoperative anemia and intraoperative blood loss, and may make surgery less technically difficult [15–17]. That said, GnRHa use for fibroids is controversial as some studies show no difference, and anecdotally, their use may make surgical planes of dissection less distinct during myomectomy [18].

Surgical/Procedure-Based Options

Hysterectomy remains the definitive treatment option for fibroids.

Myomectomy, compared to hysterectomy, involves higher morbidity (increased blood loss, adhesion formation and postoperative complications) and is not a definitive solution. Consequently, myomectomy is reserved for patients with desired future fertility. In women who have completed childbearing or who do not desire fertility, surgeons should encourage hysterectomy. If retention of the uterus is desired, surgeons should carefully explore with the patient what benefit she seeks from retention of her uterus, as there are significant misconceptions about risks and benefits of hysterectomy in the media and lay press. That said, ultimately, a well-informed and noncoerced patient can reasonably opt for a myomectomy even if fertility is not desired.

Importantly, there remains a possible risk of decreased fertility following myomectomy. The risk of this increases with increasing age at the time of myomectomy and with increasing number and localization (depth) of leiomyomas (greater number and deeper fibroids are worse). If the surgery results in pelvic adhesions or infection, fertility also could decrease [19].

The surgeon and patient must also consider the risk of future uterine rupture in pregnancy following myomectomy. Risk factors for this include excessive use of energy during dissection, single- versus multiple-layer closure of defect (with multiple preferred but indicative of deeper dissection and more risk of rupture) and the potential inexperience of the surgeon [20]. The literature regarding the true rate of uterine rupture after myomectomy is limited, and reliable assessment of risk ahead of surgery is near impossible. Obstetricians and laborists should be cautious following myomectomy and should assume the uterus would behave in the same way postmyomectomy as one with a prior classical cesarean section if direction from the surgeon or operative report is not available. Thus, the recommendation should be scheduled cesarean at 37–39 (37.0–38.6) weeks when pregnant after myomectomy, especially if full-thickness myometrial incision was made at the time of myomectomy [21].

Alternatives to surgical myomectomy exist but currently are not considered compatible with subsequent pregnancy. Uterine artery embolization (UAE) is an excellent alternative to hysterectomy or myomectomy for select patients. Some evidence suggests equivalent patient satisfaction to surgical excision in the short term. Longer term, patients experience a higher rate of complications (usually pain) and a relatively high likelihood of requiring future surgical excision [22, 23]. Pregnancy outcomes after UAE are not well characterized [24]. Some studies indicate possible increased spontaneous loss, as well as a risk of infertility, after UAE [25–28]. The hypothesis is that these outcomes result from decreased perfusion to the myometrium and possible ischemic damage. This, is turn, would imply poor blood supply to the endometrium (decreased fertility) and poor placentation (early loss). However, the true underlying pathophysiology of any decrease in fertility or poor obstetrical outcomes is not completely understood in this setting. Successful pregnancies post-UAE have been reported.

Magnetic resonance-guided high-intensity focused ultrasound (MRgHIFU) was approved for the treatment of fibroids by the FDA in 2004 but is not in widespread use. Where available, this is a reasonable option for women who fail medical therapy and have desired future fertility, as it does not compromise blood supply. Yet, long-term outcome data are lacking [29]. Preliminary pregnancy data following MRgFUS are encouraging, with a high rate of delivered and ongoing pregnancies [30].

Fertility Preservation with Myomectomy

The literature is not clear regarding a particular size or number of fibroids that would definitively direct a recommendation of surgery. However, in a patient with no other obvious cause of infertility, myomectomy has been shown to improve pregnancy rates [31]. Strong evidence exists showing that when submucosal fibroids are removed hysteroscopically, and only submucosal fibroids are present, pregnancy rates improve if no other cause of infertility is identified [32].

In the setting of multiple fibroids, determining how many fibroids to remove to enhance fertility is difficult and driven primarily by experience and expertise. There are no specific studies that address this question. Expert opinion would counsel surgeons to remove all fibroids that are greater than 3–4 cm in largest diameter and are easily accessible through a minimal number of incisions. The goal is always to minimize damage to the myometrium. Typically, this would involve removing as many fibroids through as few incisions as possible. Every case is unique. MRI can be helpful in planning number and location of incisions but is an expensive modality and should be used sparingly.

Laparoscopy in general carries a number of benefits when compared to open surgery; specifically, less blood loss, less adhesion formation, less infection, fewer thrombotic events and shorter recovery period with less postoperative pain [33]. Yet, a randomized controlled trial found no significant differences between laparoscopic and open myomectomy infertile patient groups in terms of pregnancy rate (55.9% after laparotomy, 53.6% after laparoscopy), abortion rate (12.1% versus 20%), preterm delivery (7.4% versus 5%) and rate of cesarean section (77.8% versus 65%). There were no cases of uterine rupture in either group [34].

In experienced hands, using limited electrosurgical energy, laparoscopic myomectomy and open myomectomy have similar improved pregnancy rates and low uterine-rupture rates post-myomectomy [35–38]. Thus, if technically feasible, laparoscopic myomectomy should be preferred given the benefits listed earlier.

The choice of approach will necessarily be based upon the experience of the surgeon and the patient's preference as informed by adequate and accurate counseling, as well as the size, number and location of fibroid(s) of interest. Cervical fibroids, extremely large (i.e., >20 cm) fibroids and multiple (>5) fibroids located far from one another usually require open surgery. Under certain circumstances and with surgical expertise, a minilaparotomy may combine advantages of both open and laparoscopic approaches in the right case [39].

When proceeding laparoscopically with removal of a larger number of fibroids, it is essential to keep track of the number of fibroids with notations made by the circulator in writing. The fibroids can be placed on a suture and then secured to the upper abdomen in a string-of-pearls fashion. It is essential that all fibroids are removed from the abdomen so as to avoid necrosis and potential infection or seeding postoperatively.

When a combination of fibroids exists, one should target submucosal fibroids as the most likely to impact fertility. When planning surgery for submucosal fibroids, it is essential to take careful account of how much normal myometrium is available, as this may direct the mode of surgery. If very little myometrium (less than 5 mm, for example) stands between the edge of a submucosal fibroid and the serosa, that fibroid likely should be approached laparoscopically. A small case series found that laparoscopic myomectomy for intramural fibroids penetrating the uterine cavity (partially submucosal) is a potentially safe approach. Among 23 of the 32 patients attempting pregnancy during the follow-up period, 9 (39%) conceived within 1 year; 7 pregnancies went to term without complications [34].

In a case with both submucosal and intramural fibroids requiring resection, surgeons should proceed first with hysteroscopy. There are no studies that specifically address this. However, once the myometrium is breeched through an abdominal myomectomy (whether laparoscopic or open), hysteroscopy becomes next to impossible.

Regardless of the number or location of incisions made, it is essential to close the defect in the myometrium completely. This typically will require a multiple-layer closure to prevent subsequent dehiscence. This is especially important in patients who seek subsequent pregnancy. A systematic review of laparoscopic myomectomy for symptomatic fibroids found that the risk of uterine rupture is very low when the myometrium is repaired "appropriately" (i.e., multilayer myometrial repair by an experienced surgeon) [40]. Various studies support this conclusion. A report of seven uterine rupture cases after laparoscopic myomectomy found that a multilayer closure with suture of the myometrium was performed in just 14.3% of cases [20]. Another small case series found that laparoscopic suturing and repair of the myometrium in three layers above the endometrium when entered at the time of myomectomy doesn't prevent future pregnancies. The pregnancies in this case series, when desired, progressed to term [41]. Most experts would advise a purse-string stitch over the endometrial cavity defect with vicryl to preserve and protect the cavity and then layers of locking running stiches to follow with either vicryl or barbed suture.

Minimizing Blood Loss during Myomectomy

The most common method used to decrease blood loss at myomectomy is intramyometrial injection of vasopressin. The solution is injected into the planned uterine incision site, and by constricting the smooth muscle in the walls of capillaries, small arterioles and venules, it reduces blood loss during the procedure. Randomized trial data show that blood loss during myomectomy with vasopressin is significantly less than with placebo or the use of a tourniquet [42].

There is minimal evidence to suggest that Cell Saver technology is of benefit. However, it may be useful in select patients who refuse blood transfusions or in instances when excessive blood loss is anticipated. As described previously, GnRHa can also decrease blood loss.

Conclusion

Fibroids represent a difficult and fairly ubiquitous surgical problem for women and their physicians. Current research is not adequate to provide reliable guidance for surgeons and reproductive endocrinologists who seek to assist women in addressing infertility arising from fibroids, despite a fairly large library of published articles reviewed. Further study by randomized controlled trial as appropriate would be exceedingly beneficial in advancing this area.

REFERENCES

1. Payson M, Leppert P, and Segars J. Epidemiology of myomas. *Obstet Gynecol Clin North Am.* 2006;33(1):1–11.
2. Casini ML, Rossi F, Agostini R, and Unfer V. Effects of the position of fibroids on fertility. *Gynecol Endocrinol.* 2006;22(2):106–9.
3. Pritts EA. Fibroids and infertility: A systematic review of the evidence. *Obstet Gynecol Surv.* 2001;56(8):483–91.
4. Klatsky PC, Tran ND, Caughey AB, and Fujimoto VY. Fibroids and reproductive outcomes: A systematic literature review from conception to delivery. *Am J Obstet Gynecol.* 2008;198(4):357–66.
5. Benecke C, Kruger TF, Siebert TI, Van der Merwe JP, and Steyn DW. Effect of fibroids on fertility in patients undergoing assisted reproduction. A structured literature review. *Gynecol Obstet Invest.* 2005;59(4):225–30.
6. Sunkara SK, Khairy M, El-Toukhy T, Khalaf Y, and Coomarasamy A. The effect of intramural fibroids without uterine cavity involvement on the outcome of IVF treatment: A systematic review and meta-analysis. *Hum Reprod.* 2010;25(2):418–29.
7. Guven S, Kart C, Unsal MA, and Odaci E. Intramural leoimyoma without endometrial cavity distortion may negatively affect the ICSI - ET outcome. *Reprod Biol Endocrinol.* 2013;11(1):102.
8. Eldar-Geva T, Meagher S, Healy DL, MacLachlan V, Breheny S, and Wood C. Effect of intramural, subserosal, and submucosal uterine fibroids on the outcome of assisted reproductive technology treatment. *Fertil Steril.* 1998;70(4):687–91.
9. Healy DL. Impact of uterine fibroids on ART outcome. *Environ Health Perspect.* 2000;108(S5):845–7.
10. Khalaf Y, Ross C, El-Toukhy T, Hart R, Seed P, and Braude P. The effect of small intramural uterine fibroids on the cumulative outcome of assisted conception. *Hum Reprod.* 2006;21(10):2640–4.
11. Jenabi E and Fereidooni B. The uterine leiomyoma and placenta previa: A meta-analysis. *J Matern Fetal Neonatal Med.* 2017 November 21:1–5.
12. Jenabi E and Ebrahimzadeh Zagami S. The association between uterine leiomyoma and placenta abruption: A meta-analysis. *J Matern Fetal Neonatal Med.* 2017 November;30(22):2742–6.
13. Jenabi E and Khazaei S. The effect of uterine leiomyoma on the risk of malpresentation and cesarean: A meta-analysis. *J Matern Fetal Neonatal Med.* 2018 January;31(1):87–92.
14. Sundermann AC, Velez Edwards DR, Bray MJ, Jones SH, Latham SM, and Hartmann KE. Leiomyomas in pregnancy and spontaneous abortion: A systematic review and meta-analysis. *Obstet Gynecol.* 2017 November; 130(5):1065–72.
15. Lethaby A, Vollenhoven B, Sowter MC. Pre-operative GnRH analogue therapy before hysterectomy or myomectomy for uterine fibroids. In: Lethaby A, ed. *Cochrane Database of Systematic Reviews.* Chichester, UK: John Wiley & Sons, Ltd; 2001. p. CD000547.
16. Zhang Y, Sun L, Guo Y et al. The impact of preoperative gonadotropin-releasing hormone agonist treatment on women with uterine fibroids. *Obstet Gynecol Surv.* 2014;69(2):100–8.
17. Liu CH, Lin YS, Lin CC, Tzeng CC, and Chou CY. Medical treatment of uterine myoma with long-acting gonadotropin-releasing hormone agonist prior to myomectomy. *J Formos Med Assoc.* 1993;92(6):536–9.
18. Campo S and Garcea N. Laparoscopic myomectomy in premenopausal women with and without preoperative treatment using gonadotrophin-releasing hormone analogues. *Hum Reprod.* 1999;14(1):44–8.
19. Kasum M. Fertility following myomectomy. *Acta Clin Croat.* 2009;48(2):137–43.
20. Pistofidis G, Makrakis E, Balinakos P, Dimitriou E, Bardis N, and Anaf V. Report of 7 uterine rupture cases after laparoscopic myomectomy: Update of the literature. *J Minim Invasive Gynecol.* 2012;19(6):762–7.
21. Spong CY, Mercer BM, D'Alton M, Kilpatrick S, Blackwell S, and Saade G. Timing of indicated late-preterm and early-term birth. *Obstet Gynecol.* 2011;118(2, Part 1):323–33.
22. Hamoda H, Pepas L, Tasker F, Reidy J, and Khalaf Y. Intermediate and long-term outcomes following uterine artery fibroid embolization. *Eur J Obstet Gynecol Reprod Biol.* 2015;191:33–8.
23. Narayan A, Lee AS, Kuo GP, Powe N, and Kim HS. Uterine artery embolization versus abdominal myomectomy: A long-term clinical outcome comparison. *J Vasc Interv Radiol.* 2010;21(7):1011–7.
24. Gupta JK, Sinha A, Lumsden MA, and Hickey M. Uterine artery embolization for symptomatic uterine fibroids. *Cochrane Database Syst Rev.* 2012;5:CD005073.
25. Homer H, and Saridogan E. Uterine artery embolization for fibroids is associated with an increased risk of miscarriage. *Fertil Steril.* 2010;94(1):324–30.
26. Mohan PP, Hamblin MH, and Vogelzang RL. Uterine artery embolization and its effect on fertility. *J Vasc Interv Radiol.* 2013;24(7):925–30.
27. Holub Z, Mara M, Kuzel D, Jabor A, Maskova J, and Eim J. Pregnancy outcomes after uterine artery occlusion: Prospective multicentric study. *Fertil Steril.* 2008;90(5):1886–91.
28. Torre A, Paillusson B, Fain V, Labauge P, Pelage JP, and Fauconnier A. Uterine artery embolization for severe symptomatic fibroids: Effects on fertility and symptoms. *Hum Reprod.* 2014;29(3):490–501.
29. Pron G. Magnetic resonance-guided high-intensity focused ultrasound (MRgHIFU) treatment of symptomatic uterine fibroids: An evidence-based analysis. *Ont Health Technol Assess Ser.* 2015;15(4):1–86.
30. Rabinovici J, David M, Fukunishi H, Morita Y, Gostout BS, and Stewart EA. Pregnancy outcome after magnetic resonance–guided focused ultrasound surgery (MRgFUS) for conservative treatment of uterine fibroids. *Fertil Steril.* 2010;93(1):199–209.
31. Samejima T, Koga K, Nakae H et al. Identifying patients who can improve fertility with myomectomy. *Eur J Obstet Gynecol Reprod Biol.* 2015;185:28–32.
32. Shokeir TA. Hysteroscopic management in submucous fibroids to improve fertility. *Arch Gynecol Obstet.* 2005;273(1):50–4.
33. Jin C, Hu Y, Chen X et al. Laparoscopic versus open myomectomy—a meta-analysis of randomized controlled trials. *Eur J Obstet Gynecol Reprod Biol.* 2009;145(1):14–21.
34. Seracchioli R, Colombo FM, Bagnoli A, Govoni F, Missiroli S, and Venturoli S. Laparoscopic myomectomy for fibroids penetrating the uterine cavity: Is it a safe procedure? *BJOG.* 2003;110(3):236–40.
35. Desai P and Patel P. Fibroids, infertility and laparoscopic myomectomy. *J Gynecol Endosc Surg.* 2011;2(1):36.

36. Rossetti A, Sizzi O, Chiarotti F, and Florio G. Developments in techniques for laparoscopic myomectomy. *JSLS J Soc Laparoendosc Surg*. 2007;11(1):34–40.
37. Sizzi O, Rossetti A, Malzoni M et al. Italian multicenter study on complications of laparoscopic myomectomy. *J Minim Invasive Gynecol*. 2007;14(4):453–62.
38. Tian Y, Long T, and Dai Y. Pregnancy outcomes following different surgical approaches of myomectomy. *J Obstet Gynaecol Res*. 2015;41(3):350–7.
39. Księżakowska-Łakoma K, Żyła M, and Wilczyński J. Removal of uterine fibroids by mini-laparotomy technique in women who wish to preserve their uterus and fertility. *Wideochirurgia I Inne Tech Maloinwazyjne=Videosurgery Other Miniinvasive Tech* 2016;10(4):561–6.
40. Hurst B, Matthews M, and Marshburn P. Laparoscopic myomectomy for symptomatic uterine myomas. *Fertil Steril*. 2005;83(1):1–23.
41. Stringer NH, Strassner HT, Lawson L et al. Pregnancy outcomes after laparoscopic myomectomy with ultrasonic energy and laparoscopic suturing of the endometrial cavity. *J Am Assoc Gynecol Laparosc*. 2001;8(1):129–36.
42. Kongnyuy EJ, Wiysonge CS. Interventions to reduce haemorrhage during myomectomy for fibroids. In: Kongnyuy EJ, ed. *Cochrane Database Syst Rev*. Chichester, UK: John Wiley & Sons, Ltd; 2014. p. CD005355.

22

Manual or Hand Morcellation in Minimally Invasive Surgery

Janelle K. Moulder, Tarek Toubia, and Michelle Louie

The benefits of minimally invasive surgery (MIS) have been widely documented in gynecology and include faster recovery, fewer complications, smaller scars [1–3] and reduced mortality [4] compared with laparotomy. Morcellation is required to remove large tissue specimens during MIS. In 1995, power or electromechanical morcellation was approved by the United States Food and Drug Administration (FDA), which increased the availability of MIS for women with large uteri [5]. In April and November 2014, the FDA issued safety communications regarding the potential dissemination of undiagnosed uterine sarcoma during power morcellation, which worsens patient long-term survival [6]. Following the 2014 FDA safety communication, use of power morcellation by gynecologists has significantly decreased [7], and up to 84% of gynecologists have changed their surgical approaches for hysterectomies and myomectomies [8]. Furthermore, since 2014, the rate of laparotomy has increased in 46% of cases [7], which has been associated with an increase in major surgical complications and rates of hospital readmission [9]. Almost half of the gynecologists in the United States have reported that their hospitals have banned power morcellation [7]. Gynecologists have since started to use alternative morcellation techniques such as manual or hand morcellation and in-bag or contained morcellation.

Tissue extraction by manual or hand morcellation is performed by general surgery and urology in addition to gynecology [10–14]. In gynecology, morcellation should be avoided in cases of known malignancy and in patients at high risk for uterine sarcoma, such as those who are postmenopausal, have 5 or more years of tamoxifen exposure, a history of pelvic irradiation, hereditary leiomyomatosis and renal cell carcinoma syndrome or childhood retinoblastoma [5,15]. Additionally, patient counseling and appropriate preoperative evaluation, including endometrial sampling, should be performed prior to surgery in which morcellation is anticipated.

Methods of Manual Morcellation

Manual or hand morcellation may be performed transvaginally through a colpotomy or culdotomy or transabdominally through a minilaparotomy. Route of morcellation is predominantly determined by surgeon experience. No significant differences exist between perioperative outcomes or operative times following transvaginal or transabdominal morcellation when comparing specimen weight, pathology, patient habitus and patient anatomy; complications are exceedingly rare with either approach [16,17]. When considering contained or in-bag morcellation, transabdominal morcellation has been associated with a significantly lower proportion of bag puncture or breach of bag integrity compared with the transvaginal approach [17–20].

Transvaginal Morcellation

Uterine extraction by transvaginal morcellation has been performed since the 1800s [21]. Contained or uncontained morcellation may be performed transvaginally, either through the colpotomy following total hysterectomy or through a culdotomy following supracervical hysterectomy or myomectomy. The creation of a posterior culdotomy can be facilitated by using a colpotomy cup or ring as a guide. Several techniques for uncontained vaginal morcellation have been previously described [16,22–24]. All techniques use self-retaining or assistant-held vaginal retractors to facilitate exposure, visualization and protection of the vaginal walls, urethra, bladder and rectum. Trendelenburg position is decreased to 15°–30°. Following completion of the hysterectomy, the cervix is grasped and brought down to the vaginal introitus. The uterine body is then debulked by wedge resection [21], coring or bivalving with a scalpel [24]. The "paper roll" technique has been used to morcellate uteri as large as 1690 g [22]. The "paper roll" technique is performed by starting the myometrial incision with a scalpel posteriorly and continuing circumferentially in a counterclockwise direction while simultaneously applying clockwise counter traction on the cervix with the nondominant hand [22]. The constant rotation of the specimen as it is being extracted allows the intra-abdominal portion of the uterus to roll, as if unwinding a roll of paper. The "helical incision" technique is a similar method of transvaginal morcellation which has also been successful at removing large uteri up to 1350 g [23]. The cervix is pulled directly toward the surgeon and, using an 11 blade, an incision is made starting at ten o'clock, moving clockwise to six o'clock and carried down to half the thickness of the specimen. The uterus is then rotated clockwise until the uncut portion is positioned at ten o'clock and another clockwise incision is made. Rotation and incision are repeated until the specimen is completely extricated.

To perform vaginal morcellation in a contained fashion, following completion of the hysterectomy, the bag is inserted through the colpotomy with the opening oriented cephalad to facilitate laparoscopic placement of the specimen into the bag. Laparoscopically, the specimen is placed into the bag with the uterine fundus at the bottom of the bag so that when the bag is brought through the vagina, the cervix is the presenting part of the specimen. Vaginal retractors are then placed between the specimen and the bag to protect the bag from puncture during morcellation. The same morcellation techniques applied to uncontained vaginal morcellation can be implemented with contained or in-bag morcellation. Mean time for contained morcellation has been documented as 5 minutes (range 4–19 minutes) in a study with an average uterine weight of 370 g (range 240–510 g) and no intraoperative or postoperative complications [20].

Transabdominal Morcellation

Manual or hand morcellation may also be performed through a minilaparotomy of 2–4 cm following laparoscopic or robotic-assisted supracervical hysterectomy, total hysterectomy or myomectomy [17,18,25–27]. To reduce postoperative pain and optimize incision appearance, the minilaparotomy is made in the umbilicus or 2 cm above the pubic symphysis, as opposed to laterally. To reduce the number of abdominal incisions, one of the existing port sites may be extended to form the minilaparotomy. To safely perform manual morcellation, the specimen is brought up to the minilaparotomy with penetrating clamps so that the incisions into the specimen are made extraperitoneally at the surface of the abdominal wall. The scalpel blade is oriented 45° to the abdominal wall, and the incision is made in the specimen starting at seven o'clock, moving clockwise, and ending at five o'clock. The specimen is then rotated counterclockwise to expose the uncut portion of the uterus and the next incision is made. Alternating clockwise incisions and counterclockwise rotation ideally results in a continuous spiral of tissue in a time-efficient manner.

An alternative technique is to insert a laparoscopic knife or long-handle scalpel through a 1-cm suprapubic incision or trocar site [25]. Placing the knife through a lateral port site increases the risk for iliac vessel injury. The uterus is held anteriorly by both surgeons, and the knife is drawn through the longitudinal axis of the specimen, posteriorly to anteriorly and cranially to caudally.

Transabdominal manual morcellation may be performed in a specimen containment bag to minimize the risk of tissue dissemination [28–30]. When performing contained morcellation, the specimen containment bag is passed into the peritoneal cavity through the colpotomy or through the minilaparotomy incision so that the specimen (i.e., uterus or myoma) may be placed into the bag under laparoscopic visualization. To maintain pneumoperitoneum during specimen containment, closure of the vaginal cuff, vaginal occlusion, penetrating towel clamps applied to the abdominal incision or an appropriately sized trocar may be used. Additionally, colpotomy closure prior to morcellation can reduce blood loss. The specimen containment bag is oriented parallel to the long axis of the body with the opening facing cephalad and the bottom directed caudally. To facilitate specimen placement in large bags, a sterile marking pen may be used to identify the inside of the bag and the direction of the opening. The bag is first oriented under laparoscopic guidance, and the specimen is then placed inside the bag with laparoscopic graspers. Trendelenburg position may be decreased to 30° to aid with specimen placement. With one surgeon holding the specimen against the bag opening, the other surgeon uses laparoscopic graspers to pull the edge of the bag anteriorly over the specimen. The opening of the bag is then pulled through the planned minilaparotomy site by either using the built-in tab or string or with the aid of the laparoscopic grasper. Once the opening of the bag is completely pulled through the incision, the trocar site is enlarged to the planned minilaparotomy length of 2–4 cm. Maintaining pneumoperitoneum during manual morcellation helps to distance the scalpel blade from bowel and major vessels. A number of different specimen containment bags exist, each with their own advantages and disadvantages. Compared to other available materials, ripstop nylon bags are more durable; however, bag puncture is rare with transabdominal morcellation [17–19]. To increase visualization and exposure, and protect surrounding soft tissue during morcellation, a self-retaining retractor is placed into the minilaparotomy [19]. In cases of very large uterine size, preoperative administration of a gonadotropin-releasing hormone agonist at least 3 months prior to surgery can reduce specimen size to not only facilitate a minimally invasive approach, but also to allow placement of the specimen in a bag and reduce intraoperative blood loss.

Risks and Complications Related to Hand Morcellation

Specimen morcellation can create diagnostic challenges for pathologists. Identification of endometrial tissue among numerous fragments of non-oriented tissue is difficult [31]. Even if the endometrium is identified, a malignancy could be missed and staging may be impossible [32]. Compared to electromechanical morcellation, hand morcellation has the potential to maintain more normal uterine architecture to help attain a correct diagnosis [32]. Staining the endometrium with methylene blue dye [33] or trypan blue dye [31] also facilitates identification and orientation of the endometrium.

Overall, data are suggestive of worse prognosis, survival and recurrence rate with power morcellation compared with other methods of morcellation in the setting of uterine sarcoma. Both disease-free survival (DFS) and overall survival were significantly worse in patients with sarcoma who had power, abdominal or vaginal morcellation [34]. DFS is differentially affected by type of morcellation: DFS was 6.3 months with power morcellation, 11.9 months with vaginal morcellation and 149.9 months without any morcellation [28]. Morcellation is associated with more frequent sarcoma recurrences [28,34,35]. The risk of sarcoma recurrence is higher with power morcellation compared with no morcellation; however, no difference in recurrence was found between nonpower morcellation and no morcellation [29]. Dissemination of benign tissue may cause peritoneal leiomyomatosis, parasitic myomas and retained cervical and endometrial tissue, which may only become evident remote from surgery [27].

Morcellation within a specimen-containment system (Figure 22.1) may reduce the risk of benign or malignant tissue dissemination. Contained morcellation may mediate recurrence rates in cases of occult malignancy: in two studies, there was no evidence of local recurrence after a median follow-up time of 18 months and

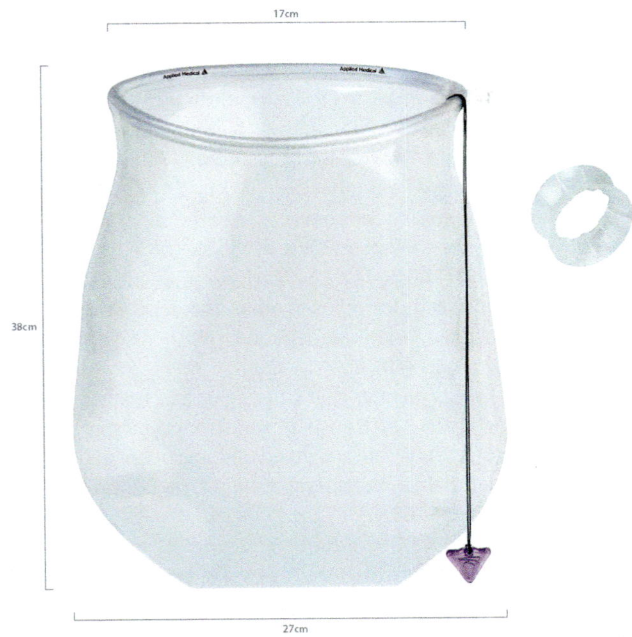

Alexis Contained Extraction System

MODEL NO.	BAG VOLUME	BAG DIMENSIONS	RING DIAMETER
GTB17	6500mL	27cm x 38cm	17cm

© 2016 Applied Medical Resources Corporation. All rights reserved. 1912INT0816

FIGURE 22.1 Alexis contained Extraction System (By courtesy of Applied Medical Resources Corp., Rancho Santa Margarita, CA.)

20 months [36,37] and overall survival was 100% at 12 months and 73% at 24 months [36]. Of note, uncontained transvaginal morcellation following hysterectomy has not been associated with sarcoma recurrence after a mean follow-up period of 25 months (range 16–36 months) [30]. More long-term data are needed to better understand the effect of contained morcellation on prognosis.

During uncontained morcellation, tissue and fluid dissemination can be mitigated by decreasing the degree of Trendelenburg to limit migration of fragments to the upper abdomen, copious irrigation to wash small fragments into the cul-de-sac [38], and extraction of the specimen in one continuous piece. All morcellated fragments should be retrieved by the surgeon if continuous extraction is not possible.

In addition to risks related to morcellation of occult malignancy, inherent risks exist with both contained and uncontained hand morcellation. Both contained and uncontained morcellation carry a risk of injury to surrounding structures. During vaginal morcellation, use of self-retaining or assistant-held vaginal retractors can minimize the risk of injury to the vagina, urethra and rectum. When considering options for vaginal morcellation, myometrial coring has higher rates of debulking failure and postoperative fever [24] compared with specimen bisection. Specific to contained vaginal morcellation, bag disruption may occur in up to one-third of cases [20]. During transabdominal hand morcellation, the viscera and major vessels are at risk of injury if careful technique is not employed. In order to distance the scalpel blade from viscera and major structures, we advocate maintaining pneumoperitoneum during manual morcellation.

Conclusion

Hand or manual morcellation extends the benefits of MIS to women with large uterine pathology and has been increasingly adopted for extraction of uterine leiomyoma. As with all surgical techniques, surgeon comfort and familiarity with the procedure will optimize patient outcome. Several techniques for manual morcellation exist for both vaginal and abdominal tissue extraction. Contained morcellation may minimize the risk of postoperative sequelae related to benign or malignant disease.

REFERENCES

1. AAGL Advancing Minimally Invasive Gynecology Worldwide. AAGL position statement: Route of hysterectomy to treat benign uterine disease. *J Minim Invasive Gynecol.* 2011 January–February;18(1):1–3.
2. Nieboer TE, Johnson N, Lethaby A et al. Surgical approach to hysterectomy for benign gynaecological disease. *Cochrane Database Syst Rev.* 2009 July 8;(3):CD003677.
3. American College of Obstetricians and Gynecologists. ACOG Committee Opinion No. 444: Choosing the route of hysterectomy for benign disease. *Obstet Gynecol.* 2009 November;114(5):1156–8.
4. Wiser A, Holcroft CA, Tulandi T, and Abenhaim HA. Abdominal versus laparoscopic hysterectomies for benign diseases: Evaluation of morbidity and mortality among 465,798 cases. *Gynecol Surg.* 2009;114:1156–8.
5. Tissue Extraction Task Force. Morcellation During Uterine Tissue Extraction. 2014; Available at: http://www.aagl.org/wp-content/uploads/2014/05/Tissue_Extraction_TFR.pdf
6. United States Food and Drug Administration. *Laparoscopic Uterine Power Morcellation in Hysterectomy and Myomectomy.* FDA Safety Communication. 2014; Available at: https://www.fda.gov/media/88703/download. (Accessed 01 July 2016).
7. Lum DA, Sokol ER, Berek JS et al. Impact of the 2014 Food and Drug Administration warnings against power morcellation. *J Minim Invasive Gynecol.* 2016 May–June; 23(4):548–56.
8. Desai VB, Guo XM, and Xu X. Alterations in surgical technique after FDA statement on power morcellation. *Am J Obstet Gynecol.* 2015 May;212(5):685–7.
9. Harris JA, Swenson CW, Uppal S et al. Practice patterns and postoperative complications before and after US Food and Drug Administration safety communication on power morcellation. *Am J Obstet Gynecol.* 2016 January;214(1):98.e1–e13.
10. Camargo AH, Rubenstein JN, Ershoff BD, Meng MV, Kane CJ, and Stoller ML. The effect of kidney morcellation on operative time, incision complications, and postoperative analgesia after laparoscopic nephrectomy. *Int Braz J Urol.* 2006 May–June;32(3):273–9; discussion 279–80.
11. Gabr AH, Gdor Y, Strope SA, Roberts WW, and Wolf JS, Jr. Approach and specimen handling do not influence oncological perioperative and long-term outcomes after laparoscopic radical nephrectomy. *J Urol.* 2009 September; 182(3):874–80.
12. Greene AK and Hodin RA. Laparoscopic splenectomy for massive splenomegaly using a Lahey bag. *Am J Surg.* 2001 June;181(6):543–6.

13. Hernandez F, Rha KH, Pinto PA et al. Laparoscopic nephrectomy: Assessment of morcellation versus intact specimen extraction on postoperative status. *J Urol.* 2003 August;170(2 Pt 1):412–5.
14. Luo JH, Zhou FJ, Xie D et al. Analysis of long-term survival in patients with localized renal cell carcinoma: Laparoscopic versus open radical nephrectomy. *World J Urol.* 2010 June;28(3):289–93.
15. Singh SS, Scott S, Bougie O et al. SOGC Clinical Practice-Gynaecology Committee. Technical update on tissue morcellation during gynaecologic surgery: Its uses, complications, and risks of unsuspected malignancy. *J Obstet Gynaecol Can.* 2015 January;37(1):68–81.
16. Clark Donat L, Clark M, Tower AM et al. Transvaginal morcellation. *JSLS.* 2015 April–June;19(2):10.4293/JSLS.2014.00255.
17. Serur E, Zambrano N, Brown K, Clemetson E, and Lakhi N. Extracorporeal manual morcellation of very large uteri within an enclosed endoscopic bag: Our 5-year experience. *J Minim Invasive Gynecol.* 2016 April 4;23.
18. Serur E and Lakhi N. Laparoscopic hysterectomy with manual morcellation of the uterus: An original technique that permits the safe and quick removal of a large uterus. *Am J Obstet Gynecol.* 2011 June;204(6):566.e1–e2.
19. Takeda A, Watanabe K, Hayashi S, Imoto S, and Nakamura H. In-bag manual extraction of excised myomas by surgical scalpel through suprapubic mini-laparotomic incision in laparoscopic-assisted myomectomy. *J Minim Invasive Gynecol.* 2016 March 3;23.
20. Solima E, Scagnelli G, Austoni V et al. Vaginal uterine morcellation within a specimen containment system: A study of bag integrity. *J Minim Invasive Gynecol.* 2015 November–December;22(7):1244–6.
21. Pelosi MA, 3rd and Pelosi MA. The Pryor technique of uterine morcellation. *Int J Gynaecol Obstet.* 1997 September;58(3):299–303.
22. Wong WS, Lee TC, and Lim CE. Novel vaginal "paper roll" uterine morcellation technique for removal of large (>500 g) uterus. *J Minim Invasive Gynecol.* 2010 May-June;17(3):374–8.
23. Lin YS. New helical incision for removal of large uteri during laparoscopic-assisted vaginal hysterectomy. *J Am Assoc Gynecol Laparosc.* 2004 Nov;11(4):519–24.
24. Nazah I, Robin F, Jais JP et al. Comparison between bisection/morcellation and myometrial coring for reducing large uteri during vaginal hysterectomy or laparoscopically assisted vaginal hysterectomy: Results of a randomized prospective study. *Acta Obstet Gynecol Scand.* 2003 November;82(11):1037–42.
25. Montella F, Cosma S, Riboni F, Dealberti D, Benedetto C, and Abate S. A safe and simple laparoscopic cold knife section technique for bulky uterus removal. *J Laparoendosc Adv Surg Tech A.* 2015 September;25(9):755–9.
26. Moawad GN, Abi Khalil ED, Opoku-Anane J et al. Comparison of methods of morcellation: Manual versus power. *Acta Obstet Gynecol Scand.* 2016 January;95(1):52–4.
27. Stine JE, Clarke-Pearson DL, and Gehrig PA. Uterine morcellation at the time of hysterectomy: Techniques, risks, and recommendations. *Obstet Gynecol Surv.* 2014 July;69(7):415–25.
28. Cusido M, Fargas F, Baulies S et al. Impact of surgery on the evolution of uterine sarcomas. *J Minim Invasive Gynecol.* 2015 September–October;22(6):1068–74.
29. Raine-Bennett T, Tucker LY, Zaritsky E et al. Occult uterine sarcoma and leiomyosarcoma: Incidence of and survival associated with morcellation. *Obstet Gynecol.* 2016 January;127(1):29–39.
30. Zhang J, Li T, Zhang J, Zhu L, Lang J, and Leng J. Clinical characteristics and prognosis of unexpected uterine sarcoma after hysterectomy for presumed myoma with and without transvaginal scalpel morcellation. *Int J Gynecol Cancer.* 2016 March;26(3):456–63.
31. Tam T, Harkins G, Caldwell T, Zaino R, and Hazard D. Endometrial dye instillation: A novel approach to histopathologic evaluation of morcellated hysterectomy specimens. *J Minim Invasive Gynecol.* 2013 September–October;20(5):667–71.
32. Rivard C, Salhadar A, and Kenton K. New challenges in detecting, grading, and staging endometrial cancer after uterine morcellation. *J Minim Invasive Gynecol.* 2012 May–June;19(3):313–6.
33. Pavlakis K, Vrekoussis T, Pistofidis G, Gavresea T, and Panoskaltsis T. Methylene blue: How to visualize the endometrium in uterine morcellation material. *Int J Gynecol Pathol.* 2014 March;33(2):135–9.
34. Park JY, Park SK, Kim DY et al. The impact of tumor morcellation during surgery on the prognosis of patients with apparently early uterine leiomyosarcoma. *Gynecol Oncol.* 2011 August;122(2):255–9.
35. Seidman MA, Oduyebo T, Muto MG, Crum CP, Nucci MR, and Quade BJ. Peritoneal dissemination complicating morcellation of uterine mesenchymal neoplasms. *PLOS ONE.* 2012;7(11):e50058.
36. Favero G, Miglino G, Kohler C et al. Vaginal morcellation inside protective pouch: A safe strategy for uterine extration in cases of bulky endometrial cancers: Operative and oncological safety of the method. *J Minim Invasive Gynecol.* 2015 September–October;22(6):938–43.
37. Montella F, Riboni F, Cosma S et al. A safe method of vaginal longitudinal morcellation of bulky uterus with endometrial cancer in a bag at laparoscopy. *Surg Endosc.* 2014 June;28(6):1949–53.
38. Sepilian V, and Della Badia C. Iatrogenic endometriosis caused by uterine morcellation during a supracervical hysterectomy. *Obstet Gynecol.* 2003 November;102(5 Pt2):1125–7.

23

Uterine Leiomyosarcoma

Roni Nitecki and J. Alejandro Rauh-Hain

Introduction

Mesenchymal tumors are comprised of uterine sarcomas (leiomyosarcomas and endometrial stromal sarcoma) and mixed epithelial/stromal tumors (carcinosarcomas and adenosarcomas) [1]. While rare, the rate of uterine sarcoma diagnosis appears to be increasing; from 1988 to 2001, their incidence rose from 7.6% to 9.1% of all uterine cancers [2]. The most common type of uterine sarcoma is uterine leiomyosarcoma (ULMS). The annual incidence of ULMS is 0.64 per 100,000 women [3] and represents only 1%–2% of uterine malignancies [1]. The median age at diagnosis is 55 years old [2]. These tumors are large myometrial masses, which typically spread hematogenously. The diagnosis is challenging because patients present with vague symptoms similar to those of patients with uterine leiomyomas. ULMSs are notorious for their aggressive nature; several studies support survival rates near 50% for stage I–II disease and 0%–28% for stage III–IV disease [4–5]. Prior studies have identified prognostic factors at the time of primary diagnosis, such as stage and mitotic count. Other factors, such as age, tumor size and tumor grade, have all similarly been investigated, but there is no clear association that has been replicable and statistically significant [2–6].

Risk Factors

Risk factors for ULMS have not been fully elucidated. A risk factor that is common to both leiomyomas and ULMS is African-American race [7]. A retrospective cohort of 12,079 cases showed that while African-American women were less likely to have uterine cancer, they were at higher risk for having a sarcoma [8]. There are some factors that should make a clinician consider ULMS when evaluating a uterine mass. Increasing age is a significant risk factor for ULMS, whereas benign leiomyomas develop primarily in the reproductive years. However, young age does not exclude the possibility of diagnosing a sarcoma, and a significant percentage of patients diagnosed with ULMS are in fact premenopausal. Moreover, tamoxifen use for over 5 years is also associated with increased risk of developing a uterine sarcoma [9]. Pelvic irradiation was previously noted to be a risk factor for developing a uterine sarcoma, but the association was most prevalent in carcinosarcomas, which are now classified as epithelial carcinomas. Furthermore, in a series of women with ULMS, only 0.5% of them had a previous history of pelvic irradiation [5]. Patients who have a history of a sarcoma at a different site (retinoblastoma, in particular) are at higher risk for developing a second sarcoma, including ULMS [10].

Increasing use of minimally invasive approaches for the management of leiomyomas may result in inadvertently morcellated ULMS, with resultant intraperitoneal dissemination of tumor. In a single-institution series of 58 patients with ULMS, including 39 who underwent a total abdominal hysterectomy and 19 who underwent intraperitoneal morcellation, intraperitoneal morcellation was associated with a significantly increased risk of abdominal/pelvic recurrences and with significantly shorter median recurrence-free survival (10.8 months vs. 39.6 months; $P = 0.002$). A multivariate adjusted model demonstrated a >3 times increased risk of recurrence associated with morcellation [11].

Pathology

Similar to sarcomas from other sites, on gross inspection, ULMS has a fleshy consistency. It is usually quite large with a median tumor diameter of 6 cm. The cut surface of the mass does not have the typical "whorled" appearance of a benign leiomyoma, but instead displays a mottled appearance with foci of hemorrhage and/or necrosis [12,13]. Most leiomyomas appear well delineated, and when they contain a combination of irregularity, hemorrhage and necrosis, a concern should be raised for ULMS [13].

As opposed to epithelial neoplasms, where invasion is synonymous with malignancy, it is more challenging to classify smooth muscle neoplasms as benign versus malignant [14]. In 1994, a group from Stanford coined the "Stanford criteria" for diagnosis of ULMS: prominent cellular atypia, abundant mitoses (>10 per 10 high-power field [HPF]) and coagulative necrosis. In the report that described these criteria, the presence of two or more of these features was associated with a risk of metastatic spread of >10% [15]. In general, mitotic count helps differentiate benign etiologies with good prognosis (which may initially appear to be malignant) such as cellular leiomyoma and bizarre leiomyoma. These entities typically contain less than five mitoses per 10 HPF. When smooth muscle tumors contain 5–9 mitoses per 10 HPF, they are given the designation of STUMP (smooth muscle tumors of uncertain malignant potential) and can exhibit inconsistent behavior. These can be further categorized by their degree of cellular atypia [16]. There is, however, extensive discussion about the pathologic diagnosis of ULMS. Some experts contend that the number of mitoses is the most important feature [17], while others argue that coagulative necrosis in the presence of significant atypia would classify the lesion as ULMS regardless of the mitotic count [18]. Infiltrative border and hypercellularity are additional features that may help determine the diagnosis. It is important to note that both leuprolide and uterine artery embolization can lead to the appearance of necrosis that may be similar to coagulative (tumor-related) necrosis and may make the diagnosis even more challenging [13].

Pathogenesis

While uterine leiomyomas can often be found concurrently with a ULMS, it is extremely rare for ULMS to arise from a benign leiomyoma. There are data from MicroRNA expression profiles that uterine leiomyomas and ULMS are, in fact, separate entities, with uterine leiomyomas being closely related to smooth muscle cells and ULMS being more consistent with mesenchymal stem cells [19–20]. The molecular pathway that leads to development of ULMS has not been elucidated. However, some studies have identified factors that might be implicated in the pathogenesis of these tumors such as p16, p53 and a high proliferative index (ki-67) [1,21]. Importantly, the absence of staining for any one of these features does not exclude ULMS. The literature supports genetic instability as a key aspect of tumor formation given the frequent finding of complex chromosomal abnormalities [22]. A promising vein of research for further elucidation of ULMS pathogenesis involves epigenetic mechanism and MicroRNA expression [23].

Clinical Presentation and Diagnosis

ULMS usually presents with vaginal bleeding, an enlarged uterus, and symptoms of pelvic pressure, pelvic pain or abdominal distention. In a study of 208 women with ULMS treated in a single institution, 56% of the women presented with abnormal bleeding, followed by the presence of a pelvic mass in 54% patients, and pain was cited as a presenting symptom in 22% of the study population [5]. Only 41% of these patients were postmenopausal. In a different study of 148 patients, premenopausal abnormal uterine bleeding was the most common presenting symptom (30.4%), followed by postmenopausal bleeding (27.7%) and pelvic pressure or pain (17%) [24]. There have been descriptions of rare presentations in the literature, including hemoperitoneum in the case of a ruptured ULMS and various presentations of distant metastases. As ULMS disseminates both hematogenously and locally, these tumors may present with gastrointestinal, urinary or respiratory symptoms, but most commonly, the primary tumor itself leads to symptoms before metastases become symptomatic [25].

Rapid growth of a uterine mass was associated with ULMS in the past. However, recent data have challenged this belief. In a study of 1331 women, the incidence of ULMS in those with a rapidly enlarging uterus by clinical examination or ultrasound imaging was compared to patients that did not experience a rapid growth. Only one woman of the 371 patients with a rapidly enlarging uterus had a ULMS [26]. West et al. [27] studied 91 women undergoing an abdominal myomectomy for uterine size equal or greater than 16 weeks, of which none were found to have a sarcoma despite extremely large-sized uteri in the study population. Studies consistently show that increased age is associated with increased risk of finding an occult malignancy regardless of the rate of growth or the size of the mass [28]. Thus, clinicians should maintain suspicion for malignancy in postmenopausal woman with either a new uterine mass or one that is growing, regardless of the rate of growth.

Frequently, the diagnosis of ULMS is made by the pathologic examination of a gross specimen postoperatively. Endometrial sampling, which is used for preoperative diagnosis of endometrial carcinomas, has not been thoroughly studied in ULMS. Hinchcliff et al. [25] examined 148 patients with ULMS, of which 45% underwent preoperative endometrial sampling. Among women who underwent sampling, 51% correctly reported either malignancy or suspicion for malignancy, and 35% accurately detected ULMS. This study highlights the importance of endometrial sampling in women with abnormal premenopausal bleeding or any postmenopausal bleeding.

There is some discrepancy in the literature regarding the risk of finding a malignant sarcoma in a woman who is planning surgery for a presumed benign leiomyoma. The FDA's literature review notes that the prevalence in this scenario is 1 in 352. For ULMS specifically, the estimated prevalence is 1 in 498 [29–30]. This statistic has been challenged as an overestimate due to the inclusion of mixed patient populations and heterogeneous studies. Another calculation presented at the FDA hearing reported an incidence of ULMS of 1 in 7450 [31]. Other studies have also reported a lower incidence. Bojar et al. [32] reported on 10,731 women undergoing a supracervical hysterectomy and found a risk of uterine sarcoma of 1 in 5400. Although not all of their patients underwent surgery for a uterine mass, in 80% of the patients, the indication for surgery was in fact symptomatic leiomyoma, making the data overall relevant. Finally, Pritts et al. [33] published a meta-analysis of prospective cohorts, retrospective cohorts and randomized trials of women undergoing surgery for a uterine mass encompassing 30,193 women. An occult ULMS rate of 1 for every 2000 procedures was reported.

Imaging

The role of imaging in the diagnosis and management of ULMS continues to evolve. Almost all women undergoing surgery for a uterine mass will undergo preoperative imaging. However, there are no pathognomonic radiologic findings for ULMS. Pelvic ultrasound is the first-line imaging modality, and there are features that have been proposed as suggestive of ULMS, such as bizarre internal echo pattern, heterogeneous echotexture and irregular vessel distribution. Yet these features can also be found in leiomyomas and are thus not reliable for diagnosis [34]. Computed tomography (CT) has not been shown to be useful in the diagnosis of ULMS, but it does have a role in identifying extrauterine disease. Magnetic resonance imaging (MRI), in comparison, has shown some promise. ULMSs manifest as large infiltrating heterogeneous myometrial masses that are hypointense on T1 and hyperintense on T2. They are also noted to have irregular margins [35]. A degenerating leiomyoma, however, is difficult to distinguish from ULMS as it may also have areas of hemorrhage and necrosis. A retrospective MRI study showed that the most sensitive and specific criteria for differentiating atypical-appearing benign neoplasms from ULMS were "ill-defined margins" and "reader gestalt," both with quite low sensitivities at 56% and 44%, respectively. Diffusion-weighted imaging (DWI) may be better able to delineate malignancy given that ability to quantify the hyperintensity of the lesion [36], but this imaging modality has not been adequately studied yet. Despite these advances, ULMS is not a disease that is amenable to radiographic diagnosis at this point in time [37].

Treatment

Total hysterectomy (TH) and bilateral salpingo-oophorectomy (BSO) are recommended for patients with ULMS grossly confined to the uterus [26]. The recommendation for BSO in premenopausal women with ULMS should be individualized. In a case-control study of 25 women who underwent BSO and 25 who opted for ovarian preservation, both recurrence-free and disease-free survival were comparable [5]. In the presence of metastatic disease, complete surgical cytoreduction should be attempted when feasible. Risk for nodal involvement without obvious extra-uterine extension is low [26,38], and lymphadenectomy does not seem to alter survival for early-stage patients; therefore, lymphadenectomy should be performed only in patients with nodes suspected of harboring metastatic disease and as part of a cytoreductive effort [1,5,26].

There are conflicting data to support adjuvant chemotherapy or radiation therapy for early-stage disease. Early studies suggested no change in overall or progression-free survival with chemotherapy for this group of patients [26]. However, in a recent study, 25 patients with high-grade and completely resected ULMS were treated with gemcitabine plus docetaxel; 59% of the patients with stage I–II ULMS remained progression-free at 3 years [39]. However, this study is limited by small patient size and the lack of a control arm. The Gynecologic Oncology Group (GOG), in collaboration with Cancer Research UK and the European Organisation for Research and Treatment of Cancer, conducted a follow-up study comparing gemcitabine plus docetaxel followed by doxorubicin to observation only in patients with high-grade, completely resected, stage I ULMS [40]. This trial closed prematurely due to slow accrual. An analysis of the enrolled patients failed to show any benefit. At this point, there is no evidence to suggest a significant clinical benefit of adjuvant chemotherapy in early-stage disease.

Treatment of recurrent ULMS depends on surgical resectability of the tumor. ULMS has a propensity to recur in the lungs, liver, abdomen, pelvis and pelvic/para-aortic lymph nodes [41]. Patients with disease recurrence amenable to surgical resection should be considered for secondary surgery. Data supporting this approach are limited to small studies [42]. In a study reporting on the role of lung resection among 31 patients with recurrent pulmonary metastases, the procedure resulted in a 70-month overall survival (OS) [43]. In a study by Leitao et al. [44], 41 patients who underwent surgical resection for recurrent ULMS were identified. The disease-specific 2-year survival for all 41 patients was 71.2%.

Optimal treatment for patients with advanced-stage and recurrent disease generally involves systemic chemotherapy; however, there is limited prospective data regarding the most effective chemotherapy regimen. Initial studies showed that in metastatic and/or loco-regional advanced ULMS, the most active drugs are gemcitabine, docetaxel, doxorubicin, ifosfamide and dacarbazine, with response rates ranging from 17% to 42% [45–48]. Of these agents, the combination of gemcitabine and docetaxel is usually recommended based on its relatively high objective response rate and favorable toxicity profile. The efficacy of this regimen has been evaluated both in the first-line and in the second- or greater-line setting in multiple phase II trials, with response rates ranging from 27% to 53% [49–52]. A GOG study reported that gemcitabine combined with docetaxel induced an objective response in 35.8% of metastatic chemo-naive ULMS patients; a lower response rate of 27% was observed when an identical regimen was used for recurrent disease [49,52]. Some studies have also demonstrated improved response rates in advanced or recurrent disease with a multi-agent chemotherapy with doxorubicin and ifosfamide. However, a phase III trial of the combination of doxorubicin and ifosfamide as first-line therapy for patients with advanced or metastatic soft tissue sarcoma (STS), including ULMS, failed to significantly improve survival and was considerably more toxic than doxorubicin alone [53]. A phase III trial compared gemcitabine plus docetaxel versus doxorubicin as first-line treatment for STS, including 27% of patients with ULMS. The regimens were similar in terms of response rates and progression free survival [54]. These studies suggest that either gemcitabine plus docetaxel or doxorubicin (with or without ifosfamide) are reasonable first-line options for unresectable disease and/or recurrent disease.

REFERENCES

1. D'Angelo E and Prat J. Uterine sarcomas: A review. *Gynecol Oncol.* 2010;116(1):131–9.
2. Ueda SM, Kapp DS, Cheung MK et al. Trends in demographic and clinical characteristics in women diagnosed with corpus cancer and their impact on the increasing number of deaths. *Am J Obstet Gynecol.* 2008:198(2):218.e1–6.
3. Harlow BL, Weiss NS, and Lofton S. The epidemiology of sarcomas of the uterus. *J Natl Cancer Inst.* 1986;76:399–402.
4. American Cancer Society. *Cancer Facts & Figures 2012.* Atlanta: American Cancer Society, 2012.
5. Giuntoli RL 2nd, Metzinger DS, DiMarco CS et al. Retrospective review of 208 patients with leiomyosarcoma of the uterus: Prognostic indicators, surgical management, and adjuvant therapy. *Gynecol Oncol.* 2003;89:460–9.
6. Rauh-Hain JA, Oduyebo T, Diver EJ et al. Uterine leiomyosacroma: An updated series. *Int J Gynecol Cancer.* 2013;23(6):1036–43.
7. Brooks SE, Zhan M, Cote T, and Baquet CR. Surveillance, epidemiology, and end results analysis of 2677 cases of uterine sarcoma 1989–1999. *Gynecol Oncol.* 2004;93(1):204–8.
8. Madison T, Schottenfeld D, and Baker V. Cancer of the corpus uteri in white and black women in Michigan, 1985–1994: An analysis of trends in incidence and mortality and their relation to histologic subtype and stage. *Cancer.* 1998;83(8):1546–54.
9. Wickerham DL, Fisher B, Wolmark N et al. Association of tamoxifen and uterine sarcoma. *J Clin Oncol.* 2002;20(11):2758–60.
10. Yu C, Tucker MA, Abramson DH et al. Cause-specific mortality in long-term survivors of retinoblastoma. *J Natl Cancer Inst.* 2009;101(8):581–91.
11. George S, Barysauskas C, Serrano C et al. Retrospective cohort study evaluating the impact of intraperitoneal morcellation on outcomes of localized uterine leiomyosarcoma. *Cancer.* 2014;120(20):3154–8.
12. Barter JF, Smith EB, Szpak CA et al. Leiomyosarcoma of the uterus: Clinocopathologic study of 21 cases. *Gynecol Oncol.* 1985;21:220–7.

13. Moinfar F, Azodi M, and Tavassoli FA. Uterine sarcomas. *Pathology*. 2007;39(1):5.
14. Chiang S and Oliva E. Recent developments in uterine mesenchymal neoplasms. *Histopathology*. 2013;62:124–37.
15. Bell SW, Kempson RL, and Hendrickson MR. Problematic uterine smooth muscle neoplasms. A clinicopathologic study of 213 cases. *Am J Surg Pathol*. 1994;18(6):535–58.
16. Dall'Asta A, Gizzo S, Musarò A et al. Uterine smooth muscle tumors of uncertain malignant potential (STUMP): Pathology, follow-up and recurrence. *Int J Clin Exp Pathol*. 2014;7(11):8136–42.
17. O'Connor DM and Norris HJ. Mitotically active leiomyomas of the uterus. *Hum Pathol*. 1990;21:223–7.
18. Toledo G and Oliva E. Smooth muscle tumors of the uterus: A practical approach. *Arch Pathol Lab Med*. 2008;132:595–605.
19. Brany D, Dvorska D, Nachajova M et al. Malignant tumors of the uterine corpus: Molecular background of their origin. *Tumour Biol*. 2015;36(9):6615–21.
20. Karmon AE, Cardozo ER, Rueda BR, and Styer AK. MicroRNAs in the development and pathobiology of uterine leiomyomata: Does evidence support future strategies for clinical intervention? *Hum Reprod Update*. 2014;20(5):670–87.
21. Mills AM, Ly A, and Balzer BL. Cell cycle regulatory markers in uterine atypical leiomyoma and leiomyosarcoma: Immunohistochemical study of 68 cases with clinical follow-up. *Am J Surg Pathol*. 2013;37:634–42.
22. Packenham JP, du Manoir S, Schrock E et al. Analysis of genetic alterations in uterine leiomyomas and leiomyosarcomas by comparative genomic hybridization. *Mol Carcinog*. 1997;19(4):273–9.
23. Danielson LS, Menendez S, Attolini CS et al. A differentiation-based microRNA signature identifies leiomyosarcoma as a mesenchymal stem cell-related malignancy. *Am J Pathol*. 2010;177(2):908–17.
24. Hinchcliff EM, Esselen KM, Watkins JC et al. The role of endometrial biopsy in the preoperative detection of uterine leiomyosarcoma. *J Minim Invasive Gynecol*. 2016;23(4):567–72.
25. Gockley AA, Rauh-Hain JA, and del Carmen MG. Uterine leiomyosarcoma: A review article. *Int J Gynecol Cancer*. 2014;24(9):1538–42.
26. Parker WH, Fu YS, and Berek JS. Uterine sarcoma in patients operated on for presumed leiomyoma and rapidly growing leiomyoma. *Obstet Gynecol*. 1994;83(3):414–8.
27. West S, Ruiz R, and Parker WH. Abdominal myomectomy in women with very large uterine size. *Fertil Steril*. 2006;85(1):369.
28. Leibsohn S, d'Ablaing G, Mishell DR Jr, and Schlaerth JB. Leiomyosarcoma in a series of hysterectomies performed for presumed uterine leiomyomas. *Am J Obstet Gynecol*. 1990;162(4):968–74.
29. Quantitative assessment of the prevalence of unsuspected uterine sarcoma in women undergoing treatment of uterine fibroids-summary and key findings. https://www.fda.gov/media/88703/download.
30. Wright JD, Tergas AI, Burke WM et al. Uterine pathology in women undergoing minimally invasive hysterectomy using morcellation. *JAMA*. 2014;312(12):1253–5.
31. FDA-2014-N-0736: Comments on laparoscopic power morcellation devices. Available at https://www.fda.gov/medical-devices/surgery-devices/laparoscopic-power-morcellators. (Accessed on 16 February 2015).
32. Bojahr B, De Wilde RL, and Tchartchian G. Malignancy rate of 10,731 uteri morcellated during laparoscopic supracervical hysterectomy (LASH). *Arch Gynecol Obstet*. 2015; 292(3):665–72.
33. Pritts EA, Vanness DJ, Berek JS et al. The prevalence of occult leiomyosarcoma at surgery for presumed uterine fibroids: A meta-analysis. *Gynecol Surg*. 2015;12:165–77.
34. Amant F, Coosemans A, Debiec-Rychter M et al. Clinical management of uterine sarcomas. *Lancet Oncol*. 2009; 10(12):1188–98.
35. Santos P and Cunha TM. Uterine sarcomas: Clinical presentation and MRI features. *Diagn Interv Radiol*. 2015;21(1):4–9.
36. Sato K, Yuasa N, Fujita M, and Fukushima Y. Clinical application of diffusion-weighted imaging for preoperative differentiation between uterine leiomyoma and leiomyosarcoma. *Am J Obstet Gynecol*. 2014;210(4):368.e1–8.
37. Hall T, Lee SI, Boruta DM, and Goodman A. Medical device safety and surgical dissemination of unrecognized uterine malignancy: Morcellation in minimally invasive gynecologic surgery. *Oncologist*. 2015;20(11):1274–82.
38. Major FJ, Blessing JA, Silverberg SG et al. Prognostic factors in early-stage uterine sarcoma: A Gynecologic Oncology Group study. *Cancer*. 1993;71:1702–9.
39. Hensley ML, Ishill N, Soslow R et al. Adjuvant gemcitabine plus docetaxel for completely resected stages I–IV high grade uterine leiomyosarcoma: Results of a prospective study. *Gynecol Oncol*. 2009;112:563–7.
40. Hensley ML, Enserro D, Hatcher H, et al. Adjuvant Gemcitabine Plus Docetaxel Followed by Doxorubicin Versus Observation for High-Grade Uterine Leiomyosarcoma: A Phase III NRG Oncology/Gynecologic Oncology Group Study. https://www.ncbi.nlm.nih.gov/pmc/articles/PMC6241678/ *J Clin Oncol*. 2018; 36(33):3324–3330.
41. Anraku M, Yokoi K, Nakagawa K et al. Pulmonary metastases from uterine malignancies: Results of surgical resection in 133 patients. *J Thorac Cardiovasc Surg*. 2004;127:1107–11.
42. Clavero JM, Deschamps C, Cassivi SD et al. Gynecologic cancers: Factors affecting survival after pulmonary metastasectomy. *Ann Thorac Surg*. 2006;81:2004–9.
43. Burt BM, Ocejo S, Mery CM et al. Repeated and aggressive pulmonary resections for leiomyosarcoma metastases extends survival. *Ann Thorac Surg*. 2011;92:1202–7.
44. Leitao MM, Brennan MF, Hensley M et al. Surgical resection of pulmonary and extrapulmonary recurrences of uterine leiomyosarcoma. *Gynecol Oncol*. 2002;87(3):287–94.
45. Gershenson DM, Kavanagh JJ, Copeland LJ et al. High-dose doxorubicin infusion therapy for disseminated mixed mesodermal sarcoma of the uterus. *Cancer*. 1987;59:1264–7.
46. Sutton G, Blessing J, Barrett R, and McGehee R. Phase II trial of ifosfamide and mesna in leimyosarcoma of the uterus: A Gynecologic Oncologic Group study. *Am J Obstet Gynecol*. 1992;166:556–9.
47. Thigpen JT, Blessing JA, Beecham J et al. Phase II trial of cisplatin as first line chemotherapy in patients with advanced or recurrent uterine sarcomas: A Gynecologic Oncologic Group study. *J Clin Oncol*. 1991;9:1962–6.
48. Gallup DG, Blessing JA, Andersen W, and Morgan MA. Evaluation of paclitaxel in previously treated leiomyosarcoma of the uterus: A Gynecologic Oncology Group study. *Gynecol Oncol*. 2003;89:48–51.

49. Hensley ML, Maki R, Venkatraman E et al. Gemcitabine and docetaxel in patients with unresectable leiomyosarcoma: Results of a phase II trial. *J Clin Oncol.* 2002;20:2824–31.
50. Hensley ML, Blessing JA, Degeest K et al. Fixed-dose rate gemcitabine plus docetaxel as second-line therapy for metastatic uterine leiomyosarcoma: A Gynecologic Oncology Group phase II study. *Gynecol Oncol.* 2008;109:323–8.
51. Hyman DM, Grisham RN, and Hensley ML. Management of advanced uterine leiomyosarcoma. *Curr Opin Oncol.* 2014;26(4):422–7.
52. Hensley ML, Blessing JA, Mannel R, and Rose PG. Fixed-dose rate gemcitabine plus docetaxel as first-line therapy for metastatic uterine leiomyosarcoma: A Gynecologic Oncology Group phase II trial. *Gynecol Oncol.* 2008;109:329–34.
53. Judson I, Verweij J, Gelderblom H et al. Doxorubicin alone versus intensified doxorubicin plus ifosfamide for first-line treatment of advanced or metastatic soft-tissue sarcoma: a randomised controlled phase III trial. *Lancet Oncol* 2014;15:415–423.
54. Seddon BM, Strauss SJ, Whelan J et al. Gemcitabine and docetaxel versus doxorubicin as first-line treatment in previously untreated advanced unresectable or metastatic soft-tissue sarcomas (GeDDiS): A randomised controlled phase 3 trial. *Lancet Oncol.* 2017;18(10):1397–410.

24

Minimizing Blood Loss

Elise Bardawil and Jessica B. Spencer

Abdominal Myomectomy

The most common route of myomectomy for patients with a large tumor burden is an abdominal myomectomy. Many surgeons feel comfortable with this route as it allows for both adequate visualization and a tactile approach to removing the myomas. Unfortunately, this route of myoma removal is associated with the highest blood loss. This high blood loss can be managed both preoperatively and intraoperatively.

Preoperative Management

Preoperative considerations should focus on decreasing either the size of the myomas or disrupting their blood supply. GnRH agonists can be used for 2–3 months preoperatively in order to shrink each individual fibroid, thus decreasing the overall size of the uterus. This pretreatment should be considered in patients where decreasing the preoperative size of the uterus will mean the difference between a midline vertical skin incision and a low transverse skin incision. The average decrease in fundal height accomplished by this pretreatment is 2 cm [1]. GnRH agonists have severe side effects mimicking the symptoms of menopause, so many patients cannot tolerate them. The evidence about whether GnRH agonists decrease intraoperative blood loss is mixed. Although the medication has been proven to decrease the size of the uterus, it also makes it harder to distinguish between the myoma capsule and the surrounding myometrium. In terms of blood loss, this loss of clear surgical planes may counteract the benefit granted by starting the surgery with smaller myomas. One large, randomized controlled trial of 100 patients comparing 8 weeks of pretreatment with a GnRH agonist versus immediate myomectomy did not show a statistically significant difference in intraoperative blood loss [2].

Uterine artery embolization (UAE) temporarily disrupts some of the blood flow to the uterus. This is accomplished by fluoroscopy-guided introduction of resorbable embolization material into the uterine arteries and is typically completed by an interventional radiology team. This decreases blood flow to the uterus and thus to the fibroids as well. There have been several small retrospective studies investigating the utility of preoperative UAE in decreasing intraoperative blood loss. All of these studies examined bilateral UAE completed on the day of, within 48 hours, or 1 week prior to surgery. The average intraoperative blood loss associated with a preoperative UAE ranged from 56.5 to 147 mL [3–5]. None of the patients in these studies required intraoperative blood transfusions.

There are several prostaglandin-derived medications that can minimize intraoperative blood loss. They act by causing vasoconstriction of the uterine arteries. They also cause myometrial contraction, which in turn causes contraction of vascular structures in the uterus, thus decreasing blood flow to myomas [6]. These medications, like misoprostol and dinoprostone, are easy to administer and can be given on the day of surgery in the preoperative holding area. Misoprostol has been well studied due to its common use in obstetrics and is considered a safe medication with few side effects. Misoprostol can be administered orally, buccally, sublingual, rectally and vaginally. The mode of delivery with the quickest onset of action, less than 30 minutes, is oral and sublingual. Vaginal misoprostol has more bioavailability at 6 hours than oral or sublingual. Rectal misoprostol has a longer half-life than oral [6]. A review article examining studies that compared misoprostol administration with placebo demonstrated a significant difference in blood loss, with a mean estimated blood loss (EBL) of 347.5 mL when using misoprostol versus 539.3 mL when using placebo [6]. A small randomized controlled trial illustrated similar results. Women who received 400 mcg of misoprostol 1 hour before surgery had a mean EBL of 574 mL versus the placebo group's 874 mL [7].

A final preoperative consideration is whether or not to use an autologous cell-salvage device. Cell-salvage devices collect the patient's blood lost throughout the case in hopes of being able to provide reinfusion of this blood during or at the end of the case. The use of cell salvage is quite costly, so research has focused on how to identify patients preoperatively who will benefit the most from its use. Clearly, patients with the highest EBL would benefit the most from this type of device. These patients usually have a large uterus, multiple fibroids, a low starting hemoglobin or decline allogenic transfusions. One article looking retrospectively at 607 abdominal myomectomy patients found that the use of cell salvage was only cost-effective 20% of the time. The authors were able to provide statistically significant characteristics that patients shared that were most commonly associated with cell-salvage setup. These included vaginal bleeding as the indication for the myomectomy, low preoperative hematocrit, uterine size greater than 15 weeks, gestation on exam and more than 5 fibroids seen on preoperative imaging [8].

Intraoperative Management

The use of a pericervical tourniquet to compress the uterine arteries is a technique that has been successfully used since the

1950s to decrease intraoperative blood loss at the time of abdominal myomectomy [9]. Many surgeons use a Foley catheter, making small windows in the anterior and posterior aspects of the broad ligament at the level of the internal os in order to facilitate placement. The catheter is then clamped tightly in place and is removed at the end of the case. Newer research has examined the efficacy of triple tourniquets. Triple tourniquets further obstruct blood flow to the uterus by compressing the ovarian arteries along with the uterine arteries. A small, randomized controlled trial with 28 participants compared triple tourniquet use to patients without tourniquets. In this study, a number 1 polyglactin suture was threaded through the windows created in the broad ligament and a Roeder slip knot was tied. Then plastic tubing was placed around the infundibulopelvic ligament lateral to the fallopian tube and ovary. A Foley catheter was then threaded over the tubing to provide cushioning. These tourniquets were clamped into place. The mean EBL in the control group without tourniquets was 1870 mL higher than the control group [10].

Vasopressin is frequently injected intraoperatively in order to cause vasoconstriction of vessels and myometrial contraction. A dilute formulation of 20 units of vasopressin diluted with 30–100 mL of normal saline is injected just below the serosa along the plane of the planned uterine incision [11]. Studies from the 1990s compared serosal injection of vasopressin with placebo and proved that there was a decrease in intraoperative blood loss. More recent studies have looked at combining the use of perivascular vasopressin with other proven techniques to see if blood loss can be further reduced. One such study compared the use of perivascular vasopressin against the combination of a single dose of preoperative rectal misoprostol and intraoperative perivascular vasopressin. A statistically significant difference in intraoperative blood loss was found when the rectal misoprostol was used along with the vasopressin [12]. It follows that vasopressin likely reduces intraoperative blood loss when paired with other previously discussed methods like tourniquet or uterine artery embolization.

Tranexamic acid has been studied as a means of decreasing blood loss through inhibition of fibrinolysis. One review concluded that perioperative intravenous use of tranexamic acid did decrease intraoperative blood loss. Physicians may be wary of using this medication as it may increase the risk of embolism, owing to its anti-fibrinolytic properties. None of the participants in the reviewed studies, however, experienced these severe side effects [13].

FLOSEAL is a type of gelatin-thrombin matrix that promotes hemostasis by working synergistically to form a clot at the site where it is placed [14]. Although it has been available for use in gynecologic surgeries for years, there is only one prospective randomized trial investigating its utility in open myomectomies. This single small trial enrolled 50 women. The surgeons in this trial used dilute vasopressin, proceeded with their myomectomy and, before closing the defects in the myometrium, either placed FLOSEAL or a sodium chloride solution into the bleeding defect. The results of this study showed that the average intraoperative blood loss in the FLOSEAL group was 85 mL versus 625 mL in the control group [15]. Further studies are needed to determine whether routine use of FLOSEAL is supported and whether it has effects on fertility or adhesion formation.

The location of a myoma plays a large role in intraoperative blood loss. Cervical and lower uterine segment fibroids are challenging to remove because of their location near the uterine arteries. The location of the fibroid can impact which tool the surgeon chooses to use to reduce blood loss. Frequently, cervical fibroids distort the normal anatomy, making a tourniquet difficult to place safely. In this case, preoperative medications in addition to vasopressin may be the wisest route to minimize blood loss.

There is little information about whether or not one incision versus several uterine incisions increases blood loss. In our institution, effort is made to use a single, well-placed incision in order to access fibroids instead of approaching myoma removal through multiple incisions. There is a similar lack of research about whether to close incisions as you make them or to remove all fibroids and then close en masse. This decision should be made on a case-by-case basis. If a certain incision is bleeding profusely, it likely should be closed before all fibroids have been removed. Some surgeons find that packing areas of bleeding myometrium with a laparotomy sponge can help to staunch heavy bleeding until the surgeon is ready to close their incisions.

Hysteroscopy

The total intraoperative blood loss from hysteroscopic myomectomies is much less than that from abdominal myomectomies. However, strategies for minimizing blood loss are critical because even a small intraoperative blood loss can completely obscure the surgeon's field in hysteroscopy.

Preoperative Management

Pretreatment with GnRH agonists can be used for patients undergoing hysteroscopic myomectomy. Research about this topic focuses on ease of surgery, decreasing fluid deficits, and patient satisfaction. Few studies look at limiting blood loss, likely because blood loss is quite minimal in these cases. One randomized controlled trial compared the use of vaginal danazol 200 mg twice a day for 30 days preoperatively with intramuscular diphereline given twice, 28 days apart. The outcomes were impressive, showing that 78.1% of the danazol group had no intraoperative bleeding versus 19.4% in the diphereline group. Unfortunately, this study did not have a control population [16]. A multicenter, prospective, randomized trial looked at immediate hysteroscopic myomectomy versus a 2-month trial of GnRH analogues preoperatively. Although this study did not examine intraoperative blood loss, the authors did report a shorter operative time with less difficulty of procedures in the pretreatment group [17]. One can extrapolate that the GnRH agonists influence the operative time by decreasing the starting size of the submucosal fibroids and by reducing their blood supply. Both of these factors likely decrease the intraoperative blood loss during these surgeries. As previously mentioned though, GnRH agonists are expensive and have several side effects, so they are not routinely used in our practice.

Intraoperative Management

Intracervical injections of dilute vasopressin have been proven to decrease blood loss during hysteroscopy [18]. The majority of research into intracervical injection of vasopressin occurred in the 1990s. One such study examined whether or not adding intracervical vasopressin injections to patients already pretreated with depot leuprolide acetate would further decrease intraoperative blood loss. The results of this small, randomized, double-blinded study showed that the patients treated with intracervical vasopressin had a lower intraoperative blood loss of 20.3 mL versus the 33.4 mL experienced by the placebo group who did not receive vasopressin. Although this difference in blood loss is numerically small, it was statistically significant [19]. Newer research on vasopressin examines its use when injected directly into the submucosal fibroid. A small, prospective, randomized, double-blinded study used dilute vasopressin, which was injected into the myoma using a single-lumen ovum aspiration needle connected to a 10 mL syringe. The vasopressin was injected until blanching was observed or 10 mL of solution was used. For the control group, normal saline was injected. This study showed that the vasopressin group had a blood loss of 5 mL versus 20 mL in the control group [20]. The difference was significant and the authors noted improved visual clarity.

Laparoscopy and Robotic Surgery

Minimally invasive techniques like laparoscopy and robotic surgery often increase operative time but have the benefit of decreased intraoperative blood loss [21]. Many of the techniques to reduce blood loss during open and hysteroscopic myomectomies can be used during laparoscopic and robotic surgery.

Preoperative Management

Uterine artery embolization was previously discussed in the Abdominal Myomectomy section. A small retrospective case-control study compared same-day uterine artery embolization with subsequent laparoscopic myomectomy with laparoscopic myomectomy alone. A non-significant trend was seen in reduced intraoperative blood loss. There are two retrospective studies that show statistically significant decreases in intraoperative blood loss with uterine artery embolization, either the day of laparoscopic myomectomy or within 48 hours of surgery. The mean perioperative blood loss reported in these studies was 90 mL and 147 mL, respectively [3,4]. However, the data for open and laparoscopic myomectomy were combined. Further study is needed to identify which patient population most benefits from UAE prior to laparoscopic or robotic-assisted surgery.

Preoperative use of misoprostol has been shown to decrease intra-abdominal blood loss during abdominal myomectomy. A meta-analysis of misoprostol use in myomectomies identified a single paper examining its use before laparoscopic myomectomy. This study compared 400 μg of vaginal misoprostol preoperatively versus placebo. The decrease in intraoperative blood loss in this single study was significant, 126 mL versus 217 mL in the control group [6].

Letrozole is an aromatase inhibitor that blocks estrogen synthesis. It has been used to decrease the size of myomas, and thus potentially decrease intraoperative blood loss. One prospective, randomized study looking at laparoscopic myomectomy gave 40 patients 3 months of daily oral letrozole and norethindrone acetate and compared outcomes with patients who were not pretreated. The authors found a significant decrease in intraoperative blood loss in the pretreated arm, with a mean of 271 mL. However, they reported that the tissue plane between the myoma capsule and surrounding myometrium was better defined in the arm that was not pretreated [22]. In this, letrozole is similar to a GnRH agonist. This potential increased intraoperative difficulty must be weighed against the decreased intraoperative blood loss when considering this method of treatment.

Intraoperative Management

Intraoperative management for decreasing blood loss is similar for laparoscopic and open cases. To our knowledge, pericervical tourniquets during laparoscopic myomectomy have not been studied. There are two studies, however, that examined outcomes associated with occluding the uterine arteries. In one retrospective case-control study, a single surgeon placed endoscopic vascular clips on the bilateral uterine arteries. This surgeon then completed the laparoscopic myomectomy and removed the clips. The intraoperative blood loss was 119 mL versus 203 mL in the control group, a significant difference [23]. An observational study examined whether laparoscopic uterine artery occlusion performed at the time of laparoscopic myomectomy or minilaparotomy was better. This study did not show a statistically significant difference in intraoperative blood loss for either technique. Yet, the average blood loss cited was 61.5 mL for the laparoscopic group and 47.6 mL for the minilaparotomy groups [24]. This article is mentioned as the low estimated blood losses further demonstrate the utility of this technique.

One of the most unique and challenging aspects of laparoscopic myomectomy is laparoscopic suturing. The advent of barbed suture that does not require intracorporeal knot tying has made laparoscopic suturing easier. Several studies have examined its utility and whether or not it can decrease intraoperative blood loss. One such study compared V-Loc, a barbed suture, with traditional suture and found that V-Loc was associated with less intraoperative blood loss. The V-Loc surgeries had an EBL of 113 mL versus 168 mL. The V-Loc was also associated with shorter mean operative time [25]. A second study examined barbed-suture use in single-site laparoscopic myomectomy. This study also found barbed sutures to be associated with less operative bleeding [26]. A meta-analysis also found a statistically significant decrease in intraoperative blood loss when barbed sutures were used to close the myometrium [27].

Vasopressin can be used in laparoscopic myomectomies in the same manner as in abdominal myomectomy. There are few studies examining whether or not this would lead to a clinically significant decrease in intraoperative blood loss. As the mechanism of action and even dose of the medication is the same as in an open myomectomy, one may assume that vasopressin would work just as well to decrease blood loss laparoscopically as it does during an open case.

REFERENCES

1. Lethaby A, Vollenhoven B, and Sowter M. Efficacy of preoperative gonadotrophin hormone releasing analogues for women with uterine fibroids undergoing hysterectomy or myomectomy: A systematic review. *BJOG Int J Obstet Gynaecol.* 2002 October;109(10):1097–108.

2. Vercellini P, Trespìdi L, Zaina B, Vicentini S, Stellato G, and Crosignani PG. Gonadotropin-releasing hormone agonist treatment before abdominal myomectomy: A controlled trial. *Fertil Steril.* 2003 June;79(6):1390–5.
3. Dumousset E, Chabrot P, Rabischong B et al. Preoperative uterine artery embolization (PUAE) before uterine fibroid myomectomy. *Cardiovasc Intervent Radiol.* 2008 June;31(3):514–20.
4. Butori N, Tixier H, Filipuzzi L et al. Interest of uterine artery embolization with gelatin sponge particles prior to myomectomy for large and/or multiple fibroids. *Eur J Radiol.* 2011 July;79(1):1–6.
5. McLucas B and Voorhees WD. The effectiveness of combined abdominal myomectomy and uterine artery embolization. *Int J Gynaecol Obstet Off Organ Int Fed Gynaecol Obstet.* 2015 September;130(3):241–3.
6. Iavazzo C, Mamais I, and Gkegkes ID. Use of misoprostol in myomectomy: A systematic review and meta-analysis. *Arch Gynecol Obstet.* 2015 December;292(6):1185–91.
7. Abdel-Hafeez M, Elnaggar A, Ali M, Ismail AM, and Yacoub M. Rectal misoprostol for myomectomy: A randomised placebo-controlled study. *Aust N Z J Obstet Gynaecol.* 2015 August;55(4):363–8.
8. Son M, Evanko JC, Mongero LB et al. Utility of cell salvage in women undergoing abdominal myomectomy. *Am J Obstet Gynecol.* 2014 July;211(1):28.e1–8.
9. Bieren R and Mckelway W. The use of a tourniquet in uterine surgery. *Am J Obstet Gynecol.* 1956 February;71(2):433–5.
10. Taylor A, Sharma M, Tsirkas P, Di Spiezio Sardo A, Setchell M, and Magos A. Reducing blood loss at open myomectomy using triple tourniquets: A randomised controlled trial. *BJOG Int J Obstet Gynaecol.* 2005 March;112(3):340–5.
11. White MS. *Te Linde's Operative Gynecology.* Woodruff Health Sciences Center Library eBooks. [cited 2016 Jul 11]. Available from: https://scholarblogs.emory.edu/whscl-ebooks/te-lindes-operative-gynecology/
12. Frederick S, Frederick J, Fletcher H, Reid M, Hardie M, and Gardner W. A trial comparing the use of rectal misoprostol plus perivascular vasopressin with perivascular vasopressin alone to decrease myometrial bleeding at the time of abdominal myomectomy. *Fertil Steril.* 2013 October;100(4):1044–9.
13. Peitsidis P and Koukoulomati A. Tranexamic acid for the management of uterine fibroid tumors: A systematic review of the current evidence. *World J Clin Cases.* 2014 December 16;2(12):893–8.
14. Oz MC, Rondinone JF, and Shargill NS. Floseal Matrix: New generation topical hemostatic sealant. *J Card Surg.* 2003 November 1;18(6):486–93.
15. Raga F, Sanz-Cortes M, Bonilla F, Casañ EM, and Bonilla-Musoles F. Reducing blood loss at myomectomy with use of a gelatin-thrombin matrix hemostatic sealant. *Fertil Steril.* 2009 July;92(1):356–60.
16. Sayyah-Melli M, Bidadi S, Taghavi S et al. Comparative study of vaginal danazol vs diphereline (a synthetic GnRH agonist) in the control of bleeding during hysteroscopic myomectomy in women with abnormal uterine bleeding: A randomized controlled clinical trial. *Eur J Obstet Gynecol Reprod Biol.* 2016 January;196:48–51.
17. Muzii L, Boni T, Bellati F et al. GnRH analogue treatment before hysteroscopic resection of submucous myomas: A prospective, randomized, multicenter study. *Fertil Steril.* 2010 September;94(4):1496–9.
18. Corson SL, Brooks PG, Serden SP, Batzer FR, and Gocial B. Effects of vasopressin administration during hysteroscopic surgery. *J Reprod Med.* 1994 June;39(6):419–23.
19. Phillips DR, Nathanson HG, Milim SJ, Haselkorn JS, Khapra A, and Ross PL. The effect of dilute vasopressin solution on blood loss during operative hysteroscopy: A randomized controlled trial. *Obstet Gynecol.* 1996 November;88(5):761–6.
20. Wong ASW, Cheung CW, Yeung SW, Fan HL, Leung TY, and Sahota DS. Transcervical intralesional vasopressin injection compared with placebo in hysteroscopic myomectomy: A randomized controlled trial. *Obstet Gynecol.* 2014 November;124(5):897–903.
21. Iavazzo C, Mamais I, and Gkegkes ID. Robotic assisted vs laparoscopic and/or open myomectomy: Systematic review and meta-analysis of the clinical evidence. *Arch Gynecol Obstet.* 2016 July;294(1):5–17.
22. Maggiore ULR, Scala C, Venturini PL, and Ferrero S. Preoperative treatment with letrozole in patients undergoing laparoscopic myomectomy of large uterine myomas: A prospective non-randomized study. *Eur J Obstet Gynecol Reprod Biol.* 2014 October;181:157–62.
23. Kwon Y-S, Jung D-Y, Lee S-H, Ahn JW, Roh HJ, and Im KS. Transient occlusion of uterine arteries with endoscopic vascular clip preceding laparoscopic myomectomy. *J Laparoendosc Adv Surg Tech A.* 2013 Aug;23(8):679–83.
24. Wang P-H, Liu W-M, Fuh J-L, Chao H-T, Yuan C-C, and Chao K-C. Symptomatic myoma treated with laparoscopic uterine vessel occlusion and subsequent immediate myomectomy: Which is the optimal surgical approach? *Fertil Steril.* 2009 August;92(2):762–9.
25. Angioli R, Plotti F, Montera R et al. A new type of absorbable barbed suture for use in laparoscopic myomectomy. *Int J Gynecol Obstet.* 2012 June;117(3):220–3.
26. Song T, Kim T-J, Kim WY, and Lee S-H. Comparison of barbed suture versus traditional suture in laparoendoscopic single-site myomectomy. *Eur J Obstet Gynecol Reprod Biol.* 2015 February;185:99–102.
27. Iavazzo C, Mamais I, and Gkegkes ID. The role of knotless barbed suture in gynecologic surgery: Systematic review and meta-analysis. *Surg Innov.* 2015 October1;22(5):528–39.

25

Fibroid Adhesions

Eleni Greenwood Jaswa and Evelyn Mok-Lin

Introduction

Intrauterine adhesions or synechiae may develop as a result of uterine surgery, and vary in severity from thin and filmy to innumerable dense bands obliterating the cavity. The extent of disease may manifest as a spectrum of symptoms. Many patients are asymptomatic. Others experience menstrual abnormalities, amenorrhea, dysmenorrhea, infertility or recurrent pregnancy loss.

The pathogenesis of infertility and abnormalities in uterine bleeding are attributed in part to changes observed in the vasculature of the endometrium in adhesive disease [1]. Symptomatic uterine adhesions are termed Asherman's syndrome [2–4].

There are several grading systems for severity of adhesive disease. In the United States, the most commonly used system is from the American Fertility Society (today, the American Society for Reproductive Medicine, ASRM) [5]. This classification takes into account proportion of cavity involvement, adhesion character and menstrual pattern (Table 25.1).

Awareness of the pathogenesis, prevention and management of adhesive disease is a crucial component of the surgical repertoire.

Prognostic Classification

Stage I (Mild): 1 to 4

Stage II (Moderate): 5 to 8

Stage III (Severe): 9 to 12

TABLE 25.1

American Fertility Society Classification of Intrauterine Adhesions

Extent of cavity involved	<1/3	1/3 to 2/3	>2/3
	1	2	4
Type of adhesions	Filmy	Filmy and dense	Dense
	1	2	4
Menstrual pattern	Normal	Hypomenorrhea	Amenorrhea
	0	2	4

Source: The American Fertility Society classifications of adnexal adhesions, distal tubal occlusion, tubal occlusion secondary to tubal ligation, tubal pregnancies, Müllerian anomalies and intrauterine adhesions. *Fertil Steril.* 1988;49(6):944–55.

Epidemiology

The overall prevalence of intrauterine adhesions is unknown, as the condition is often asymptomatic. Adhesions are incidentally noted in about 1.5% of patients sent for hysterosalpingogram [4].

The prevalence of adhesions has been reported for various clinical diagnoses: 6.9% of women with infertility [6] are estimated to have intrauterine adhesions. In women presenting with secondary amenorrhea, 1.7% have adhesive disease [7]. Incidence estimates following various puerperal procedures range from 2.8% following cesarean delivery to 40% following curettage for retained products of conception. Adhesions following hysteroscopic myomectomy also range widely (Table 25.2).

TABLE 25.2

Incidence of Intrauterine Adhesions Following Various Procedures

Procedure	%	References
Gynecologic		
Hysteroscopic myomectomy	40%	Yang et al. [8]
	7.5%	Touboul et al. [9]
Single myoma	31.3%	Taskin et al. [10]
	4.5%	Mazzon et al. [11]
	1.5%	Yang et al. [12]
Multiple myomas	45.5%	Taskin et al. [10]
	3.2%	Mazzon et al. [11]
Apposing submucous position	78%	Yang et al. [12]
Hysteroscopic polypectomy	3.6%	Taskin et al. [10]
	0%	Yang et al. [8]
Hysteroscopic septum resection	88%	Yang et al. [8]
	25%	Guida et al. [13]
	5.3%	Tonguc et al. [14]
	6.5%	Roy et al. [15]
	6.7%	Taskin et al. [10]
Hysteroscopic adhesiolysis	76%	Yang et al. [8]
Puerperal		
Early SAB D&C	6.4%	Adoni et al. [16]
Late SAB D&C	30.9%	Adoni et al. [16]
Missed abortion	35%	Schenker and Margalioth [17]
Postpartum D&C (any time)	3.7%	Bergman [18]
Postpartum D&C (2nd to 4th week)	23.4%	Eriksen and Kaestel [19]
Retained products of conception	40%	Westendorp et al. [20]

Risk Factors

Trauma to the regenerative basalis layer of the endometrium predisposes the development of intrauterine adhesions. The gravid uterus is particularly vulnerable to such injury. Adhesions are most frequently associated with instrumentation for complications of pregnancy, including postpartum hemorrhage, spontaneous or missed abortion and retained products of conception [21]. In the puerperal setting, timing of instrumentation is a clear risk factor. Adhesions are more common following curettage for spontaneous abortion at later, compared with earlier, gestational ages [16] and delayed postpartum hemorrhage (2–4 weeks postpartum) compared with earlier procedures [19]. Risk of adhesion formation following uterine instrumentation increases with repeated procedures [22].

Surgery for gynecologic conditions unrelated to pregnancy may also be complicated by adhesions [10,23]. Rates of adhesion formation following operative hysteroscopy vary by procedure and are overall lower following polypectomy and septoplasty versus myomectomy and adhesiolysis (Table 25.1). It is proposed that endometrial healing differs based on treated pathology [8].

A variety of risk factors predisposing to adhesions following hysteroscopic myomectomy have been cited. Apposing distribution of fibroids is one risk factor [12]. While size of myoma has not been demonstrated to directly affect risk of adhesions [11], diameter >3.5 cm has been associated with reduced fertility rates [9]. Certain authors report increased risk for adhesions after removal of numerous fibroids compared with a solitary lesion [10,12], while others contest this observation [11]. Preoperative GnRH therapy and degree of intramural involvement have not been found as risk factors [11].

Endometrial injury may vary by operative technique and subsequently predispose to adhesion formation following myomectomy. Monopolar electrocautery is likely more harmful than bipolar resection. Avoiding energy at the level of the myometrium altogether (i.e., cold loop technique) may further reduce risk [9,11,24].

Infection contributes risk in certain situations. The role of concurrent puerperal infection at time of instrumentation is controversial, with no clear increase in risk for adhesions [25]. In the developing world, chronic endometritis due to tuberculosis infection is a cause of intrauterine adhesions [26].

It is not known why certain women develop intrauterine adhesions after a given procedure while others do not. An individual constitutional factor has been postulated [23].

Prevention

Data establishing effective measures to prevent adhesions are limited. In the puerperal setting, avoidance of instrumentation in the management of spontaneous abortion is associated with lower risk [27]. In the gynecologic setting, several postoperative measures, such as Foley catheters, estrogen or intrauterine devices, and barrier gels are commonly employed. However, efficacy of these practices following hysteroscopic myomectomy is controversial [28].

Surgical Technique

A variety of surgical techniques for hysteroscopic myomectomy are practiced. Resectoscopic slicing is suggested as the gold standard for safe and effective removal of intracavitary (G0) fibroids; however, no single superior approach for fibroids with an intramural component (G1, G2) has been established [24]. Bipolar electrocautery with the resectoscope is believed to reduce synechiae formation compared with monopolar techniques, owing to reduced thermal spread [9]. The use of the "cold loop" technique, in which the intramural component is removed bluntly without energy, may further reduce the incidence of adhesions [11].

Newer techniques using morcellators such as the MyoSure device (Hologic, Marlborough, MA) are safe and effective [29]. No direct comparisons of risk for adhesions following resectoscopic versus morcellation techniques have been published.

There are very limited data regarding surgical approach when treating intramural myomas. In a nonrandomized interventional trial of laparotomy and laparoscopy, Asgari et al. reported the same incidence of intrauterine adhesions 3 months following surgery in both groups (19% and 21%, respectively) [30]. In this trial, no difference in risk was noted based on type or location of fibroid; however, size and location of largest myoma were identified as risk factors, with the greatest occurrence of adhesions after removal of fibroids located on the lateral aspects of the uterus. While there was a higher incidence of adhesions when the cavity was entered, this was not significant [30]. A prospective observational study of open myomectomy reported a 50% incidence of intrauterine adhesions after surgery. Number of fibroids removed was a significant risk factor, but entry into the cavity was not [31]. Breach of the endometrial cavity was also not identified as a risk factor in a prospective study including laparoscopic myomectomy; the incidence of adhesions in this experience was 22% [32]. While robotic-assisted laparoscopic myomectomy has been described as safe and effective [33], there are no data regarding occurrence of intrauterine adhesions following this approach. These reports are limited by small patient numbers and single center experience, limiting the ability to draw conclusive results.

Mechanical

Insertion of devices to mechanically stent the cavity following operative hysteroscopy are proposed to reduce adhesion formation. Data support use of a balloon (e.g., bladder catheter with a 5 cc balloon or Malecot catheter) after hysteroscopic adhesiolysis. A retrospective cohort study of 107 women with Asherman's syndrome demonstrated significant reduction in adhesive disease on second-look hysteroscopy using an intrauterine balloon compared with controls. The balloon was more effective than an intrauterine device (IUD) and gel [34]. Adjunctive use of a pediatric Foley catheter was similarly shown to be more effective than loop IUD in restoration of normal menses and subsequent conception [35]. Generally, a Foley catheter is left in for 7–10 days following surgery with concurrent administration of prophylactic antibiotics (100 mg doxycycline PO bid).

Data regarding utility of IUD insertion is conflicting. IUD effect may vary by type. The copper IUD is postulated to have a detrimental inflammatory effect. The T-shaped IUD may provide inadequate surface area as a physical barrier. The larger loop IUD (e.g., the Lippes loop) is not available in all countries [36]. The Lippes loop [35] and cooper coil IUD [34] were inferior to the intrauterine balloon system in two observational studies. However, similar efficacy was demonstrated using heart-shaped balloon and IUDs for prevention of adhesion recurrence in a randomized controlled trial of 201 women with Asherman's syndrome in China [37]. IUDs are typically removed 3 months after insertion.

Hormonal

Postoperative estrogen or combined estrogen/progestin is thought to promote endometrial growth with repair of epithelialization, thus preventing postoperative adhesion formation. A review of Asherman cases showed an association of severity of disease with hypoestrogenic state at time of dilation and curettage [38]. Estrogen is commonly used following uterine instrumentation. However, no definitive evidence supports this practice.

Several investigators have examined the utility of estrogen following hysteroscopic metroplasty. A prospective study of 46 patients receiving postoperative conjugated estrogen and progesterone found no benefit to hormonal treatment in restoring normal uterine contour following hysteroscopic septal incision [39]. In a 2009 trial, 100 women in Turkey were randomized to four groups following septal resection with the resectope: 1—estrogen + progesterone (2 mg of estradiol valerate and 0.5 mg of norgestrel), 2—Copper IUD, 3—hormones + IUD, and 4—no treatment (control). At the 2-month follow-up, adhesions developed in none of the estrogen + progesterone group, compared with 12% of the estrogen + IUD group, 10.5% of the IUD-only group and 5.3% of control women. These differences were not significant [14]. A 2014 prospective trial of 90 women in India randomized to a 30-day course of daily estrogen (2 mg estradiol valerate PO) versus control (5 mg folate PO) after hysteroscopic septum resection revealed adhesion formation in 6.9% of patients in the control group versus none in the estrogen group at 2-month follow-up hysteroscopy, a difference which was also not significant [40].

No studies have compared dosage, administration or combination of hormones [4]. Pooled analyses report varying conclusions. A 2014 systematic review of 26 studies suggested postoperative estrogen combined with ancillary measures (e.g., Foley catheter, IUD) was beneficial for menstrual and fertility outcomes; however, heterogeneity among studies precluded a meta-analysis [41]. On the other hand, both a 2015 Cochrane review [36] and a 2016 NIH meta-analysis [42] found no evidence of reduction in adhesion formation with estrogen after operative hysteroscopy.

Barrier Gels

The use of biodegradable surgical gel barriers is an emerging strategy to prevent postoperative adhesions. Like balloons, barriers are based on the principle of mechanical separation of adjacent wound surfaces during healing [43]. Many gels are derivatives of hyaluronic acid, a water-soluble polysaccharide with viscoelastic properties.

One clinical controlled trial of 54 women in France did not find a difference in rates of adhesions following operative hysteroscopy with the use of auto-crosslinked polysaccharide (ACP) gel, a hyaluronic acid derivative [44].

Newer studies support the use of barrier gels. An Italian study of 143 patients randomized to ACP versus no gel following hysteroscopic myomectomy found a significant reduction in incidence (33.3% vs. 16%), as well as severity of adhesions [13]. Another investigation of 110 women undergoing operative hysteroscopy found a reduction in *de novo* adhesion formation (6% vs. 22%) with the use of a polyethylene oxide-sodium carboxymethylcellulose gel (Intercoat) [45]. A 2014 systematic review and meta-analysis of five randomized trials including 372 women found reduced adhesions at second-look hysteroscopy at 1–3 months following operative hysteroscopy (RR 0.65%, 95% CI 0.45 to 0.93, P=0.02), with a number needed to treat to benefit of nine. When adhesions did occur, they were more likely to be mild. However, the level of evidence was deemed very low quality [46].

A 2016 meta-analysis demonstrated a significant reduction of intrauterine adhesion with both hyaluronic acid gel and polyethylene oxide-sodium carboxymethylcellulose gel, although notably all the positive data came from a single research group [42]. There are presently no data regarding pregnancy outcome after gels.

Management

There are no randomized trials addressing management of intrauterine adhesions. Treatment is based on small case series and expert opinion. Historically, dilation and curettage was implemented, but this is no longer recommended. Current treatment strategies include hysteroscopic lysis of adhesions followed by mechanical (Foley balloon, IUD) and/or estrogen therapy to prevent reformation of adhesions. Treatment is indicated only for symptomatic women or those desiring pregnancy [47].

The goal of hysteroscopic adhesiolysis is to restore normal cavity contour and endometrial function. Care must be taken to avoid creation of a false passage during cervical dilation in patients with severe disease. Strategies to minimize this risk include intraoperative ultrasound guidance and use of a small (3–7 mm) rigid hysteroscope to traverse the cervical canal under direct visualization. Maintenance of orientation during the procedure is important to avoid inadvertent damage to the myometrium. Techniques to achieve this include careful attention to maintaining the camera upright, identifying landmarks such as the tubal ostia and internal os, and the use of simultaneous ultrasonography or laparoscopy [48]. Fluoroscopic guidance has been employed in severe cases with success [49].

Most authors prefer sharp dissection with hysteroscopic scissors. This avoids potential for thermal injury, which may be a risk factor for adhesion reformation [50]. Adhesive bands are clipped at their junction with the endometrium to excise the tissue. This is in contrast to the technique for septum resection, in which the band is incised at its center. Blunt dissection and electrosurgery with bipolar energy have also been described [51].

Various techniques are available for troubleshooting with severe disease in which the cavity is obliterated. Dissection starting centrally and moving laterally under ultrasound or laparoscopic guidance may enhance safety. In cases in which the cavity may not be entered hysteroscopically, hysterotomy via laparotomy or laparoscopy may be performed, though it is uncommon today [47].

Overall recurrence is high, estimated between 33% and 66% [47]. Various methods have been employed to reduce this risk.

Expert opinion recommends postoperative placement of an intrauterine bladder catheter (e.g., Malecot catheter or pediatric size 8 Foley with 5 cc balloon) with estrogen therapy to provide mechanical stenting and stimulation of endometrial growth. The balloon is typically left in place for 7–10 days with concurrent administration of prophylactic antibiotics, such as doxycycline. Various hormonal regimens exist. Common courses include 2.5 mg conjugated equine estrogen or 2 mg estradiol PO twice daily for 30 days, plus 10 mg of medroxyprogesterone acetate or 2.5 mg of norethindrone acetate PO daily during the last 10 days to induce a withdrawal bleed.

Sequential hysteroscopies may have a role in prevention of adhesion reformation. Early intervention to remove filmy adhesions bluntly has been reported with good success [52,53]. Shorter interval hysteroscopy (i.e., 1 week after initial sharp dissection) compared to traditional 2-month follow-up is suggested to have superior outcomes [52]. Similarly, following hysteroscopic resection of multiple apposing submucosal myomas, a reduction of adhesion formation from 78% to 0% after the addition of 1–2 week follow-up hysteroscopy has been reported [12].

REFERENCES

1. Chen Y, Chang Y, Yao S. Role of angiogenesis in endometrial repair of patients with severe intrauterine adhesion. *Int J Clin Exp Pathols.* 2013;6(7):1343–50.
2. Asherman JG. Amenorrhoea traumatica (atretica). *J Obstet Gynaecol British Empire.* 1948;55(1):23–30.
3. Asherman JG. Traumatic intra-uterine adhesions. *J Obstet Gynaecol British Empire.* 1950;57(6):892–6.
4. Deans R and Abbott J. Review of intrauterine adhesions. *J Minimally Invasive Gynecol.* 2010;17(5):555–69.
5. The American Fertility Society classifications of adnexal adhesions, distal tubal occlusion, tubal occlusion secondary to tubal ligation, tubal pregnancies, Müllerian anomalies and intrauterine adhesions. *Fertil Steril.* 1988;49(6):944–55.
6. Nawroth F, Foth D, and Schmidt T. Minihysteroscopy as routine diagnostic procedure in women with primary infertility. *J Am Assoc Gynecologic Laparoscopists.* 2003;10(3):396–8.
7. Jones WE. Traumatic intrauterine adhesions. A report of 8 cases with emphasis on therapy. *Am J Obstet Gynecol.* 1964;89:304–13.
8. Yang JH, Chen MJ, Chen CD, Chen SU, Ho HN, and Yang YS. Optimal waiting period for subsequent fertility treatment after various hysteroscopic surgeries. *Fertil Steril.* 2013;99(7):2092–6.e3.
9. Touboul C, Fernandez H, Deffieux X, Berry R, Frydman R, and Gervaise A. Uterine synechiae after bipolar hysteroscopic resection of submucosal myomas in patients with infertility. *Fertil Steril.* 2009;92(5):1690–3.
10. Taskin O, Sadik S, Onoglu A et al. Role of endometrial suppression on the frequency of intrauterine adhesions after resectoscopic surgery. *J Am Assoc Gynecologic Laparoscopists.* 2000;7(3):351–4.
11. Mazzon I, Favilli A, Cocco P et al. Does cold loop hysteroscopic myomectomy reduce intrauterine adhesions? A retrospective study. *Fertil Steril.* 2014;101(1):294–8.e3.
12. Yang JH, Chen MJ, Wu MY, Chao KH, Ho HN, and Yang YS. Office hysteroscopic early lysis of intrauterine adhesion after transcervical resection of multiple apposing submucous myomas. *Fertil Steril.* 2008;89(5):1254–9.
13. Guida M, Acunzo G, Di Spiezio Sardo A et al. Effectiveness of auto-crosslinked hyaluronic acid gel in the prevention of intrauterine adhesions after hysteroscopic surgery: A prospective, randomized, controlled study. *Human Reprod (Oxford, England).* 2004;19(6):1461–4.
14. Tonguc EA, Var T, Yilmaz N, and Batioglu S. Intrauterine device or estrogen treatment after hysteroscopic uterine septum resection. *Int J Gynecol Obstet.* 2010;109(3):226–9.
15. Roy KK, Singla S, Baruah J, Kumar S, Sharma JB, and Karmakar D. Reproductive outcome following hysteroscopic septal resection in patients with infertility and recurrent abortions. *Arch Gynecol Obstet.* 2011;283(2):273–9.
16. Adoni A, Palti Z, Milwidsky A, and Dolberg M. The incidence of intrauterine adhesions following spontaneous abortion. *Int J Fertility.* 1982;27(2):117–8.
17. Schenker JG and Margalioth EJ. Intrauterine adhesions: An updated appraisal. *Fertil Steril.* 1982;37(5):593–610.
18. Bergman P. Traumatic intra-uterine lesions. *Acta Obstetricia et Gynecologica Scandinavica Supplement.* 1961;40(Suppl 4):1–39.
19. Eriksen J and Kaestel C. The incidence of uterine atresia after post-partum curettage. A follow-up examination of 141 patients. *Danish Med Bull.* 1960;7:50–1.
20. Westendorp IC, Ankum WM, Mol BW, and Vonk J. Prevalence of Asherman's syndrome after secondary removal of placental remnants or a repeat curettage for incomplete abortion. *Human Reprod (Oxford, England).* 1998;13(12):3347–50.
21. Schenker JG. Etiology of and therapeutic approach to synechia uteri. *Eur J Obstet Gynecol Reprod Biol.* 1996;65(1):109–13.
22. Hooker AB, Lemmers M, Thurkow AL et al. Systematic review and meta-analysis of intrauterine adhesions after miscarriage: Prevalence, risk factors and long-term reproductive outcome. *Human Reprod Update.* 2014;20(2):262–78.
23. Al-Inany H. Intrauterine adhesions. An update. *Acta Obstet Gynecol Scand.* 2001;80(11):986–93.
24. Di Spiezio Sardo A, Mazzon I, Bramante S et al. Hysteroscopic myomectomy: A comprehensive review of surgical techniques. *Human Reprod Update.* 2008;14(2):101–19.
25. Polishuk WZ, Anteby SO, and Weinstein D. Puerperal endometritis and intrauterine adhesions. *Int Surg.* 1975;60(8): 418–20.
26. Sharma JB, Roy KK, Pushparaj M et al. Genital tuberculosis: An important cause of Asherman's syndrome in India. *Arch Gynecol Obstet.* 2008;277(1):37–41.
27. Tam WH, Lau WC, Cheung LP, Yuen PM, and Chung TK. Intrauterine adhesions after conservative and surgical management of spontaneous abortion. *J Am Assoc Gynecologic Laparoscopists.* 2002;9(2):182–5.
28. Carranza-Mamane B, Havelock J, Hemmings R et al. The management of uterine fibroids in women with otherwise unexplained infertility. *J Obstet Gynaecol Canada.* 2015; 37(3):277–85.
29. Lee MM and Matsuzono T. Hysteroscopic intrauterine morcellation of submucosal fibroids: Preliminary results in Hong Kong and comparisons with conventional hysteroscopic monopolar loop resection. *Hong Kong Med J=Xianggang yi xue za zhi/Hong Kong Acad Med.* 2016;22(1):56–61.
30. Asgari Z, Hafizi L, Hosseini R, Javaheri A, and Rastad H. Intrauterine synechiae after myomectomy; laparotomy versus laparoscopy: Non-randomized interventional trial. *Iranian J Reprod Med.* 2015;13(3):151–8.

31. Conforti A, Krishnamurthy GB, Dragamestianos C et al. Intrauterine adhesions after open myomectomy: An audit. *Eur J Obstet Gynecol Reprod Biol.* 2014;179:42–5.
32. Bhandari S, Ganguly I, Agarwal P, Singh A, and Gupta N. Effect of myomectomy on endometrial cavity: A prospective study of 51 cases. *J Human Reprod Sci.* 2016;9(2):107–11.
33. Cheng HY, Chen YJ, Wang PH et al. Robotic-assisted laparoscopic complex myomectomy: A single medical center's experience. *Taiwanese J Obstet Gynecol.* 2015;54(1):39–42.
34. Lin X, Wei M, Li TC et al. A comparison of intrauterine balloon, intrauterine contraceptive device and hyaluronic acid gel in the prevention of adhesion reformation following hysteroscopic surgery for Asherman syndrome: A cohort study. *Eur J Obstet Gynecol Reprod Biol.* 2013;170(2):512–6.
35. Orhue AA, Aziken ME, and Igbefoh JO. A comparison of two adjunctive treatments for intrauterine adhesions following lysis. *Int J Gynaecol Obstet: Off Organ Int Fed Gynaecol Obstet.* 2003;82(1):49–56.
36. Bosteels J, Weyers S, Kasius J, Broekmans FJ, Mol BW, and D'Hooghe TM. Anti-adhesion therapy following operative hysteroscopy for treatment of female subfertility. *Cochrane Database Syst Rev.* 2015(11):Cd011110.
37. Lin XN, Zhou F, Wei ML et al. Randomized, controlled trial comparing the efficacy of intrauterine balloon and intrauterine contraceptive device in the prevention of adhesion reformation after hysteroscopic adhesiolysis. *Fertil Steril.* 2015;104(1):235–40.
38. Buttram VC, Jr and Turati G. Uterine synechiae: Variations in severity and some conditions which may be conducive to severe adhesions. *Int J Fertility.* 1977;22(2):98–103.
39. Dabirashrafi H, Mohammad K, Moghadami-Tabrizi N, Zandinejad K, and Moghadami-Tabrizi M. Is estrogen necessary after hysteroscopic incision of the uterine septum? *J Am Assoc Gynecologic Laparoscopists.* 1996;3(4):623–5.
40. Roy KK, Negi N, Subbaiah M, Kumar S, Sharma JB, and Singh N. Effectiveness of estrogen in the prevention of intrauterine adhesions after hysteroscopic septal resection: A prospective, randomized study. *J Obstet Gynaecol Res.* 2014; 40(4):1085–8.
41. Johary J, Xue M, Zhu X, Xu D, and Velu PP. Efficacy of estrogen therapy in patients with intrauterine adhesions: Systematic review. *J Minimally Invasive Gynecol.* 2014;21(1):44–54.
42. Healy MW, Schexnayder B, Connell MT et al. Intrauterine adhesion prevention after hysteroscopy: A systematic review and meta-analysis. *Am J Obstet Gynecol.* 2016 Sep;215(3):267–75.e7.
43. Renier D, Bellato P, Bellini D, Pavesio A, Pressato D, and Borrione A. Pharmacokinetic behaviour of ACP gel, an autocrosslinked hyaluronan derivative, after intraperitoneal administration. *Biomaterials.* 2005;26(26):5368–74.
44. Ducarme G, Davitian C, Zarrouk S, Uzan M, and Poncelet C. Interest of auto-cross-linked hyaluronic acid gel in the prevention of intrauterine adhesions after hysteroscopic surgery: A case-control study. *J de Gynecologie, Obstetrique et Biologie de la Reprod.* 2006;35(7):691–5.
45. Di Spiezio Sardo A, Spinelli M, Bramante S et al. Efficacy of a polyethylene oxide-sodium carboxymethylcellulose gel in prevention of intrauterine adhesions after hysteroscopic surgery. *J Minimally Invasive Gynecol.* 2011;18(4):462–9.
46. Bosteels J, Weyers S, Mol BW, and D'Hooghe T. Anti-adhesion barrier gels following operative hysteroscopy for treating female infertility: A systematic review and meta-analysis. *Gynecol Surg.* 2014;11:113–27.
47. AAGL practice report: Practice guidelines for management of intrauterine synechiae. *J Minimally Invasive Gynecol.* 2010;17(1):1–7.
48. Berman JM. Intrauterine adhesions. *Semin Reprod Med.* 2008;26(4):349–55.
49. Hanstede MM, van der Meij E, Goedemans L, and Emanuel MH. Results of centralized Asherman surgery, 2003–2013. *Fertil Steril.* 2015;104(6):1561–8.e1.
50. March CM and Miller C. Hysteroscopic lysis of intrauterine adhesions. *Obs Gynecol News.* 2006;41:36–7.
51. Fernandez H, Gervaise A, and de Tayrac R. Operative hysteroscopy for infertility using normal saline solution and a coaxial bipolar electrode: A pilot study. *Human Reprod (Oxford, England).* 2000;15(8):1773–5.
52. Pabuccu R, Onalan G, Kaya C et al. Efficiency and pregnancy outcome of serial intrauterine device-guided hysteroscopic adhesiolysis of intrauterine synechiae. *Fertil Steri..* 2008;90(5):1973–7.
53. Robinson JK, Colimon LM, Isaacson KB. Postoperative adhesiolysis therapy for intrauterine adhesions (Asherman's syndrome). *Fertil Steril.* 2008;90(2):409–14.

26

How Long Does it Take Uterine Scar(s) to Heal?

Hope Y. Yu and Gary N. Frishman

Uterine Anatomy

The uterus is a fibromuscular hollow organ located between the bladder and rectum that consists of an inner layer of mucosa called the endometrium, a thick muscular wall known as the myometrium, and the peritoneal serosa that overlies the outer wall. The blood supply to the uterus arises from the ascending branch of the uterine artery and from the medial or uterine branch of the ovarian artery [1].

Biochemistry of Healing

The normal healing process can be divided into three phases. The first phase is the inflammatory phase that lasts up to 72 hours after the time of injury. In muscular injuries, peripheral muscle fiber contraction occurs within the first 2 hours of injury. Edema and anoxia result in cell damage and death within the first 24 hours. Phagocytosis then rids the area of cell debris and edema.

The second phase is known as the fibro-elastic or collagen-forming phase and lasts between 48 hours to 6 weeks after injury. During this phase, muscular regeneration and repair occur. Fibroblast cells begin to produce type III collagen. Capillary budding facilitates nutrient delivery to the site of injury and collagen cross-linking begins. Toward the end of this phase, wound contracture begins with shortening of the margins in the injured area.

The final phase of normal healing is known as the remodeling phase, which lasts between 3 weeks and 12 months after injury. During this period, final aggregation, cross-linking and shortening of the collagen fibers takes place to promote formation of a strong scar [2]. However, foreign bodies (such as suture, mesh material, etc.) and adequate blood supply (which may be diminished by suture or thermal injury from energy sources) may both impact healing.

Assessment of Uterine Healing

There are currently no standardized methods of assessing uterine healing. However, several methods, including ultrasound, Doppler studies and MRI, have been utilized in assessing healing and scar formation. Baranov et al. demonstrated that transvaginal ultrasound is a validated tool to evaluate uterine scars, specifically to quantify the severity of the uterine defect by comparing the myometrium thickness at the incision with that of the surrounding tissue [3]. Observational studies employing Doppler to assess the change in resistance index with healing have reported confounding findings. Chang et al. showed a decrease in the resistance index in the uterine arteries up to 7 days after laparoscopic myomectomy [4]. On the other hand, Tinelli et al. showed an increase in the resistance index until 7 days postoperatively, followed by a decrease also in women undergoing laparoscopic myomectomy [2]. MRI has been compared with transvaginal ultrasound as a modality for uterine scar assessment. Singh et al. used each of these two modalities to measure scar thickness on the day of a patient's elective repeat cesarean section. They found that MRI is a costlier modality and that ultrasound has a better correlation coefficient with actual scar thickness as measured with calipers at the time of surgery [6].

Table 26.1 outlines the types of uterine surgery with associated healing times.

Polypectomy

Polypectomy is a common surgery of the endometrium performed for both infertility and abnormal uterine bleeding. A study by Yang et al. used serial hysteroscopy to assess the endometrium for healing after polypectomy and found that 86% of patients had a fully healed endometrium 1 month after the procedure [7]. Consistent with this, Pereira et al. reported that in women undergoing IVF after polypectomy, ovarian stimulation can be initiated after the next menses with comparable pregnancy rates compared with longer time periods [8].

Uterine Septoplasty

A uterine septum is the most common congenital uterine anomaly. The American Society for Reproductive Medicine (ASRM) uterine septum practice committee guidelines published grade C evidence that hysteroscopic septum incision is associated with a reduction in subsequent miscarriage rates and an improvement in live-birth rates in patients with a history of recurrent pregnancy loss. In terms of uterine healing, available evidence suggests that the uterine cavity is healed by 2 months postoperatively, although there is insufficient evidence to advocate a specific length of time before a woman should conceive [9,7,11,12].

Adhesiolysis

Intrauterine adhesions (IUAs) remain a challenge in modern day gynecology. Yang et al. used office hysteroscopy to assess

TABLE 26.1

Common Surgical Procedures with Associated Healing Times and Recommendations

Surgery	Rates of Complete Healing	Recommended Waiting Time for Fertility Treatment
Polypectomy	86% at 1 month (Yang et al. 2013)	2 months (Yang et al. 2013)
Uterine septoplasty	50% at 1 month (Yang et al. 2013)	2 months (Yang et al. 2013), however insufficient evidence to advocate a specific length of time (ASRM Practice Committee Guidelines)
Intrauterine adhesiolysis	67% at 1 month (Yang et al. 2013)	3 months (Yang et al. 2013)
Resectoscopic myomectomy	80% at 2 months (Yang et al. 2008)	2 months (Yang et al. 2013)
Abdominal myomectomy	86% at 3 months; 100% at 6 months (Tsuji et al. 2006) 93% at 1 month; 100% at 6 months (Darwish et al. 2005)	6 months (Tsuji et al. 2006)
Cesarean section	3 months for scar maturation, 6 months for restoration of zonal anatomy (Dicle et al. 1997)	18-month interconceptual period (Shipp et al. 2001)

Note: There are no long-term data or even pregnancy outcomes but rather the majority of studies use measurements and other sonographic features of the uterine scar or absence of intrauterine adhesions as their end point.

healing after hysteroscopic adhesiolysis. This was performed 10–14 days after the hysteroscopic procedure. They suggested that healing can take anywhere between 1 and 3 months [24].

Myomectomy

Myomectomy involves surgical removal of leiomyomas from their surrounding tissue. The depth of the uterine incision depends on the number, location and size of the leiomyomas and will invariably affect scar formation and healing. Tsuji et al. used MRI to evaluate uterine changes following abdominal myomectomy on women with a single intramural fibroid. They found that uterine volume and length were stabilized by 6 weeks postoperatively, as was the myometrium as assessed by analyzing the junctional zone. Using hematoma or edema formation as an end point, endometrial healing was typically complete at 12 weeks. However, 2 out of 14 cases (14.2%) had incomplete healing at that time, with these cases being resolved by 6 months [14]. Darwish et al. found similar results using monitoring with transvaginal ultrasound after abdominal myomectomy, reporting 7% of patients with hematomas at the myomectomy scar at 4 weeks but that all 169 women scanned had complete resolution of any hematomas by 3 months postoperatively [15]. Therefore, it is reasonable to consider imaging such as ultrasound to assess the status of healing after 12 weeks. Alternatively, healing is very likely to be complete at 6 months.

Cesarean Section

Cesarean section incisions are an example of a full-thickness uterine wall incision. Multiple studies have been published to assess methods of uterine closure to minimize risk of uterine rupture with future pregnancies. There is currently no consensus on the method of uterine closure of a low transverse incision following cesarean delivery in terms of use of one or two layers, locking or not with the first layer and whether the decidua should be included or excluded [16,17,18].

In terms of healing time, a study performed by Dicle et al. used MRI to examine the healing period of cesarean section incisions. They found that there was complete involution and recovery of the zonal anatomy after 6 months [19]. Multiple studies have also evaluated the relationship of short interconceptual periods with risk of uterine rupture in trial of labor after cesarean section (TOLAC), which can provide insight to the amount of time needed for cesarean section incision healing (see "Complications of Healing" section). This is independent of other maternal and fetal benefits of avoiding short interconception intervals.

Complications of Healing

Complications of healing that can occur following uterine surgery include IUA, extrauterine (abdominal) adhesions, uterine rupture, fistula tracts and postmenstrual bleeding or discharge as a result of cesarean section defects.

Intrauterine adhesions, also known as Asherman's syndrome, are defined as the presence of adhesions inside the uterine cavity and/or endocervix. Clinical manifestations include amenorrhea, hypomenorrhea, recurrent pregnancy loss, infertility and abnormal placentation. Conforti et al. reviewed the risk factors associated with Asherman's syndrome and identified curettage after miscarriage to have the highest incidence of Asherman's syndrome [25]. Extrauterine adhesions following abdominal myomectomies may similarly cause problems with fertility as well as pain. There are many anti-adhesion adjuvants but there is no one accepted standard of care, and careful surgical technique is highly recommended.

Uterine rupture is a complication most commonly associated with cesarean section scars [20,21,22]. However, it can also follow other surgeries such as myomectomy or metroplasty. Parker et al. analyzed 19 case reports of uterine rupture and found no commonality in surgical technique; however, the results of their analysis suggested avoiding electrosurgery and to close with multiple layers [23]. There have also been studies performed to assess the relationship between the interconceptual period and risk of uterine rupture. A retrospective study by Shipp et al. showed that an interconceptual interval of less than 18 months was associated with an increased risk of symptomatic uterine rupture during TOLAC [10].

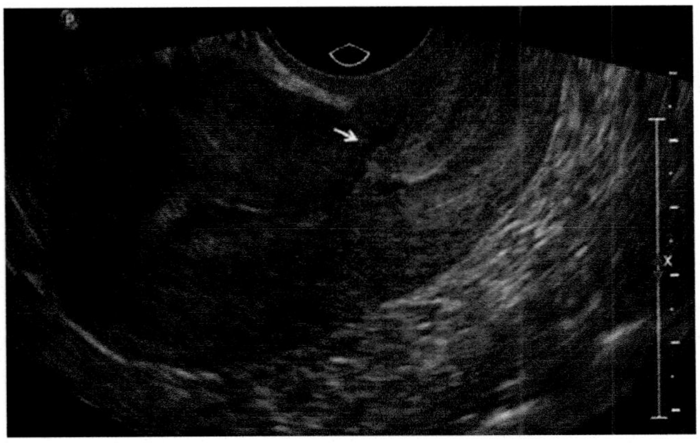

FIGURE 26.1 Cesarean scar defect (arrow) on transvaginal ultrasound scan. (Courtesy of Tower and Frishman, 2013.)

Thermal injury or improper suturing may lead to a fistula formation at the surgical site. Similar to the risk of uterine rupture noted previously, this adverse outcome can be minimized by judicious use of energy sources and proper surgical technique.

Cesarean scar defects (CSDs) following cesarean section incisions have been associated with other major obstetrical complications such as ectopic scar pregnancies and placenta accreta, as well as numerous gynecological problems including postmenstrual spotting, dysmenorrhea and pelvic pain [13]. There is currently no consensus as to how to make the diagnosis of CSD, with some suggested techniques utilizing transvaginal ultrasound, sonohysterogram and hysteroscopy (Figure 26.1). There have been multiple approaches documented to repair these CSDs including hysteroscopic, laparoscopic, transvaginal and robotic-assisted laparoscopic. In a prospective study of 41 women with secondary infertility and postmenstrual bleeding, Gubbini et al. treated the CSD hysteroscopically. Although there was no control group, 100% of women had resolution of their irregular bleeding, and all became pregnant within 24 months after surgery [5].

Conclusions

Multiple factors impact uterine healing including type of energy source, volume of tissue treated, number of incisions or lesions treated, etc. Although not definitively studied, many surgeons advocate minimizing the use of electrosurgery and attention to careful surgical technique. No surgical adjuvants have been shown to improve uterine healing (as opposed to bleeding, adhesion formation, etc.). It appears, and makes sense clinically, that hysteroscopic techniques lead to faster healing than an abdominal approach but there are no data comparing open and endoscopic abdominal routes. All myomectomy studies are limited by variations in technique, number of fibroids and location of fibroids and other variables limiting the ability to make comparisons and draw definitive conclusions.

Imaging studies of uterine scars are considered proxies for uterine healing and, even within this area of study, there are no standardized assessment scales or tools. Thickness of the scar can be used as a surrogate for strength but other factors likely play a role and the relationship of hematoma formation and resolution to strength is not clear. However, uterine healing by imaging is likely a reasonable lower limit with 1–2 months recommended prior to attempting pregnancy for most hysteroscopic procedures and 3–6 months for an abdominal myomectomy.

REFERENCES

1. Hoffman B, Schorge J, Schaffer J, Halvorson L, Bradshaw K, Cunningham G. *Williams Gynecology*. 2nd ed. McGraw Hill; 2012.
2. Tinelli A, Hurst BS, Mettler L, Tsin DA, Pellegrino M, Nicolardi G, Dell'Edera D, and Malvasi A. Ultrasound evaluation of uterine healing after laparoscopic intracapsular myomectomy: An observational study. *Human Reproduction*. 2012 September 1;27(9):2664–70.
3. Baranov A, Gunnarsson G, Salvesen KÅ, Isberg PE, and Vikhareva O. Assessment of Cesarean hysterotomy scar in non-pregnant women: Reliability of transvaginal sonography with and without contrast enhancement. *Ultrasound Obstet Gynecol*. 2016 April;47(4):499–505.
4. Chang WC, Chang DY, Huang SC, Shih JC, Hsu WC, Chen SY, and Sheu BC. Use of three-dimensional ultrasonography in the evaluation of uterine perfusion and healing after laparoscopic myomectomy. *Fertil Steril*. 2009 Sep 30;92(3):1110–5.
5. Gubbini G, Centini G, Nascetti D, Marra E, Moncini I, Bruni L, Petraglia F, and Florio P. Surgical hysteroscopic treatment of cesarean-induced isthmocele in restoring fertility: Prospective study. *J Minim Invasive Gynecol*. 2011 April 30;18(2):234–7.
6. Singh N, Tripathi R, Mala YM, Dixit R, Tyagi S, and Batra A. Comparison of scar thickness measurements using trans-vaginal sonography and MRI in cases of pregnancy with previous caesarean section. Do they correlate with actual scar thickness? *J Obstet Gynaecol*. 2013 November 1;33(8):810–3.
7. Yang JH, Chen MJ, Chen CD, Chen SU, Ho HN, and Yang YS. Optimal waiting period for subsequent fertility treatment after various hysteroscopic surgeries. *Fertil Steril*. 2013 June 30;99(7):2092–6
8. Pereira N, Amrane S, Estes JL, Lekovich JP, Elias RT, Chung PH, and Rosenwaks Z. Does the time interval between hysteroscopic polypectomy and start of *in vitro* fertilization affect outcomes?. *Fertil Steril*. 2016 February 29;105(2):539–44.
9. Practice Committee of the American Society for Reproductive Medicine. *Uterine septum: a guideline. Fertility and sterility*. 2016 May 25.
10. Shipp TD, Zelop CM, Repke JT, Cohen A, and Lieberman E. Interdelivery interval and risk of symptomatic uterine rupture. *Obstet Gynecol*. 2001 February 28;97(2):175–7.
11. Candiani GB, Vercellini P, Fedele L, Carinelli SG, Merlo D, and Arcaini L. Repair of the uterine cavity after hysteroscopic septal incision. *Fertil Steril*. 1990 December 31;54(6):991–4.
12. Berkkanoglu M, Isikoglu M, Arici F, and Ozgur K. What is the best time to perform intracytoplasmic sperm injection/embryo transfer cycle after hysteroscopic surgery for an incomplete uterine septum? *Fertil Steril*. 2008 December 31;90(6):2112–5.
13. Tower AM and Frishman GN. Cesarean scar defects: An underrecognized cause of abnormal uterine bleeding and other gynecologic complications. *J Minim Invasive Gynecol*. 2013 October 31;20(5):562–72.

14. Tsuji S, Takahashi K, Imaoka I, Sugimura K, Miyazaki K, and Noda Y. MRI evaluation of the uterine structure after myomectomy. *Gynecol Obstet Investig.* 2006 February 17;61(2):106–10.
15. Darwish AM, Nasr AM, and El-Nashar DA. Evaluation of postmyomectomy uterine scar. *J Clin Ultrasound.* 2005 May 1;33(4):181–6.
16. Brocklehurst P, Quigley M, Ayers S, and Juszczak E. Caesarean section surgical techniques: A randomised factorial trial (CAESAR). *BJOG.* 2010;117(11):1366–76.
17. Bujold E, Goyet M, Marcoux S et al. The role of uterine closure in the risk of uterine rupture *Obstet Gynecol.* 2010 July 1;116(1):43–50.
18. Roberge S, Demers S, Girard M, Vikhareva O, Markey S, Chaillet N, Moore L, Paris G, and Bujold E. Impact of uterine closure on residual myometrial thickness after cesarean: A randomized controlled trial. *Am J Obstet Gynecol.* 2016 April 30;214(4):507–e1.
19. Dicle O, Küçükler C, Pirnar T, Erata Y, and Posaci C. Magnetic resonance imaging evaluation of incision healing after cesarean sections. *Eur Radiol.* 1997 January 1;7(1):31–4.
20. Ofili-Yebovi D, Ben-Nagi J, Sawyer E, Yazbek J, Lee C, Gonzalez J, and Jurkovic D. Deficient lower-segment Cesarean section scars: Prevalence and risk factors. *Ultrasound Obstet Gynecol.* 2008 January 1;31(1):72–7.
21. Roberge S, Boutin A, Chaillet N, Moore L, Jastrow N, Demers S, and Bujold E. Systematic review of cesarean scar assessment in the nonpregnant state: Imaging techniques and uterine scar defect. *Am J Perinatol.* 2012 June;29(06):465–72.
22. Vikhareva Osser O, Jokubkiene L, and Valentin L. High prevalence of defects in Cesarean section scars at transvaginal ultrasound examination. *Ultrasound Obstet Gynecol.* 2009 July 1;34(1):90–7.
23. Parker WH, Einarsson J, Istre O, and Dubuisson JB. Risk factors for uterine rupture after laparoscopic myomectomy. *J Minim Invasive Gynecol.* 2010 October 31;17(5):551–4.
24. Yang JH, Chen MJ, Wu MY, Chao KH, Ho HN, Yang YS. Office hysteroscopic early lysis of intrauterine adhesion after transcervical resection of multiple apposing submucous myomas. *Fertil Steril.* 2008;89(5):1254–9. doi:10.1016/j.fertnstert.2007.05.027
25. Conforti A, Alviggi C, Mollo A, De Placido G, Magos A. The management of Asherman syndrome: A review of literature. *Reprod Biol Endocrinol.* 2013;11:118. doi:10.1186/1477-7827-11-118

27

When to Recommend a Cesarean Section

Matthew S. Smith and Joan M. Mastrobattista

Key Terms

Cesarean delivery: Birth of the fetus through an abdominal incision, excluding abdominal or ectopic pregnancies [1]

VBAC (vaginal birth after cesarean delivery): Vaginal birth after 1 or more previous cesarean births [1]

TOLAC (trial of labor after previous cesarean delivery): Labor after 1 or more previous cesarean births [1]

Uterine dehiscence: Asymptomatic rupture of a uterine scar (scar separation with intact serosa) noted at repeat cesarean or scar separation noted after manual exploration after vaginal delivery [2,3]

Uterine rupture: Symptomatic rupture of uterine scar with through-and-through disruption of uterine layers [2,3]

Noncesarean uterine surgery/surgical scar: Surgery/injury and healing of the myometrium prior to birth other than cesarean birth [1]

The dramatic rise in the cesarean delivery (CD) rate in the United States from 5% in the early 1970s to present-day practice is concerning. This may be explained in part by the introduction of electronic fetal monitoring, decreasing practices of vaginal breech and operative vaginal deliveries, and fewer women and providers opting to pursue a TOLAC. [4] The latest National Vital Statistics report published in 2015 describes a decline in the CD rate to 32.2% of the 3,988,076 registered births in the US [5]—but this represents almost 1 in 3 women.

Descriptions of CD dates back to 1790, when French obstetrician Baudelocque defined the procedure as the "operation by which any way is opened for the child than that destined for by nature" [6]. A primary CD is classified as delivery of one or more fetuses through an abdominal incision in a woman without a prior CD—this definition does not apply to ectopic or abdominal pregnancies. [1] The decision to proceed with a primary CD is an important one as it has repercussions for the initial surgery including hemorrhage, infection, venous thromboembolism, mortality and repeat CDs; future pregnancies may be complicated by placenta previa, scar ectopic and placenta accreta spectrum [7]. In this chapter, suggested maternal and fetal indications for CD will be reviewed with the understanding of individual practice styles and differing availability of resources in labor and delivery units.

Obstetric and Maternal Indications

Overlap exists between obstetric, maternal and fetal indications for CD [8]. Zhang and colleagues, for the Consortium on Safe Labor, collected labor and delivery data on 228,668 electronic medical records from 19 hospitals in the United States between 2002 and 2008 with the goal of describing contemporary CD practice [9]. The increased CD rate today in part reflects a decrease in TOLAC, an increase in cesarean by maternal request, reluctance of lesser-experienced physicians to perform operative vaginal deliveries and external cephalic versions and the current medico-legal climate. The consortium of centers lists a previous uterine scar (45.1%) as the most common indication for CD *before labor*, with the next most common (excluding elective) being fetal malpresentation (17.1%). The most frequently reported *intrapartum indication* was failure to progress/cephalopelvic disproportion (47.1%) followed by non-reassuring fetal testing/fetal distress (27.3%) [9]. The authors concluded that important strategies to decrease the CD rate in the United States include reducing primary CDs, increasing VBACs and avoiding CD for dystocia before active labor (cervix of 6 cm) especially in nulliparous women [9]. The continued increase in the CD rate in the United States (>1/3 of pregnancies) compelled our societies (NICHD, ACOG, SMFM) to address the concept of preventing the first CD in a workshop convened in February 2012 [10]. Specific areas were identified to assist in reduction of the initial CD. Following this publication, an Obstetric Care Consensus Document developed jointly by the ACOG and SMFM in 2014 focused on the key points of the NICHD conference; the document lists suggested approaches for the safe prevention of the primary CD (Table 27.1) [11].

Specific Maternal/Obstetric Indicators for Cesarean Delivery

Obstetric, maternal and fetal indications for CD are listed in Table 27.2. In women with worsening hypertensive disorders including severe preeclampsia or HELLP syndrome remote from delivery or at a gestational age <28 weeks, a CD may be indicated [8]. Labor dystocia is a common indication for CD but is often a subjective diagnosis that may vary between providers [8]. Fetal malpresentation is another indication for primary CD. In

TABLE 27.1

Recommendations for the Safe Prevention of the Primary Cesarean Delivery

Recommendations	Grade of Recommendations
First Stage of Labor	
A prolonged latent phase (e.g., >20 h in nullipara & >14 h in multipara) should not be an indication for CD.	1B Strong recommendation, moderate-quality evidence
Slow but progressive labor in the first stage of labor should not be an indication for CD.	1B Strong recommendation, moderate-quality evidence
Cervical dilation of 6 cm should be considered the threshold for the active phase of most women in labor. Thus, before 6 cm of dilation is achieved, standards of active-phase progress should not be applied.	1B Strong recommendation, moderate-quality evidence
CD for active-phase arrest in the first stage of labor should be reserved for women ≥6 cm of dilation with ruptured membranes who fail to progress despite 4 hours of adequate uterine activity or at least 6 hours of oxytocin administration with inadequate uterine activity and no cervical change.	1B Strong recommendation, moderate-quality evidence
Second Stage of Labor	
A specific absolute maximum length of time spent in the second stage of labor beyond which all women should undergo operative delivery has not been identified.	1C Strong recommendation, low-quality evidence
Before diagnosing arrest of labor in the second stage, if the maternal and fetal conditions permit, allow for the following: • At least 2 h of pushing in multiparous women (1B) • At least 3 h of pushing in nulliparous women (1B) Longer durations may be appropriate on an individualized basis (e.g., with the use of epidural analgesia or with fetal malposition) as long as progress is being documented (1B).	1B Strong recommendation, moderate-quality evidence
Operative vaginal delivery in the second stage of labor by experienced and well-trained physicians should be considered a safe, acceptable alternative to CD. Training in, and ongoing maintenance of, practical skills related to operative vaginal delivery should be encouraged.	1B Strong recommendation, moderate-quality evidence
Manual rotation of the fetal occiput in the setting of fetal malposition in the second stage of labor is a reasonable intervention to consider before moving to operative vaginal delivery or CD. In order to safely prevent CDs in the setting of malposition, it is important to assess the fetal position in the second stage of labor, particularly in the setting of abnormal fetal descent.	1B Strong recommendation, moderate-quality evidence
Fetal Heart Rate Monitoring	
Amnioinfusion for repetitive variable fetal heart rate decelerations may safely reduce the rate of CD.	1A Strong recommendation, high-quality evidence
Scalp stimulation can be used as a means of assessing fetal acid–base status when abnormal or indeterminate (formerly, non-reassuring) fetal heart patterns (e.g., minimal variability) are present and is a safe alternative to CD in this setting.	1C Strong recommendation, low-quality evidence
Induction of Labor	
Before 41 0/7 weeks of gestation, induction of labor generally should be performed based on maternal and fetal medical indications. Inductions at 41 0/7 weeks of gestation and beyond should be performed to reduce the risk of CD and the risk of perinatal morbidity and mortality.	1A Strong recommendation, high-quality evidence
Cervical ripening methods should be used when labor is induced in women with an unfavorable cervix.	1B Strong recommendation, moderate-quality evidence
If the maternal and fetal status allow, CDs for failed induction of labor in the latent phase can be avoided by allowing longer durations of the latent phase (up to 24 hours or longer) and requiring that oxytocin be administered for at least 12–18 hours after membrane rupture before deeming the induction a failure.	1B Strong recommendation, moderate-quality evidence
Fetal Malpresentation	
Fetal presentation should be assessed and documented beginning at 36 0/7 weeks of gestation to allow for external cephalic version to be offered.	1C Strong recommendation, low-quality evidence
Suspected Fetal Macrosomia	
CD to avoid potential birth trauma should be limited to estimated fetal weights of at least 5000 g in women without diabetes and at least 4500 g in women with diabetes. The prevalence of birth weight of 5000 g or more is rare, and patients should be counseled that estimates of fetal weight, particularly late in gestation, are imprecise.	2C Weak recommendation, low-quality evidence
Excessive Maternal Weight Gain	
Women should be counseled about the IOM maternal weight guidelines in an attempt to avoid excessive weight gain.	1B Strong recommendation, moderate-quality evidence

(Continued)

TABLE 27.1 (*Continued*)

Recommendations for the Safe Prevention of the Primary Cesarean Delivery

Recommendations	Grade of Recommendations
Twin Gestations	
Perinatal outcomes for twin gestations in which the first twin is in cephalic presentation are not improved by CD. Thus, women with either cephalic/cephalic-presenting twins or cephalic/noncephalic-presenting twins should be counseled to attempt vaginal delivery.	1B Strong recommendation, moderate-quality evidence
Other	
Individuals, organizations and governing bodies should work to ensure that research is conducted to provide a better knowledge base to guide decisions regarding CD and to encourage policy changes that safely lower the rate of primary CD.	1C Strong recommendation, low-quality evidence

Source: Adapted from Caughey AB et al. ACOG/SMFM. *Am J Obstet Gynecol.* 2014;210:179–93.
Abbreviations: CD, cesarean delivery; IOM, Institute of Medicine.

previous years, more providers offered vaginal breech delivery; however, this is much less frequent today. Multifetal gestations often undergo CD owing to a noncephalic-presenting twin, noncephalic second twin and high-order multiples. Monochorionic twins with twin transfusion or unequal placental sharing, monoamniotic twins and conjoined twins frequently undergo CD [12]. In some cases of fetal macrosomia, a CD may be warranted. For women at high risk for uterine rupture with labor, CD is recommended; these include: previous classical or T-incision, prior uterine rupture or extensive transfundal uterine surgery [4].

Additional obstetric or labor-related indicators for CD include placenta previa, placenta accreta spectrum, vasa previa and umbilical cord prolapse. CD is recommended in cases of suspected placental abruption if evidence of life-threatening hemorrhage or non-reassuring fetal heart rate (Category III) tracing [8]. Certain maternal medical conditions related to pregnancy represent additional indicators for CD. For HIV-positive women with an unknown viral load or with viral loads >1000 copies/mL and women with active genital herpes or a herpes prodrome, CD is recommended [8]. Similarly, CD may be considered in women with repaired obstetric anal sphincter injuries (OASIS) that extend into or through the anal sphincter complex [13]. Women with invasive cervical cancer, large obstructing condyloma with risk of bleeding, large fibroids and displaced pelvic fractures may warrant CD [8]. CD is also considered in women with significant cardiac disease, Marfan syndrome with aortic root dilation, inflammatory bowel disease with risk of fistula formation and those with an unrepaired cerebral aneurysm [3,8].

Uterine Rupture After Myomectomy

The risk for uterine rupture after a previous classical incision ranges from as high as 12% to as low as 1% for women undergoing a trial of labor [15–17]. A national survey in Japan over a 5-year period identified 152 cases of uterine rupture for an overall incidence of 0.015%, with those related a myomectomy occurring

TABLE 27.2

Obstetric, Maternal and Fetal Indications for Cesarean Delivery

Obstetric Indication	Maternal Indication	Fetal Indication
Dystocia (CPD/FTP), macrosomia	Cardiac disease	Open neural tube defect
Malpresentaion	Marfan's disease with aortic root dilation >4 cm	Hydrocephalus or macrocephaly
Multiple gestation: twins or higher-order multiples	Crohn's/inflammatory bowel disease	Sacrococcygeal teratoma
Non-reassuring fetal heart rate tracing	Unrepaired cerebral aneurysm	Anterior neck mass
Umbilical cord prolapse	Active genital HSV	Fetal cardiac dysrhythmias: congenital heart block, SVT
Vasa previa or funic presentation	HIV with VL>1000 copies/mL or unknown VL	
Placenta previa	HPV with obstructing condyloma	
Placenta accreta spectrum	Invasive cervical cancer	
Placental abruption with hemorrhage or non-reassuring FHR tracing	Previous OASIS	
	Previous transmural myomectomy	
	Obstructing fibroids	
	Displaced pelvic fracture	
	Abdominal cerclage	
	CD upon maternal request	

Sources: Adapted from Landon MB and Grobman WA. Cesarean delivery. In: Gabbe SG, Niebyl JR, Simpson JL et al. (eds). *Obstetrics: Normal and Problem Pregnancies*, 7th Ed. Philadelphia, PA: Elsevier, 2017; Tita ATN. *Semin Perinatol.* 2012;36:324–7; Simpson LL. *Semin Perinatol.* 2012;36:328–35; Waldman R. *Obstet Gynecol.* 2019; Anteby EY and Yagel S. *Eur J Obstet Gynecol Reprod Biol.* 2003;106(1):5–9.

Abbreviations: CD, cesarean delivery; CPD, cephalopelvic disproportion; FHR, fetal heart rate; FTP, failure to progress; HIV, human immunodeficiency virus; HPV, human papillomavirus; HSV, herpes simplex virus; OASIS, obstetric anal sphincter injuries; SVT, supraventricular tachycardia; VL, viral load.

at approximately 32 weeks vs 37 weeks for prior cesarean sections [18].

Cases of uterine rupture after a classical cesarean section, unlike low transverse cesareans, tend to rupture prior to labor without any warning signs, which has led to the practice of scheduled repeat cesarean sections at 36-37 weeks, despite a paucity of data [19].

A history of a prior myomectomy is not uncommon and of 24,739 primary cesarean sections performed during a 2-year period in the MFMU Cesarean Registry, 222 (0.9%) had previous myomectomy with a mean gestational age at delivery of 37.1 weeks [19].

The overall uterine rupture rate after an open myomectomy is approximately 1.7% compared with 0.49% for the laparoscopic approach [20]. This is comparable to the reported risk of rupture in women with a prior low transverse cesarean undergoing a trial of labor. In contrast, Kelly and colleagues conducted a retrospective review of the literature and noted that women with a prior abdominal myomectomy, who were allowed to labor and achieved vaginal delivery, had no uterine rupture [21]. Several case series after laparoscopic myomectomy report no uterine rupture before labor; however, a prior review reports on 19 cases with most uterine ruptures occurring prior to labor and 15 prior to 36 weeks [22].

A Canadian study surveyed 49 practicing obstetricians from 2012 to 2013. If an abdominal myomectomy was performed, 27% of obstetricians would allow vaginal delivery versus 76% if a laparoscopic myomectomy was performed. If the uterine cavity was entered, the percent dropped to 14% and 71%, respectively, despite no evidence to suggest that cavity entry is associated with an increased risk for uterine rupture [23]. A recent systematic review of the literature identified 23 studies with at least five cases reporting pregnancy outcomes after a prior myomectomy. The overall incidence of uterine rupture was 0.6% (11/1825). Eleven of the 23 studies reported outcomes on trial of labor, with 0.47% (2/426) women having uterine rupture during labor and 1.52% (5/330) prior to labor. Of these 7 ruptures, 5 of them occurred prior to 36 weeks [24].

A more recent retrospective cohort study evaluated all women who had either a laparoscopic or abdominal myomectomy over a 12-year period in 3 university hospitals in Italy. Overall, 469 women were identified of which 110 pregnancies were achieved that ended in deliveries after 24 weeks gestation. Over 90% of the women, who underwent a trial of labor, successfully delivered vaginally and no uterine ruptures were reported [25].

Almost all studies looking at uterine rupture after myomectomies do not account for number of fibroids, type of fibroids, depth of dissection, entry into cavity, type of dissection (cautery vs no cautery), single-layer vs multi-layer closure, post-op evaluation of healing (hematoma vs no hematoma), and number of prior myomectomies or other uterine surgeries. These factors are all critical in designing studies that can adequately address the question of when and if a cesarean section should be done after a myomectomy. Until then, here are our recommendations:

1. Every surgeon who performs a myomectomy should document, based on the amount of myometrial dissection, whether a cesarean section is indicated, to help guide their obstetrical colleagues.
2. Entry into the uterine cavity is not a validated indication for cesarean section, but rather it seems reasonable that the amount of myometrial dissection is a more important consideration.
3. Abdominal myomectomies are often performed, versus laparoscopic myomectomies, for more extensive fibroid burden, and thus it seems reasonable that these cases are higher risk for subsequent cesarean section.
4. The risk for uterine rupture after hysteroscopic myomectomy is unknown, but usually involves less myometrial dissection.
5. The risk for uterine rupture after myomectomy, regardless of the approach, is quite low and on par with what is seen with prior cesarean sections. Thus, some patients can be considered for trial of labor after extensive counseling.
6. Many uterine ruptures appear to occur prior to 36 weeks, thus requiring careful observation and diligence when managing these pregnant patients, even when a cesarean section is planned after 36 weeks gestation.

KEY POINTS

- Provider goals should include incorporation of the safe prevention of the primary CD recommendations into clinical practice [11].
- A cesarean performed without an accepted indication is labeled a "non-indicated" cesarean [10].
- Labor inductions should be performed only for medical indications; if nonmedical indication, gestational age should be 39 weeks or more [10].
- Discussion of patient and provider expectations and conduct of labor and delivery should be discussed in the office prior to hospital admission.
- External cephalic version and operative vaginal delivery are alternatives to primary CD, which should be considered, provided an experienced operator is available.
- Certain maternal infections and fetal anomalies are not amenable to vaginal delivery.

REFERENCES

1. American College of Obstetricians and Gynecologists (ACOG):reVITALize Obstetric Data Definitions. Available at https://www.acog.org/practice-management/health-it-and-clinical-informatics/revitalize-obstetrics-data-definitions (accessed August 13, 2016).
2. *Vaginal Birth after Cesarean (VBAC)*. Rockville, MD: Agency for Health Care Research and Quality;2003 (AHRQ publication no. 03-E018).
3. Landon MB and Grobman WA. Vaginal birth after cesarean delivery. In: Gabbe SG, Niebyl JR, Simpson JL et al. (eds). *Obstetrics: Normal and Problem Pregnancies*, 7th Ed. Philadelphia, PA: Elsevier, 2017.

4. ACOG Practice Bulletin No. 205: Vaginal Birth After Cesarean Delivery. *Obstet Gynecol.* 2019 Feb; 133(2):e110-e127. PMID: 30681543.
5. Hamilton BE, Martin JA, Osterman MJK et al. *Births: Final data for 2014. National Vital Statistics Reports.* December 23, 2015 (accessed July 24, 2016).
6. Mastrobattista JM. Vaginal birth after cesarean delivery. *Obstet Gynecol Clin North Am.* June 1999;26(2): 295–304.
7. Caughey AB. Safe prevention of primary cesarean delivery in the United States: Why and how? *Clin Obstet Gynecol.* 2015;58(2):207–10.
8. Tita ATN. When is primary cesarean appropriate: Maternal and obstetrical indications. *Semin Perinatol.* 2012;36:324–7.
9. Zhang J, Troendle J, Reddy UM et al. Consortium on safe labor: Contemporary cesarean delivery practice in the United States. *Am J Obstet Gynecol.* 2010;203:326.e1–e10.
10. Spong CY, Berghella V, Wenstrom KD et al. Preventing the first cesarean delivery: Summary of a joint Eunice Kennedy Shriver National Institute of Child Health and Human Development, Society for Maternal-Fetal Medicine, and American College of Obstetricians and Gynecologists Workshop. *Obstet Gynecol.* 2012;120:1181–93.
11. Caughey AB, Cahill AG, Guise JM et al. American College of Obstetricians and Gynecologists; Society for Maternal-Fetal Medicine. Safe prevention of the primary cesarean delivery. *Am J Obstet Gynecol.* 2014 Mar;210:179–93.
12. Simpson LL. When is primary cesarean appropriate: Fetal indications. *Semin Perinatol.* 2012;36:328–35.
13. Waldman R. ACOG Practice Bulletin No. 198: Prevention and Management of Obstetric Lacerations at Vaginal Delivery. *Obstet Gynecol.* 2019. PMID: 30575652
14. Anteby EY and Yagel S Route of delivery of fetuses with structural anomalies. *Eur J Obstet Gynecol Reprod Biol.* 2003;106(1):5–9.
15. Rosen MG, Dickinson JC, Westhoff CL. Vaginal birth after cesarean: A meta-analysis of morbidity and mortality. *Obstet Gynecol.* 1991;77:465–470.
16. Halperin ME, Moore DC, Hannah WJ. Classical versus low-segment transverse incision for preterm caesarean section: Maternal complications and outcome of subsequent pregnancies. *Br J Obstet Gynaecol.* 1988;95:990.
17. Douglas RG. Pregnancy and labor following cesarean section. In: Reid DE, and Barton TC (eds). *Controversy in Obstetrics and Gynecology.* Philadelphia: W. B. Saunders, 1969, pp. 308–309.
18. Makino S, Takeda S, Kondoh E, Kawai K, Takeda J, Matsubara S, Itakura A, Sago H, Tanigaki S, Tanaka M, Ikeda T, Kanayama N et al. National survey of uterine rupture in Japan: Annual report of Perinatology Committee, Japan Society of Obstetrics and Gynecology, 2018. *J Obstet Gynaecol Res.* 2019 Apr;45(4):763–765.
19. Landon MB, Lynch CD. Optimal timing and mode of delivery after cesarean with previous classical incision or myomectomy: A review of the data. *Semin Perinatol.* 2011;35(5):257–261.
20. Nahum GG and Pham KQ. Uterine rupture in pregnancy. http://emedicine.medscape.com/refarticle-srch/275854-overview. Accessed May 12, 2020.
21. Kelly BA, Bright P, MacKenzie IZ. Does the surgical approach used for myomectomy influence the morbidity in subsequent pregnancy? *J Obstet Gynaecol.* 2008;28:77.
22. Parker WH, Einarsson J, Istre O et al. Risk factors for uterine rupture after laparoscopic myomectomy. *J Minim Invasive Gynecol.* 2010;17:551.
23. Weibel HS, Jarcevic R, Gagnon R, Tulandi T. Perspectives of obstetricians on labour and delivery after abdominal or laparoscopic myomectomy. *J Obstet Gynaecol Can.* 2014;36(2):128–32.
24. Gambacorti-Passerini Z, Gimovsky AC, Locatelli A, Berghella V. Trial of labor after myomectomy and uterine rupture: A systematic review. *Acta Obstet Gynecol Scand.* 2016;95(7):724–34.
25. Gambacorti-Passerini ZM, Penati C, Carli A, Accordino F, Ferrari L, Berghella V, Locatelli A. Vaginal birth after prior myomectomy. *Eur J Obstet Gynecol Reprod Biol.* 2018;231:198–203.

28

Uterine Artery Embolization

Gloria M. Salazar and Eric Paul Wehrenberg-Klee

What is Uterine Artery Embolization?

Uterine artery embolization (UAE) is a transcatheter technique for management of uterine fibroids that represents an alternative to myomectomy or hysterectomy for select patients. Broadly, using fluoroscopy, the interventional radiologist selects the patient's bilateral uterine arteries with a catheter and injects embolic beads into the distal uterine arteries, causing the fibroid to become ischemic, leading to a gradual reduction in size and symptomatology. Patients typically have to be managed for pain control. UAE results in similar improvement in quality of life and is associated with significantly reduced recovery time and fewer complications in comparison with surgical interventions, although with a higher need for reintervention to achieve symptom resolution. For patients that desire to maintain fertility, UAE is not well studied and thus not the preferred therapy.

Which Patients Should Receive Uterine Artery Embolization?

UAE is a good alternative to surgery for patients not desiring fertility and with a wide-range of fibroid-induced symptomatology. UAE is best studied in the context of dysmenorrhea secondary to fibroids, where it is has been demonstrated in a randomized controlled trial to show similar improvement in quality of life outcomes to hysterectomy on 2-year follow-up [1]. Ten-year follow-up of this study population showed two-thirds of UAE-treated patients had avoided hysterectomy and equivalent quality-of-life scores in both UAE and hysterectomy patients [2]. An additional randomized controlled trial comparing UAE to surgery (both hysterectomy and myomectomy) with a patient population mostly comprised of people whose primary complaint was dysmenorrhea showed no difference in symptom scores between groups at 1 year. UAE was associated with a shorter hospitalization (median 1 day versus 5 days), quicker recovery and fewer complications, but a higher rate of reintervention (20%) necessary for symptom control [3]. In single-arm, nonrandomized studies and registries, the results for UAE are far better, with a secondary hysterectomy rate of less than 10% [4].

The benefit of UAE for control of bulk symptoms and pain is less well-studied. Randomized controlled trials were not powered to adequately compare UAE with surgery for their ability to improve these symptoms. However, a retrospective study including large numbers of women with bulk symptoms shows significant improvement in quality of life [5].

Traditionally, use of UAE has been limited to fibroids with relatively small diameters, owing to reports of limited results and increased complications in larger (>8 cm) fibroids. However, two recent studies showed no different clinical results or complication rates after UAE of large (>10 cm) fibroids in a total of 100 patients [6,7].

UAE also is an alternative to hysterectomy for the management of adenomyosis. Necrosis is achieved in 40%–82.5% of patients depending on the trial [8–10]. A retrospective analysis showed that 24% of patients with adenomyosis treated with UAE had recurrence of symptoms within 4 years, and that necrosis <34% on follow-up imaging was predictive of recurrence [11].

Which Patients Should Not Receive Uterine Artery Embolization?

Generally, UAE is not recommended for patients desiring fertility, and the overall fertility rate may be decreased relative to myomectomy [12], although uncomplicated pregnancies and normal deliveries have been reported after UAE [13]. Thus, if a patient desiring fertility is not a candidate for myomectomy, UAE may represent a reasonable treatment option; however, the possible impact on fertility must be discussed with the patient.

UAE is contraindicated in patients with a viable pregnancy or active infection of the uterus. UAE also is relatively contraindicated for patients with pedunculated subserosal fibroids (fibroid tumor with a stalk diameter at least 50% narrower than the diameter of the tumor) due to risk of fibroid separation from the uterus [14]. For similar reasons, submucosal fibroids with an intracavitary component with high endometrial interface to tumor diameter ratio are at increased risk of complications, including fibroid exclusion, and this risk should be discussed with the patient [15].

UAE should not be performed for primary treatment of malignancy of the uterus or ovaries, but can be an adjunct procedure to reduce operative bleeding risk or as a palliative procedure.

Patient Work-up Prior to Uterine Artery Embolization

In a patient being considered for UAE, it is critical to confirm the diagnosis of uterine leiomyomata. This is best achieved with

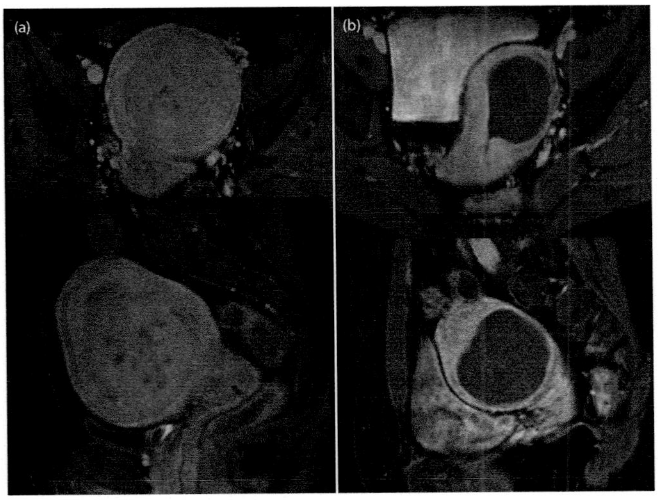

FIGURE 28.1 Evaluation of viable fibroids with MRI. (a) Preprocedure sagittal images demonstrate intramural large fibroid with avid enhancement with gadolinium. (b) Post-UAE follow-up MRI sagittal images demonstrate tissue necrosis with no residual enhancement of the fibroids consistent with good technical success.

a contrast-enhanced pelvic MRI [16], which is superior to ultrasound in the evaluation of fibroid location and characteristics, uterine blood supply, presence or absence of adenomyosis, and any incidental pathology. Administration of gadolinium contrast allows for assessment of fibroid viability, which is critical in planning treatment, as a nonviable fibroid is unlikely to respond to UAE (Figure 28.1). The inclusion of a 3D-MRA (MR angiogram) sequence in a contrast-enhanced MRI also allows for assessment of vascular supply to the uterus and ovaries, which can help with procedural planning.

A contrast-enhanced MRI is also valuable for identification and differentiation of uterine leiomyosarcoma from degenerating benign leiomyomata. Recent retrospective studies cite accuracy up to 88% in differentiating the two entities when a combination of contrast-enhanced sequences and diffusion-weighted imaging (DWI) is used [17]; however, this degree of accuracy is unlikely to be achieved in the community, as until recently authors have suggested that differentiating between the two entities can be quite challenging [18]. In a patient in whom the possibility of a uterine leiomyosarcoma is raised on imaging, we could recommend biopsy as a first diagnostic step. There is no evidence that UAE spreads uterine leiomyosarcoma, but pursuing UAE rather than surgical options in this scenario would delay the diagnosis.

Other aspects of the patient work-up prior to UAE include routine laboratory assessment, with assessment of renal function, as well as a recent complete blood count. In patients with dysmenorrhea, also consider evaluation of an underlying bleeding disorder with activated PTT, PT and INR. Patients with an IUD ideally should have it removed prior to the procedure to avoid infection [19], but in a small study, there was no significant risk of infection in patients with IUD undergoing UAE [20].

Prepping for the Procedure

Some institutions initiate patients on calcium channel blockers such as nifedipine to reduce the risk of uterine artery vasospasm secondary to catheter manipulation during the procedure. On the day of the procedure, after routine periprocedural evaluation, the patient may receive a diclofenac suppository to assist with pain control, with use varying across institutions. Antibiotic prophylaxis use across institutions also varies. Placement of a Foley catheter is standard, as the patient may have to lie flat for several hours after the procedure, depending on the arteriotomy site and whether or not a closure device is used.

Procedure in Brief

The patient is brought to the fluoroscopy suite, and the procedure performed under moderate sedation. Arterial access is usually obtained through the common femoral artery, although recent studies have shown the feasibility of using a left radial artery approach [21], which holds potential for an improved patient experience without the necessity to lie flat after the procedure. Access may be obtained bilaterally, or unilaterally, depending on operator preference and fibroid volume (Figure 28.2). The uterine artery is selected typically as the second branch of the anterior division of the internal iliac artery and catheterized with a 4 Fr or 5 Fr catheter. Once the uterine artery is selected, a microcatheter is advanced past the cervical branches to avoid vaginal necrosis, typically recognized as the horizontal portion of the uterine artery (Figure 28.3). Once appropriate catheter position has been achieved, embolic beads mixed with iodinated contrast are injected. Injection proceeds under continuous fluoroscopic guidance to ensure that embolic material does not reflux into cervical branches. The bilateral uterine arteries are embolized to stasis, with exact visual marker of adequate fibroid embolization depending on the embolic material chosen (Figure 28.4).

In 5%–10% of patients, there is collateral flow from the ovarian arteries to the fibroid. Preprocedural MRI can be helpful in identifying this supply prior to arteriography. After embolization of the bilateral uterine arteries, a contrast aortogram can be

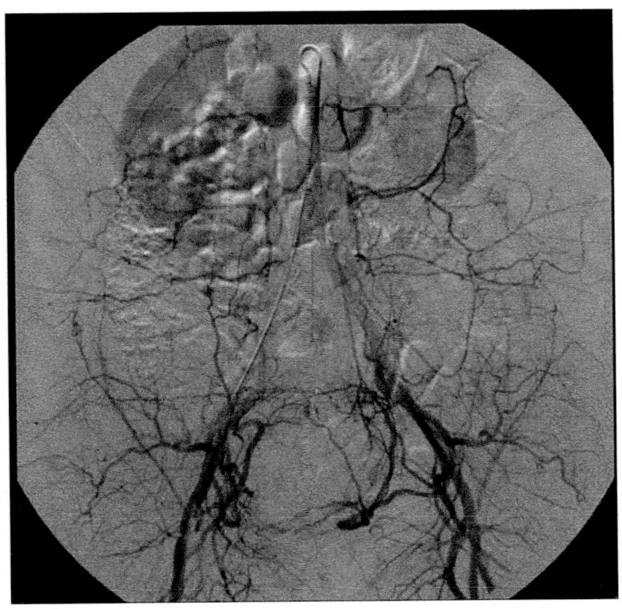

FIGURE 28.2 Aortogram demonstrating bilateral uterine artery supply of the fibroids.

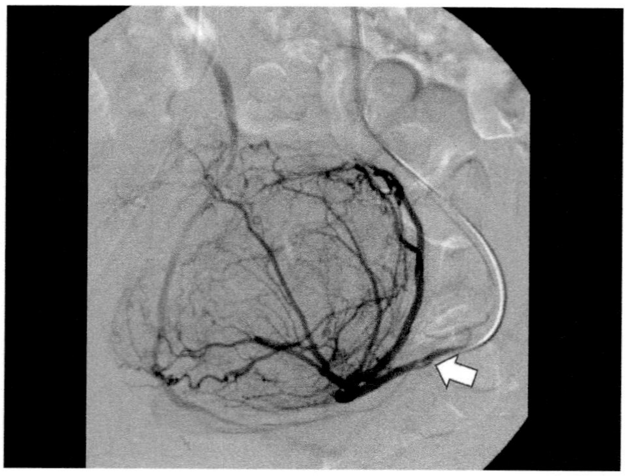

FIGURE 28.3 Transcatheter angiography demonstrating a 3 Fr microcatheter positioned at the horizontal portion of the UA (arrow) and perifibroid arterial plexus prior to embolization.

performed to identify ovarian collaterals, which tend to increase in size once fibroid ischemia is induced. Depending on the exact anatomy of the ovarian artery and ovarian-fibroid collateral supply, embolization can be considered; however, the patient needs to be informed prior to the procedure of the risk of embolization-induced menopause. A review of the FIBROID registry found that the overall risk of amenorrhea after UAE was 7%, with almost all affected patients >45 years of age [22,23] (Figure 28.5).

After embolization, catheters are removed and hemostasis of the arteriotomy site achieved with either manual compression or a closure device.

Postprocedure

Patients do not experience significant discomfort during the procedure itself, but cramping starts shortly after bilateral embolization of uterine arteries is completed and will be at its most intense for approximately 24 hours. Postprocedural pain is characterized by cramping, which is usually relieved with NSAIDs and narcotics. Our pain management protocol is a combination of intravenous ketorolac and patient-controlled analgesia pump with hydromorphone for the first 12 hours after UAE.

Tissue necrosis after embolization of the perifibroid vascular plexus leads to postembolization syndrome (PES) that affects up to 90% of patients in the first 48–72 hours [24]. Patients may experience PES for approximately a week after the procedure. These symptoms include low-grade fever, fatigue, nausea, vomiting and pain commonly described as analogous to the flu. We suggest management with oral NSAIDs such as ibuprofen for the week following the procedure.

Technical Failure

Technical failure is defined as the inability to embolize both uterine arteries to stasis. The most common cause of this is uterine artery vasospasm caused by catheter manipulation. Other causes of technical failure include atypical vascular anatomy preventing adequate embolization or ovarian artery anastomoses. The rate of technical failure is described as high as 25% in randomized studies and 10% in noncontrolled studies [25].

Complications

The overall complication rate following UAE in the REST trial was 36% [3]. By far the most common complaint was PES, which, as described earlier, includes pelvic pain, low-grade fever, nausea, vomiting, loss of appetite and fatigue in the first few days after UAE. Treatment with oral NSAIDs can be helpful for amelioration of many of these symptoms.

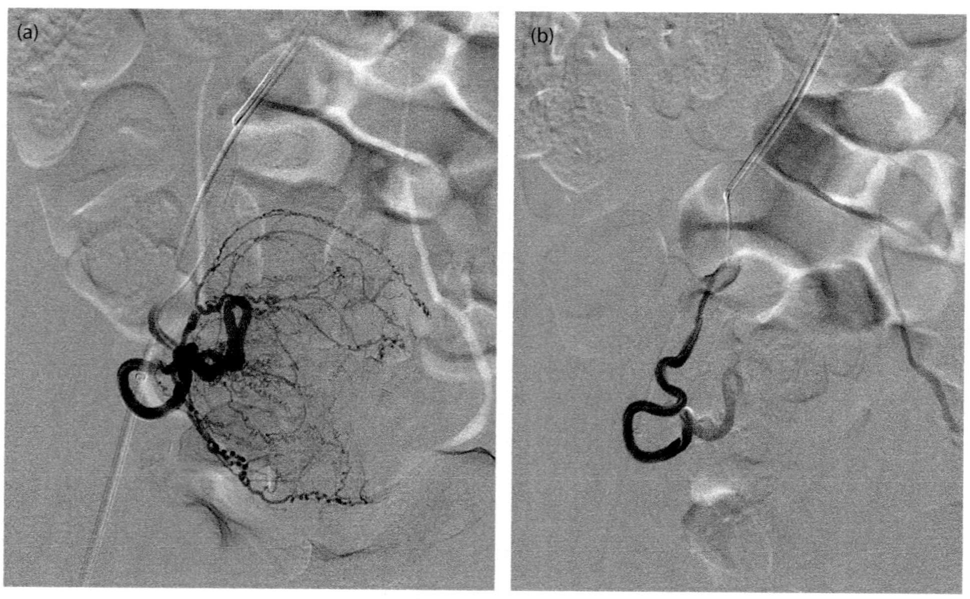

FIGURE 28.4 UAE procedure and endpoint. (a) Perifibroid vascularity pre-embolization. (b) Postembolization angiographic images demonstrating technically successful procedure and devascularized fibroid.

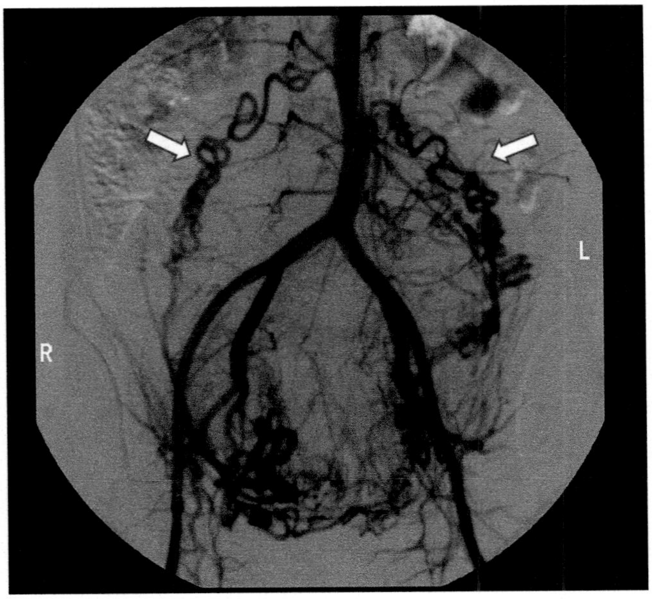

FIGURE 28.5 Bilateral ovarian artery supply to the fibroids (arrows).

The other most common adverse events include:

- Endometritis, presenting as pelvic pain with watery vaginal discharge, fever and/or leukocytosis that occur from days to weeks after the procedure and may be due to infectious or noninfectious causes.
- Fibroid infection from bacterial colonization of embolized fibroid tissue either through blood or vaginal ascent of pathogens. Symptoms and signs include abdominal or pelvic pain, fever and/or leukocytosis.
- Uterine infection, possibly as a result of necrosis of all or part of the uterus, again manifest with abdominal or pelvic pain, vaginal discharge, fever and/or leukocytosis.
- Fibroid expulsion, with detachment of a devascularized fibroid from the uterine wall and subsequent transvaginal passage. This is most common among submucosal fibroids with a narrow attachment. Fibroid expulsion is associated with uterine contractions, abdominal pain, fever, nausea, vomiting and vaginal bleeding or discharge.

These adverse events are most likely to occur within the first month following embolization.

Follow-up

As UAE does not remove but rather devascularizes the fibroid, shrinkage in size and reduction in symptoms is a gradual process. Patients may not notice any change in symptoms in the month or so after the procedure and should anticipate maximum reduction in fibroid volume and symptom resolution at approximately 6 months [1]. Routine practice is to obtain a repeat MRI at 1 month, along with a follow-up clinic visit. At this visit, overall symptomatology may not have significantly changed; however, the visit is valuable to assess for possible complications. The 1-month MRI assesses residual fibroid enhancement, as percentage devascularization is predictive of treatment success [26]. Furthermore, the 1-month MRI assesses for the rare case of a missed diagnosis of uterine sarcoma.

We schedule an additional visit and MRI at 6 months post-UAE. At this point, maximal symptomatic benefit from the embolization should have been achieved. In a successful embolization, MRI will demonstrate maximal anticipated decrease in fibroid volume at this time. Additionally, this MRI may demonstrate areas of enhancement that were not demonstrated on the 1-month MRI owing to collateral vessel recruitment and/or hypertrophy [27]. In this event, repeat embolization to remove the collateral vessels can be pursued.

REFERENCES

1. Hehenkamp WJ, Volkers NA, Birnie E, Reekers JA, and Ankum WM. Symptomatic uterine fibroids: Treatment with uterine artery embolization or hysterectomy—results from the randomized clinical Embolisation versus Hysterectomy (EMMY) Trial. *Radiology*. 2008;246:823–32.
2. de Bruijn AM, Ankum WM, Reekers JA et al. Uterine artery embolization vs hysterectomy in the treatment of symptomatic uterine fibroids: 10-year outcomes from the randomized EMMY trial. *Am J Obstet Gynecol*. 2016;215(6):745.e1–e12.
3. Edwards RD, Moss JG, Lumsden MA et al. Uterine-artery embolization versus surgery for symptomatic uterine fibroids. *N Engl J Med*. 2007;356:360–70.
4. van der Kooij SM, Bipat S, Hehenkamp WJ, Ankum WM, and Reekers JA. Uterine artery embolization versus surgery in the treatment of symptomatic fibroids: A systematic review and metaanalysis. *Am J Obstet Gynecol*. 2011;205:317 e311–8.
5. Scheurig-Muenkler C, Koesters C, Powerski MJ, Grieser C, Froeling V, and Kroencke TJ. Clinical long-term outcome after uterine artery embolization: Sustained symptom control and improvement of quality of life. *J Vasc Interv Radiol*. 2013;24:765–71.
6. Berczi V, Valcseva E, Kozics D et al. Safety and effectiveness of UFE in fibroids larger than 10 cm. *Cardiovasc Intervent Radiol*. 2015;38:1152–6.
7. Choi HJ, Jeon GS, Kim MD, Lee JT, and Yoon JH. Is uterine artery embolization for patients with large myomas safe and effective? A retrospective comparative study in 323 patients. *J Vasc Interv Radiol*. 2013;24:772–8.
8. McLucas B and Perrella R. Adenomyosis: MRI of the uterus treated with uterine artery embolization. *AJR Am J Roentgenol*. 2004;182:1084–5; author reply 1085.
9. Bratby MJ and Walker WJ. Uterine artery embolisation for symptomatic adenomyosis--mid-term results. *Eur J Radiol*. 2009;70:128–32.
10. Kim MD, Kim YM, Kim HC et al. Uterine artery embolization for symptomatic adenomyosis: A new technical development of the 1-2-3 protocol and predictive factors of MR imaging affecting outcomes. *J Vasc Interv Radiol*. 2011;22:497–502.
11. Bae SH, Kim MD, Kim GM et al. Uterine artery embolization for adenomyosis: Percentage of necrosis predicts midterm clinical recurrence. *J Vasc Interv Radiol*. 2015;26:1290–6 e1292.

12. Mara M, Maskova J, Fucikova Z, Kuzel D, Belsan T, and Sosna O. Midterm clinical and first reproductive results of a randomized controlled trial comparing uterine fibroid embolization and myomectomy. *Cardiovasc Intervent Radiol.* 2008;31:73–85.
13. Holub Z, Mara M, Kuzel D, Jabor A, Maskova J, and Eim J. Pregnancy outcomes after uterine artery occlusion: Prospective multicentric study. *Fertil Steril.* 2008; 90:1886–91.
14. Goodwin SC, Bonilla SC, Sacks D et al. Reporting standards for uterine artery embolization for the treatment of uterine leiomyomata. *J Vasc Interv Radiol.* 2003;14:S467–76.
15. Verma SK, Bergin D, Gonsalves CF, Mitchell DG, Lev-Toaff AS, and Parker L. Submucosal fibroids becoming endocavitary following uterine artery embolization: Risk assessment by MRI. *AJR Am J Roentgenol.* 2008;190:1220–6.
16. Spielmann AL, Keogh C, Forster BB, Martin ML, and Machan LS. Comparison of MRI and sonography in the preliminary evaluation for fibroid embolization. *AJR Am J Roentgenol.* 2006;187:1499–504.
17. Lin G, Yang LY, Huang YT et al. Comparison of the diagnostic accuracy of contrast-enhanced MRI and diffusion-weighted MRI in the differentiation between uterine leiomyosarcoma/smooth muscle tumor with uncertain malignant potential and benign leiomyoma. *J Magn Reson Imaging.* 2016;43:333–42.
18. Kirby JM, Burrows D, Haider E, Maizlin Z, and Midia M. Utility of MRI before and after uterine fibroid embolization: Why to do it and what to look for. *Cardiovasc Intervent Radiol.* 2011;34:705–16.
19. Andrews RT, Spies JB, Sacks D et al. Patient care and uterine artery embolization for leiomyomata. *J Vasc Interv Radiol.* 2009;20:S307–311.
20. Smeets AJ, Nijenhuis RJ, Boekkooi PF, Vervest HA, van Rooij WJ, and Lohle PN. Is an intrauterine device a contraindication for uterine artery embolization? A study of 20 patients. *J Vasc Interv Radiol.* 2010;21:272–4.
21. Resnick NJ, Kim E, Patel RS, Lookstein RA, Nowakowski FS, and Fischman AM. Uterine artery embolization using a transradial approach: Initial experience and technique. *J Vasc Interv Radiol.* 2014;25:443–7.
22. Spies JB, Myers ER, Worthington-Kirsch R et al. The FIBROID Registry: Symptom and quality-of-life status 1 year after therapy. *Obstet Gynecol.* 2005;106:1309–18.
23. Salazar GM, Gregory Walker T, Conway RF et al. Embolization of angiographically visible type I and II utero-ovarian anastomoses during uterine artery embolization for fibroid tumors: Impact on symptom recurrence and permanent amenorrhea. *J Vasc Interv Radiol.* 2013;24:1347–52.
24. Ganguli S, Faintuch S, Salazar GM, and Rabkin DJ. Postembolization syndrome: Changes in white blood cell counts immediately after uterine artery embolization. *J Vasc Interv Radiol.* 2008;19:443–5.
25. Pron G, Bennett J, Common A et al. Technical results and effects of operator experience on uterine artery embolization for fibroids: The Ontario Uterine Fibroid Embolization Trial. *J Vasc Interv Radiol.* 2003;14:545–54.
26. Kroencke TJ, Scheurig C, Poellinger A, Gronewold M, and Hamm B. Uterine artery embolization for leiomyomas: Percentage of infarction predicts clinical outcome. *Radiology.* 2010;255:834–41.
27. Schwartz LB, Panageas E, Lange R, Rizzo J, Comite F, and McCarthy S. Female pelvis: Impact of MR imaging on treatment decisions and net cost analysis. *Radiology.* 1994;192:55–60.

29

Magnetic Resonance-Guided Focused Ultrasound (MRgFUS)

Zubin Irani

What is MRgFUS?

MRgFUS is a technique of thermal ablation that uses intra-procedurally acquired MR imaging to guide ablation of a fibroid(s) using focused energy from an array of ultrasound probes and was approved in 2004. In the procedure, preliminary imaging defines the fibroid(s) to be ablated. After a procedure planning period, the fibroid is systemically ablated using an array of ultrasound probes overlying the patient's abdomen. Repeat sonications bring the treatment zone to 65°C–85°C, inducing coagulative necrosis within the treated volume. During the procedure, there is periodic assessment of the adequacy of ablation using a technique called magnetic resonance thermometry, whereby the fibroid tissue temperature is assessed noninvasively. This technique has also been approved for ablation of bone metastases, along with ablation of benign essential tremor. Other applications remain under investigation.

How is the Procedure Performed?

There is one FDA-approved MRgFUS company, INSIGHTEC (Haifa, Israel), with two MRgFUS systems on the market (Exablate 2000, Exablate 2100). These systems work in conjunction with both 1.5-tesla and 3-tesla MR systems, but are currently only compatible with General Electric MRIs (General Electric HealthCare, Milwaukee, WI). The procedure is performed as an outpatient procedure without the need for a postprocedure hospital stay. Antibiotics are not routinely administered pre-procedure. For treatment, the patient will lie on the MRI gantry as they would during a diagnostic MRI. A multiple phased-array transducer interfaces with the MRI and overlies the patient's abdomen. This transducer delivers ultrasound energy in a focal zone of targeted tissue described as the size of a jelly bean. The goal temperature in the targeted area is 65°C–85°C. It takes approximately 20 seconds to ablate a focal zone. After ablating a given focal zone, the array is refocused on an adjacent area until the entire fibroid is treated. The total procedure time varies significantly based on the volume of fibroid(s) to be treated. In one study, mean procedure duration was 03:59 hours, with procedure times varying between 01:39 and 06:36 hours [1]. Procedure times have been shown to decrease significantly with increased procedural experience. If bowel loops are in the path of the ultrasound beams, mitigation strategies such as bladder filling can be employed to generate a suitable window for sonication. Many operators will divide treatment of fibroids into two sessions and/or repeat treatment of fibroids.

Which Fibroids are Suitable for MRgFUS Treatment?

Prior to consideration of MRgFUS, a contrast-enhanced MRI should be obtained to document size and location of fibroids. There are several unique anatomic considerations that must be considered prior to proceeding with MRgFUS, owing to the use of ultrasound energy during ablation; appropriate patient selection is an important factor affecting procedure outcomes [2,3]. Due to the rapid decrease in ultrasound energy as it passes through tissue, fibroid depth from the skin surface is an important consideration impacting ablation outcome. This cannot be greater than 12 cm [1,4]. Mindjuk et al. evaluated factors associated with clinical success in a single-center experience with 252 women [1], finding that a more complete ablation could be achieved in fibroids with low-enhancement pre-procedure, as well as fibroids distant from the spine (>3 cm). Less complete ablation was seen in fibroids with a subserosal component and those further away from the skin (skin-distant fibroids) ($p < 0.001$), with the postprocedure nonperfused fraction of the fibroid decreasing by 1.5% per centimeter of distance. A single-center evaluation of the anatomic appropriateness of MRgFUS for all fibroid patients presenting for care found that only 80 of 169 (47%) patients were eligible for treatment with this technique [5], with the main reasons being obesity and inaccessibility of fibroids. Other considerations include overlying bowel loops, as ultrasound energy cannot travel through air, as well as location of fibroids close to the spine, which limit the ability to sonicate owing to risk of injury to the sacral nerve [1].

Assessing Response

The technical success of MRgFUS ablation is assessed at the end of the procedure by performing a T1-weighted gadolinium-enhanced imaging sequence. This imaging sequence is used to assess the ratio of non-enhancing myomata volume to total myomata volume, called the nonperfused volume (NPV). A higher NPV ratio corresponds with a lower need for retreatment and improved quality of life post-treatment [6]. LeBlang et al. found a mean NPV ratio of 55% immediately after treatment, which corresponded to an average volume reduction of 31%; this was associated with a wide range of outcomes [7]. At 24 months of follow-up of all patients enrolled in registration trials, Stewart et al. showed that achieving an NPV of >20% resulted in a significantly greater reduction in the symptom severity score (SSS) in comparison with fibroids in which an NPV <20% was achieved [8]. NPVs can be influenced by the technique used; a wide range have been reported, with higher NPV ratios achieved with the less restrictive protocol now approved by the FDA [6,7,9,10].

How Effective is MRgFUS?

No randomized clinical trial has compared MRgFUS for uterine fibroids to alternative treatment options; however, single-arm prospective and retrospective studies have been conducted. Of note, the early studies were conducted under an FDA protocol requiring a 1.5-cm margin from the treatment zone to the serosal and mucosal uterine borders, as well as limiting treatment volume of any single fibroid to 100 cm^3 and total volume of 150 cm^3 [11]. These restrictions resulted in, on average, only 10% of myoma volume being ablated in the approval study, which correlated with an SSS reduction of at least 10 points in 71% and 51% of women at 6 and 12 months, respectively. There was mean reduction in SSS of 39% and 36% at 6 and 12 months, respectively [11]. With relaxation of ablation criteria by the FDA, reduction in SSS has improved in more recent studies. For example, in a retrospective review of 60 patients, MRgFUS demonstrated an improvement in SSS from 50 +/− 22 to 19 +/− 12 ($P < 0.001$) at 12 months post-treatment [12]. With further refinements in the technology used for MRgFUS, much higher ablation volumes have been reported. A retrospective study using the newer version of the MRgFUS device in which 72 patients voluntarily returned SSS questionnaires showed a reduction in the mean SSS from 62.5 to 37.5 ($P < 0.001$) at an average of 6.5 months [13]. Another recent retrospective study in 40 patients demonstrated a reduction in the mean SSS from 62.2 (±16.4) to 35.0 (±9.5) at 6 months [14].

Adverse Events

All studies have reported a low rate of adverse events. In the registration trial, skin burns were seen in 5% of the women, there was a single overnight admission for nausea and there was a single event of a sciatic nerve palsy secondary to sonication of posterior fibroids [11]. In a cohort study of 280 patients, the rate of minor complications was 3.9%, with 1.1% rate of major complication, which included one skin burn, a fibroid expulsion and one case of persistent neuropathy [15].

Reintervention Rate

A retrospective study found that in a group of 138 women who had undergone MRgFUS, the reintervention rate was 19% at 36 months and 23% at 48 months [16]. This study stands in contrast to a previous retrospective study from the same institution with a smaller sample size and shorter length of follow-up, which found a reintervention rate of 44.7% [17]. In a separate retrospective study examining 5-year outcomes of 162 women, an overall reintervention rate of 58.6% was seen, decreasing to 50% in patients in whom an NPV of >50% was achieved [15].

Impact on Fertility

MRgFUS does not have an indication for treatment of fibroids in women desiring fertility, and its impact on post-treatment fertility has not been compared with alternative treatment options. However, in a study of all patients enrolled in clinical trials of MRgFUS, Rabinovici et al. reported 54 pregnancies in 51 women following MRgFUS treatment [18]. Live births occurred in 41% of these pregnancies. Spontaneous abortion was seen in 28% and elective pregnancy termination in 11%. Eleven (20%) patients had ongoing pregnancies beyond 20 gestational weeks.

MRgFUS in Clinical Practice

MRgFUS has several appealing aspects, including an entirely noninvasive approach, an outpatient procedure and minimal adverse events reported in the literature. However, the technique has not been compared with other treatment options for fibroids, is associated with a high reintervention rate in most studies and remains available at only a few centers in the United States. Adoption of the technique has likely been significantly limited by the lack of insurance coverage as the procedure has not received favorable reimbursement decisions by the large majority of payors, and thus, patients must largely pay out of pocket. Diminished prospects for reimbursement have in turn limited adoption by radiologists, whose departments must first acquire the device, which, at time of writing, costs in the range of a new diagnostic MRI scanner. Significant changes in the reimbursement environment, possibly spurred by new compelling clinical data comparing MRgFUS in a randomized clinical trial with alternative treatments options, are required to drive further implementation of the procedure.

REFERENCES

1. Mindjuk I, Trumm CG, Herzog P, Stahl R, and Matzko M. MRI predictors of clinical success in MR-guided focused ultrasound (MRgFUS) treatments of uterine fibroids: Results from a single centre. *Eur Radiol.* 2015;25:1317–28.
2. Machtinger R, Inbar Y, Cohen-Eylon S, Admon D, Alagem-Mizrachi A, and Rabinovici J. MR-guided focus ultrasound (MRgFUS) for symptomatic uterine fibroids: Predictors of treatment success. *Hum Reprod.* 2012;27:3425–31.
3. Lenard ZM, McDannold NJ, Fennessy FM et al. Uterine leiomyomas: MR imaging-guided focused ultrasound surgery—imaging predictors of success. *Radiology.* 2008;249:187–94.
4. Stewart EA, Gedroyc WM, Tempany CM et al. Focused ultrasound treatment of uterine fibroid tumors: Safety and feasibility of a noninvasive thermoablative technique. *Am J Obstet Gynecol.* 2003;189:48–54.
5. Behera MA, Leong M, Johnson L, and Brown H. Eligibility and accessibility of magnetic resonance-guided focused ultrasound (MRgFUS) for the treatment of uterine leiomyomas. *Fertil Steril.* 2010;94:1864–8.

6. Fennessy FM, Tempany CM, McDannold NJ et al. Uterine leiomyomas: MR imaging-guided focused ultrasound surgery—results of different treatment protocols. *Radiology*. 2007;243:885–93.
7. LeBlang SD, Hoctor K, and Steinberg FL. Leiomyoma shrinkage after MRI-guided focused ultrasound treatment: Report of 80 patients. *AJR Am J Roentgenol*. 2010;194:274–80.
8. Stewart EA, Gostout B, Rabinovici J, Kim HS, Regan L, and Tempany CM. Sustained relief of leiomyoma symptoms by using focused ultrasound surgery. *Obstet Gynecol*. 2007;110:279–87.
9. Hindley J, Gedroyc WM, Regan L et al. MRI guidance of focused ultrasound therapy of uterine fibroids: Early results. *AJR Am J Roentgenol*. 2004;183:1713–9.
10. Morita Y, Takeuchi S, Hikida H, Ohashi H, and Ito N. Decreasing margins to the uterine serosa as a method for increasing the volume of fibroids ablated with magnetic resonance-guided focused ultrasound surgery. *Eur J Obstet Gynecol Reprod Biol*. 2009;146:92–5.
11. Stewart EA, Rabinovici J, Tempany CM et al. Clinical outcomes of focused ultrasound surgery for the treatment of uterine fibroids. *Fertil Steril*. 2006;85:22–9.
12. Yoon SW, Cha SH, Ji YG, Kim HC, Lee MH, and Cho JH. Magnetic resonance imaging-guided focused ultrasound surgery for symptomatic uterine fibroids: Estimation of treatment efficacy using thermal dose calculations. *Eur J Obstet Gynecol Reprod Biol*. 2013;169:304–8.
13. Trumm CG, Stahl R, Clevert DA et al. Magnetic resonance imaging-guided focused ultrasound treatment of symptomatic uterine fibroids: Impact of technology advancement on ablation volumes in 115 patients. *Invest Radiol*. 2013; 48:359–65.
14. Tung SL, Chou TY, Tseng HS, and Lee CM. A retrospective study of magnetic resonance-guided focused ultrasound ablation for uterine myoma in Taiwan. *Taiwan J Obstet Gynecol*. 2016;55:646–9.
15. Quinn SD, Vedelago J, Gedroyc W, and Regan L. Safety and five-year re-intervention following magnetic resonance-guided focused ultrasound (MRgFUS) for uterine fibroids. *Eur J Obstet Gynecol Reprod Biol*. 2014;182:247–51.
16. Gorny KR, Borah BJ, Brown DL, Woodrum DA, Stewart EA, and Hesley GK. Incidence of additional treatments in women treated with MR-guided focused US for symptomatic uterine fibroids: Review of 138 patients with an average follow-up of 2.8 years. *J Vasc Interv Radiol*. 2014;25:1506–12.
17. Gorny KR, Borah BJ, Weaver AL et al. Clinical predictors of successful magnetic resonance-guided focused ultrasound (MRgFUS) for uterine leiomyoma. *J Ther Ultrasound*. 2013;1:15.
18. Rabinovici J, David M, Fukunishi H et al. Pregnancy outcome after magnetic resonance-guided focused ultrasound surgery (MRgFUS) for conservative treatment of uterine fibroids. *Fertil Steril*. 2010;93:199–209.

Index

Q

R

S

T

U

V

W

Taylor & Francis Group
an informa business

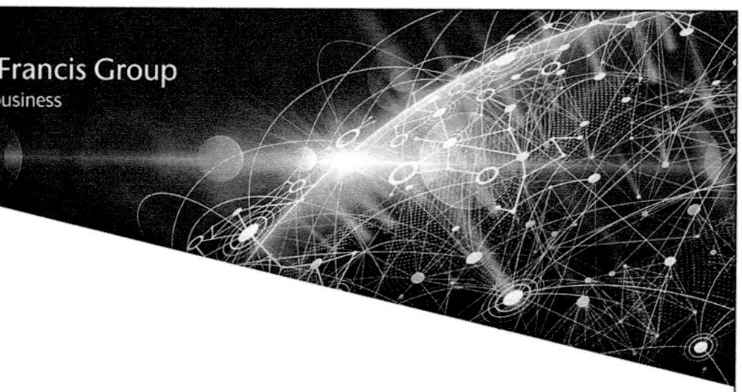

Taylor & Francis eBooks

www.taylorfrancis.com

A single destination for eBooks from Taylor & Francis with increased functionality and an improved user experience to meet the needs of our customers.

90,000+ eBooks of award-winning academic content in Humanities, Social Science, Science, Technology, Engineering, and Medical written by a global network of editors and authors.

TAYLOR & FRANCIS EBOOKS OFFERS:

- A streamlined experience for our library customers
- A single point of discovery for all of our eBook content
- Improved search and discovery of content at both book and chapter level

REQUEST A FREE TRIAL

support@taylorfrancis.com

Routledge
Taylor & Francis Group

CRC Press
Taylor & Francis Group